War and Disease

Critical Issues in Health and Medicine

Edited by Rima D. Apple, University of Wisconsin–Madison,
and Janet Golden, Rutgers University, Camden

Growing criticism of the U.S. health care system is coming from consumers, politicians, the media, activists, and health care professionals. Critical Issues in Health and Medicine is a collection of books that explores these contemporary dilemmas from a variety of perspectives, among them political, legal, historical, sociological, and comparative, and with attention to crucial dimensions such as race, gender, ethnicity, sexuality, and culture.

War and Disease

Biomedical Research on Malaria in the Twentieth Century

Leo B. Slater

Rutgers University Press

New Brunswick, New Jersey, and London

Library of Congress Cataloging-in-Publication Data

Slater, Leo Barney, 1963–
    War and disease : biomedical research on malaria in the twentieth century / Leo B. Slater.
        p. ; cm. — (Critical issues in health and medicine)
    Includes bibliographical references and index.
    ISBN 978–0–8135–4438–0 (hardcover : alk. paper)
    1. Malaria—Treatment—United States—History—20th century. 2. Malaria—Research—
United States—History—20th century. 3. Antimalarials—United States—History—20th
century. 4. Chloroquine—Therapeutic use—United States—History—20th century. I.
Title. II. Series.
    [DNLM: 1. Malaria—history. 2. Biomedical Research—history. 3. History, 20th Century.
WC 750 S631w 2009]
    RC161.A2S53 2009
    362.196'936200973—dc22

                                                                              2008013961

A British Cataloging-in-Publication record for this book is available from the British
Library

Visit our Web site: http://rutgerspress.rutgers.edu

Manufactured in the United States of America

Dedicated to my loving parents, Paul and Miriam

Contents

Acknowledgments

I have many institutions and individuals to thank for helping make this book a reality. These people are far too numerous for me to catalog without the real risk of missing someone. Please forgive my weak memory; you know who you are.

I should begin with those institutions who have materially and intellectually supported my research: the Chemical Heritage Foundation, the Institute for Applied Economics and the Study of Business Enterprise at Johns Hopkins University (JHU), the Malaria Research Institute of the Johns Hopkins Bloomberg School of Public Health, and the Max-Planck Institute for the History of Science. At each of these places, many people discussed this project with me and read and commented on its various iterations. These include Lloyd Ackert, Tara Abraham, Nancy Anderson, Susan Booker, Christina Brandt, Gert Brieger, David Brock, Arthur Daemmrich, Mary Fissell, Lou Galambos, Diane Griffin, John Haas, Bob Kargon, Sharon Kingsland, Ursula Klein, Sofie LaChapelle, Tom Lassman, Bill Leslie, Anna Maerker, Harry Marks, Tania Munz, Laura Otis, Randy Packard, Hans-Jörg Rheinberger, Christine Ruggere, Jeff Seeman, Clive Shiff, David Sicilia, Andrew Sparling, David Sullivan, Dan Todes, and Sacha Tomic. I also want to offer a special thanks to the Office of NIH History and the Laboratory of Malaria and Vector Research of the National Institute of Allergy and Infectious Disease for bringing my understanding and appreciation of malaria and biomedicine into the twenty-first century: William Chin, Bill Collins, E. Brooke Fox, Caroline Hannaway, Victoria Harden, Geoff Jeffery, Sarah Leavitt, Michele Lyons, Louis H. Miller, Buhm Soon Park, Alan Schechter, Lisa Walker, Mac Warren, and Thomas E. Wellems.

I want also to acknowledge my debt to the archives from which I drew resources: the Alan Mason Chesney Medical Archives (JHU), the American Philosophical Society, the Bayer Corporate Archives, the Bernhard Nocht Institute for Tropical Medicine, the Ferdinand Hamburger University Archives (JHU), the Hamburg State Archives, the History of Medicine Division of the National Library of Medicine, the National Academy of Science, the Rockefeller Archive Center, the Special Collections Research Center of the University of Chicago, and the U.S. National Archives and Records

Administration. Many at these repositories helped me. I can only thank few of those who helped me here: Marjorie Ciarlante, Robert S. Cox, Barbara Ebert, Charles Greifenstein, Andy Harrison, Nancy McCall, Hans-Hermann Pogarell, Thomas Rosenbaum, Jim Stimpert, and Darwin Stapleton.

There are also a number of folks with various institutional affiliations who have discussed this project with me and helped to clarify my thought. Among these are Jesse Bump, David Clyde, Angela Creager, Marcos Cueto, Wolfgang Eckart, Bernadino Fantini, Liz Fee, John Goyette, Christoph Gradmann, Jeremy Greene, Bob and Rita Gresl, Marion Hulverscheidt, Karen Masterson, Peter Morris, Carsten Reinhardt, Dominique Tobbell, Y. Alexei Veterok, and James Webb.

I thank, too, my anonymous reviewers and my editor at Rutgers University Press, Doreen Valentine.

I gratefully acknowledge the Bulletin of the History of Medicine for their permission to republish here portions of my article "Malarial Birds: Modeling Infectious Human Disease in Animals," Bulletin of the History of Medicine 79 (2005): 261–294.

And of course my loving family, Margaret, Miriam, and Paul Slater, and my lovely wife, Eden Savino.

War and Disease

Introduction

To understand the development of the military-industrial complex in the second half of the twentieth century, we look back at the Manhattan Project that built the first atomic bombs during World War II. For biomedicine in the twentieth century, the U.S. antimalarial program serves a similar role. It was a dynamic, evolving, and inventive program that spanned some seven years (1939–1946). It changed how biomedical research and development (R&D) would be funded and organized in the postwar period. World War II was a watershed for science and technology. The atomic bomb, jets and rockets, radar, and penicillin were just a few of the high-profile products of wartime R&D. Chloroquine—the drug of choice identified by the U.S. antimalarial program—was another. In debates about the purposes and nature of biomedical research, historians—and often the historical actors themselves—have cited this program's significance while neglecting the details of its actual organization and accomplishments. As with many other projects, World War II was not an end, but a beginning. For the scientists, physicians, and administrators involved, the antimalarial program was a formative experience. Many of the program's veterans went on to prominent careers and leadership positions. James A. Shannon, who made the National Institutes of Health into the foremost biomedical research organization in the world, was a leader in malaria research during World War II. Lowell Coggeshall, a Rockefeller malariologist before the war, became an innovator in medical education and science-based medicine as a postwar dean of the University of Chicago Medical School. The list goes on. For many in government, academe, and industry, the antimalarial program was a template for how biomedicine should be organized.

Today this wartime program remains an important example for those who would understand the history of the twentieth century and those who would set policy for future medical R&D and public health interventions. It was a milestone in drug development and a powerful practical and rhetorical model for the organization of research in the years following World War II. While not *the* model for future biomedical endeavors, it was both more and less than this: less for the fact that diverse resources and constraints—scientific and political—shaped postwar science; more for the way in which the program was a conduit for the research and methods—by way of the Rockefeller Institutes and Foundation, among others—of the German pharmaceutical industry and its associated academic scientists.[1] As William N. Hubbard Jr., MD, president of the Upjohn Company, wrote in 1976: "The founding of the Rockefeller Institute for Medical Research in 1902 and the remarkable achievements of research under grants begun by the Rockefeller Foundation in 1913 were important supplemental influences in the creation and expansion of industrial research laboratories that would facilitate the achievements of the 1940s."[2] Malaria was a major research area for Rockefeller investigators, and many of these scientists crossed over into wartime government work. The evolution and shape of this national program merit examination as many of its research structures and approaches survived the war. This wartime project organized and funded research on a large scale and connected many institutions in an international network. It protected millions of GIs from the worst of a terrible, debilitating, and potentially fatal disease. And it remains an excellent model for large-scale, disease-based, biomedical research that operates simultaneously on clinical and basic research questions. But the program was never designed to do more than protect elites in malarial lands. In this, it differed little from so much research and so many public health interventions, before and after, that preserved the health of colonial administrators, soldiers, and business people, yet left millions of poor people ravaged by disease. In this regard, it is a negative model, a potential example of how not to pursue public health research for impoverished civilians. The drugs that emerged from the program, especially chloroquine, proved effective and cheap enough for widespread public health use, but this benefit was not one of design. Although it had repercussions throughout the postwar period, the program was fundamentally a wartime project put together in a time of immanent national emergency.

On 7 December 1941, the Imperial Navy of Japan bombed Pearl Harbor. The Japanese attack on Hawaii was only the first of several major setbacks suffered by U.S. forces before the tide turned toward eventual U.S. victory in the Pacific. The Japanese and their Axis allies were not the U.S. military's only enemies. Malaria was a threat as significant as Imperial Japan, and one that would stalk U.S. soldiers, sailors, and marines across the islands of the Pacific, around the Mediterranean, and onto the Asian mainland. Malaria also threatened recruits in training camps across the southern and western United States. The global threat was made clear shortly after Pearl Harbor. In the days and weeks that followed, U.S. and allied troops and installations were hit hard in the Philippine islands. The Japanese took the capital, Manila, on 2 January 1942. Allied forces under General Douglas MacArthur retreated down the Bataan Peninsula. On 12 March, uttering his famous words, "I shall return," MacArthur left the Philippines. For those left behind, the future was one of siege and disease. The Japanese overran Bataan on 9 April, while the island fortress of Corregidor surrendered on 9 May. When the fortress capitulated, 85 percent of the garrison was suffering from malaria.[3] Over the next four years, malaria proved to be the number one medical problem of World War II, often accounting for more U.S. casualities than the Japanese. By the time of the surrender at Bataan, the U.S. antimalarial program was just hitting its stride after a stuttering start.

United States victory in the Pacific was tied to the fate of a number of research and development programs. Most famous of these were the Manhattan Project, which produced the atomic bombs, and the Radiation Laboratory ("Rad Lab" for short), which helped develop radar. Less famous was the antimalarial program, which would safeguard the health and lives of millions of GIs sent to malarious locations around the globe. In 1939, U.S. public health officials and malariologists began to act in response to a looming world war. The Japanese empire was already on the march in Asia, and tensions in Europe were near their breaking point. The National Research Council (NRC)—a nongovernmental body established by Congress to advise the federal government on technical and scientific matters—put together a Committee on Chemotherapy, focused first and foremost on drugs for malaria. In the United States Public Health Service (PHS), Surgeon General Thomas Parran moved chemists and pharmacologists from scattered academic laboratories to the National Institutes of Health's new campus in Bethesda, Maryland, to work on potential new antimalarials. And scientists and policy makers at the Rockefeller Foundation expanded their antimalarial programs and discussed how best to proceed in a time of national emergency. For all these concerned experts, priority would shift from issues of combating malaria in peaceful civilian populations to dealing with the disease in conditions of combat and disruption. Joined by their counterparts from the U.S. Army and Navy, they convened a series of conferences, began soliciting and exchanging research and clinical materials, and discussed again and again how best to move forward. All these efforts were dramatically accelerated by official federal action. In 1941, President Franklin D. Roosevelt first established the new federal Office of Scientific Research and Development (OSRD) and then its subsidiary Committee on Medical Research (CMR). Under OSRD and CMR, the nascent antimalarial program would receive funding and coordination and eventually develop an administrative bureaucracy characteristic to large-scale public projects. The wartime malaria work was arguably the largest biomedical research program up to this time and a model—both practical and rhetorical—for postwar biomedical research. All this was a sudden response to a disease that had been around for thousands of years.

Malaria's enormous impact on human populations during the modern era has often put this disease at the center of colonial expansion, warfare, economic transformation, and North-South global tensions. Because of the complexity of the disease—malaria is caused by several mosquito-borne protozoans—and its widespread incidence, it has been the subject of multicenter, interdisciplinary research programs on more than one occasion. For the United States, malaria's peak year was 1933, with 125,000 cases reported resulting in 5,000 deaths. The disease was essentially eliminated in the United States by the 1950s, but it drew considerable attention during World War II. While the United States has been malaria-free for most of living memory, it is instructive to recall that throughout much of modern history, including much of the twentieth century, malaria was an endemic disease in large parts of the continental United States, and a persistent problem for military and colonial personnel in many parts of the world. Yet without visible local victims of the disease, it has only been since the 1990s that efforts by NGOs and philanthropists have managed to bring this ancient scourge back into the public consciousness in the developed world. From the end of World War II to the final decade of the twentieth century, there were relatively few resources available for large-scale biomedical research on malaria. Despite such efforts such as the World Health Organization's (WHO) ill-fated and short-lived eradication program and narrowly targeted education research programs for the military, to this day millions of children continue to die of malaria every year.

With regard to the number of people killed, malaria remains one of the deadliest diseases in the world. It has been so for millennia. For every person killed by malaria, there are hundreds who are made sick by the malaria parasites. Exact numbers are hard to know because malaria's scourge is worst in some of the poorest places on earth. The WHO believes that malaria kills one to two million people each year, most of them children under the age of six in sub-Saharan Africa. Most likely a child will die of malaria while you read this paragraph. Along with HIV/AIDS and tuberculosis, malaria rounds out the top three most deadly infectious diseases in the world. Out of the hundreds of millions who are infected, the disease causes serious illness in 10 to 20 million people. These numbers are staggering; to give some perspective to these demographics, overlay the numbers on the United States: Every year malaria kills the equivalent of the entire population of Manhattan. The seriously ill equal the entire population of the New York metropolitan area, extending into Long Island, New Jersey, Connecticut, and Pennsylvania, all laid low by a debilitating, possibly fatal disease. And those afflicted each year with malaria number in the hundreds of millions, as many as the entire population of the United States. As with all infectious diseases, war and disorder can dramatically boost malaria's terrible toll on human populations. Though most in developed countries know few details about malaria, it is a disease that most everyone has heard of. It is a disease that raises visions of nineteenth-century explorers stumbling feverishly through steaming jungles. But malaria is not just a figment of our historical imaginations. It is one of the most frequent causes of sickness and death in the world today, a role it has apparently enjoyed throughout most of human history.[4]

What is malaria? Today we understand a lot about the parasites that cause malaria. In the case of the *falciparum* malaria, the most deadly kind, its DNA sequence—its genetic fingerprint—is available on the Internet. During the last 125 years, many of malaria's secrets emerged from diverse research projects in many countries. By World War II, the period on which most of this book focuses, most of malaria's basic biology was known. These single-celled protozoan parasites are larger and more complex organisms than bacteria. Taxonomically, they belong to the genus *Plasmodium*. Over 100 species of *Plasmodium* infect birds, reptiles, and mammals. For the human disease complex, there are four recognized species of *Plasmodium*: *falciparum*, *vivax*, *malariae*, and *ovale*. All four share characteristic febrile episodes—with chills, rigors, and sweating—as well as a range of other possible symptoms overlapping with those of other illnesses: nausea, headaches, body aches, and general weakness. *P. ovale* was the last to be characterized by Western medicine, as its natural range was limited to regions of sub-Saharan Africa. The other three species have long histories in Western medicine, as defined by their symptomatologies. Known as intermittent fevers or agues, these diseases were often characterized by the severity and periodicity of the fevers they induced. Tertian fevers produced high temperatures in patients every other day. "Benign" tertian fevers (*P. vivax*) were so-called because they were not associated with the severe, and often fatal, episodes of "malignant" tertian or "subtertian" fevers (*P. falciparum*). This malignant tertian variety was also known as aestivo-autumnal fever, because the number of cases often peaked in late summer and fall. *P. falciparum* can produce severe conditions involving the brain, kidneys, lungs, or liver, often resulting in death. Quartan fever (*P. malariae*) produces fever peaks on every third day. Multiple infections of any of these parasites could produce fever peaks every day, yielding a diagnosis of quotidian (daily) fever. Although there are only four species of *Plasmodium* parasite that attack humans, there are diverse genetic isolates, as recognized by variations in immune response or resistance to different drugs. In the confines of military medicine during World War II, it was *P. vivax* and *P. falciparum* that figured most prominently. For clarity, *Plasmodium* species names are used throughout this volume.

All these species of malaria are transmitted to people by mosquitoes of the genus *Anopheles*. To reproduce and negotiate these two hosts—one insect (the definitive host, where sexual reproduction takes place) and one vertebrate (the intermediate host)—the *Plasmodium* has evolved a complex life cycle. Transmitted to its human host through the bite of an infected female mosquito (only female mosquitoes bite, as the blood meal is a requisite for nourishing eggs), the *Plasmodium* enter the bloodstream, via the mosquito's saliva, in a form known as sporozoites. This small, mobile form swiftly makes its way, via the blood, to the liver, where it enters a liver cell. Ensconced in the hepatocyte, the parasite reproduces asexually, increasing its numbers by some five orders of magnitude before the cell ruptures and releases the parasites in their merozoite form to the bloodstream. Each merozoite is capable of infecting a red blood cell and reproducing itself asexually by another order of magnitude. The rupture of the red blood cells releases these new merozoites and is the cause of the malarial fever. The developmental stages within the red blood cells are called schizonts or (erythrocytic) trophozoites. After a number of cycles of reproduction, certain of the parasites, instead of growing into multiple new merozoites, grow into single gametocytes, either female or male in sex. These circulating gametocytes are infectious to the mosquito. When a female *Anopheles* mosquito bites an infected human, she ingests these gametocytes. Once inside a mosquito's gut, the female and male gametocytes burst forth and engage in sexual reproduction, yielding the ookinete. The ookinete makes its way to the outside of the gut where it becomes an oocyst that ruptures when fully developed, releasing numerous sporozoites. These then traverse the mosquito and enter the salivary glands where they stand poised to infect another human host. Much of this life cycle had been documented by 1939, although the liver stage was not discovered until after the war.[5]

The control of malaria also has a long history. Eliminating the wetlands associated with fever is an ancient approach. In the seventeenth century, cinchona bark entered the European pharmacopeia. The bark's active principal, quinine, was isolated at the beginning of the nineteenth century. Later, once the parasites and the vector mosquitoes were known, other modes of attack on malaria opened up. Killing or inhibiting the parasites and the mosquitoes at any stage of their complex life cycles were potential avenues for limiting disease. The divide between pursuit of the disease organism itself or its vector has separated environmental and biomedical approaches to malaria. Most famous on the environmental side is the use of DDT (dichloro-diphenyl-trichloroethane) to kill mosquitoes. With regard to the biomedical history of malaria control, drug development takes center stage.

The wartime program built on substantial but incomplete biological and medical knowledge. Workers in the field divided chemotherapeutic (drug) approaches to malaria into the prevention of infection—technically *chemoprophylaxis*—and the treatment of those already infected. Interventions were further divided into those that were suppressive—keeping symptoms at bay and soldiers in the field—and those that were sterilizing and would eliminate all the parasites from the body. However, an important piece of the malaria puzzle was missing, making either approach, prevention or treatment, difficult to study: None of the malarial parasites could be cultured outside of a living host. For malariologists, there were no petri dishes filled with bugs that could be dabbed with potential antibiotics. And testing on humans was difficult, expensive, and slow. What pharmacologists and others relied on were animal models of malaria, often birds or monkeys. All these models had major drawbacks. Animals could not be infected with human parasites, so both the parasite and the host of the model systems differed from the human disease state. One should remember, however, that the discovery of a relatively successful chemotherapeutic agent did not require an understanding of malaria's true cause or biology: Quinine is an old antimalarial that predates modern understandings of malaria's etiology.

The territory of malaria research is a vast one, ranging from mosquitoes in the field to parasites under the microscope to malarial canaries at pharmaceutical companies. This book looks at a select and significant portion of this territory: the use and development of drugs to treat and prevent the disease. It provides a detailed historical analysis of the background, development, organization, and legacy of the U.S. antimalarial program during World War II. When conducting research, treating patients, preventing illness, or even just thinking about disease, one has to decide where the disease is, what causes it, how one might intervene, and how it compares to other diseases and pathologies. One must choose what is in and what is out. One must decide what is the same and what is different. For example, will a drug for bacterial disease work against malaria? Are the blood parasites of common crows similar enough to human disease to make them a worthwhile model of our malarias? This book argues for the plasticity of disease concepts and of research materials—particularly chemical compounds tested as drugs against malaria and birds employed as models of human malaria—illustrating the shifting boundaries of what constitutes an adequate model of disease. It addresses chemical, animal, and organizational models in biomedical research while treating environmental models of malaria only where appropriate to primary themes.

War and Disease is centered on the U.S. government's antimalarial research program during World War II, a program administered through the Committee on Medical Research beginning in 1941. By the end of 1943, the U.S. Army, Navy, PHS, and CMR had instituted the Board for the Coordination of Malaria Studies, a body that would continue to evolve and guide antimalarial research. This institution's roots lie in a modest National Research Council chemotherapy initiative begun in 1939, an initiative that grew over the course of the war to a scale not previously seen in biomedical research, involving chemical and pharmaceutical companies, university researchers of many disciplines, and nonprofit and government laboratories. The project screened more than 14,000 compounds for activity, ratified the prewar synthetic antimalarial atabrine as the drug of choice in 1943, and, by war's end, identified another synthetic, chloroquine, as the superior compound. The NRC and others drew on a set of intellectual and organizational resources and models extending back to the German pharmaceutical and dye industries and such domestic institutions as the Rockefeller Institutes and Foundation.

The program was one of a family of projects—along with its siblings, the penicillin and synthetic rubber programs, and its colossal cousins, the radar program and the Manhattan Project—that contributed to the transformation of American science in scale and organization as well as in public expectation. As a potential postwar model for biomedicine, penicillin was distinct as it was very much a development project, emphasizing the D of R&D, while the antimalarial program took a wide-ranging, interdisciplinary approach to a narrowly defined disease area. Its later use as a model system was perhaps most clearly seen at the National Institutes of Health (NIH) generally and in the National Cancer Institute's chemotherapy screening programs. U.S. antimalarial research efforts followed the extensive German industrial antimalarial program between the two world wars. The U.S. case provides an early example of a hybrid research program—what might today be called a public–private partnership—a mix of scientists working in diverse locations, such as government laboratories, universities, and pharmaceutical and chemical companies. The wartime antimalarial program deserves attention as both an undertaking in its own right—one that helped to safeguard millions of GIs— and its position as a model for future large-scale biomedical research projects. The innovations of the U.S. wartime antimalarial program lay chiefly in three areas: administration, scale, and communication. The program produced not just research findings, novel compounds, and clinical protocols, but it developed new organizational structures for scientific cooperation and distributed research networks. Wartime work was essential to the development of NIH; the confused and faltering structures of the early war years, 1939–1943, suggest that the organizational infrastructure for large scale, multicenter cooperative research was not in place prior to World War II.

The history of malaria research can be productively divided in a number of ways. Some twenty years ago, Louis Miller—an NIH scientist who has studied malaria for many years—and his colleagues suggested a tripartite division: "There have been three major periods of scientific discovery in malaria: the first just before the turn of the century with the dual discoveries of the pathogen and the vector; the second in the 1930s and 1940s with the introduction of larvicides, synthetic antimalarial drugs and the discovery of DDT; and the third, taking place today, with the application of new techniques of immunochemistry and molecular biology for the development of malaria vaccines."[6] This book will guide the reader through the first two periods in some detail, before looking at the future of malaria research in the final chapter. The promise of a successful malaria vaccine—a holy grail in preventive medicine and public health—remains as yet unattained.

The first chapter, "Quinine and the Environment of Disease," serves as a prehistory and includes a narrative account of the development of quinine—particularly in a colonial and military context—and of the rise of the pharmaceutical industry in the late nineteenth and early twentieth centuries. Quinine—or the bark of the cinchona tree from which quinine was extracted—was valuable because of its capacity to control certain fevers. While these fevers had been referred to collectively as malaria since the middle of the eighteenth century, intermittent fevers were ancient diseases going back at least to ancient Greece and Rome. The word *malaria* derives from the Italian for "bad air," and malarial fevers were often associated with the bad or corrupt air of swamps and marshes. With the discovery of the New World, the possibility of treatment emerged in the form of the bark of the cinchona tree, native to South America. In the nineteenth century, colonial cinchona plantations were developed elsewhere in the world, most successfully by the Dutch in Java. The chapter also offers a historical discussion of the environmental aspects of malaria research and control, such as the association of malaria with wetlands, mosquito control, drainage, and DDT. Among the ecological models—or ecological conceptions of disease—were nutritional studies, drainage schemes, and chemical pest control technologies. The concept of chemotherapy—a term coined by Paul Ehrlich in 1907—is discussed in the context of malaria.

Chapter 2, "Avian Malaria," introduces the study of malaria in laboratory animals, including the famous discoverers of malaria's causes—Alphonse Laveran, Ronald Ross, and William G. MacCallum, to name three—who all employed avian malarias in their research. With the pioneering work of Wilhelm Roehl (1881–1929), avian malaria grew in prominence as a research tool. Roehl, a student of Paul Ehrlich, used canaries infected with *Plasmodium relictum*, a species of avian malaria, to screen new antimalarials at Bayer (I. G. Farben) in the 1920s and revolutionized malaria drug discovery. During the interwar period, the focus is on Bayer and the Johns Hopkins School of Hygiene and Public Health. At Johns Hopkins, the nature and limits of avian malarias were explored. Hopkins professor Robert Hegner, his students, and his collaborators did much to increase knowledge of these bird malarias. The chapter traces the development of a number of avian malarias as model systems for research. Overall, the animal models of malaria were notable for their variety and their complexity. In contrast with the drive for simplified models in fields like bacteriology, complexity remained an essential part of malaria biology. When malaria workers did capture the disease in the laboratory (when they transferred the disease, as hosts and parasites, from the field to the lab), they seemed to have had an appreciation of (or even a passion for) complexity. Those working with model organisms also had to cope with many types of hard-to-distinguish parasites; even human malaria is caused by several distinct species. Furthermore, until the 1970s, researchers could not culture the parasites and always needed live host animals.

Wilhelm Roehl and Bayer make the connection to chapter 3. "New Drugs" outlines the development of the first successful synthetic antimalarials, plasmochin and atabrine, by Roehl, his coworkers, and his successors at Bayer in the 1920s and 1930s. These German scientists molded the conception of disease around chemical shapes and structures. Bayer's chemists developed structure-activity relationships for several series of potential drug candidates. They also characterized these compounds with a therapeutic index—the ratio of the effective dose to the tolerable dose—using canaries and *Plasmodium relictum*. Here was an interface between chemical and biological models of disease, but, after the initial development of the canary model, most innovation centered on the chemical aspects of drug development while testing became routinized. In this chapter, I discuss chemical structures in disease intervention. For example, Bayer employed the natural drug quinine and the synthetic dye methylene blue as lead compounds for drug discovery. Methylene blue had first been explored in relation to malaria by Paul Ehrlich. This is a significant episode in the molecularization of medicine and biology.

The chapter continues in the United States, with a look at Bayer's marketing of their new synthetic drugs—plasmochin and atabrine—and the reactions to these drugs by the Rockefeller Foundation, the U.S. Public Health Service, and others involved in antimalarial work in the United States and its tropical possessions. The chapter also covers Bayer's work on synthetic antimalarials into the early 1940s and introduces chloroquine, a drug that would go on to be a post–World War II wonder drug.

With the German story largely complete, the focus moves to the early days of the U.S. wartime work with chapter 4, "Preparing for War." This chapter details the beginnings of the U.S. program, set against the background of Japanese expansion in Asia and the outbreak of World War II in Europe. From NRC's chemotherapy initiative in 1939 to the early days of CMR in 1941, U.S. planning for the exigencies of war and malaria were not highly organized or well funded. William Mansfield Clark (1884–1964)—

professor of physiological chemistry at the Johns Hopkins School of Medicine and wartime chairman of NRC's Division of Chemistry and Chemical Technology—characterized the early efforts as "kaleidoscopic":

> The changes in organization were sufficiently kaleidoscopic to give the impression of an unstable pattern. Indeed, a person concerned only with the superficial aspects of organization might be tempted to use the record in support of the contention that a similar emergency in the future had best be handled by a predetermined body in accordance with a pre-formed plan. But this would be to misread the record. It is a record of research in which organizational matters were continually adjusted to meet the demands of scientific advances. This aspect of the record deserves the greater emphasis.[7]

This early period, prior to U.S. entry into the war, showed some of the weaknesses and strengths of the NRC's approach to scientific research. The chapter discusses the networks of the Rockefeller Foundation, which cooperated with commercial firms such as United Fruit Company, Squibb, and Parke Davis, to test compounds for efficacy against malaria. Lowell T. Coggeshall (1901–1987)—a physician/researcher of the Rockefeller Institute, the University of Michigan, and later the University of Chicago—was a pivotal figure here, connecting Rockefeller interests directly with NRC.

Also explored are some early research goals and problems of the U.S. wartime program. Basic tests for activity and toxicity had to be established before new compounds could be usefully solicited or synthesized. The separation of activity and toxicity into different screening procedures, in different animals, by Eli Kennerly Marshall Jr. (1889–1966)—a chemist and pharmacologist at the Johns Hopkins School of Medicine—marked one of the U.S. program's departures from the interwar work of Bayer. In September 1941, OSRD money was first made available for malaria research. By year's end, the United States was at war, and quinine supplies were about to be disrupted by the Japanese offensive in Southeast Asia. With the United States preparing to send millions of troops into malarious areas of the world, the need to replace quinine became acute.

After Pearl Harbor, the antimalarial program became critical to the war effort. Java fell to the Japanese in March 1942, cutting off the United States from the source of 90 percent of the world's supply of quinine. Chapter 5, "Cooperation and Coordination," deals with sources of innovation in military medicine and drug discovery. NRC and CMR established new organizational structures for the conduct and coordination of research. For example, the Survey of Antimalarial Drugs controlled the flow of material and various classes of information—"restricted," "confidential," "secret," and "in confidence"—between workers and the committees coordinating the work. The Committee (later Panel) on Synthesis oversaw the solicitation of novel compounds. When screening had caught up with the inflow of compounds, the synthesis of new compounds and the pursuit of these leads came to play a major role in research. Other essential clinical activities included the development of dosage regimens for atabrine. In this area, researchers such as E. K. Marshall and James A. Shannon (1904–1994) addressed questions such as the potential toxicity of commercial atabrine. This work on atabrine was one of the major practical military accomplishments of the wartime program. Atabrine was the primary preventive/suppressive drug employed in the field. The testing of compounds and dosage regimens was done with prisoner volunteers, military personnel, and neurosyphilis patients. The chapter treats the organizational framing of malaria as a disease and as an expanding series of problems to be addressed. Central to the organizational evolution of the research program was the Subcommittee on (later, Board for) the Coordination of Malaria Studies.

Chapter 6, "Trust and Transition," explores the changes wrought in biomedical R&D by the large-scale involvement of the federal government. The transition from the professional ethos of the NRC to the bureaucratic realm of wartime government work was not an easy one for the antimalarial program or its protagonist, William Mansfield Clark. Clark's conflict with A. N. Richards—chairman of CMR—and others over the sharing of proprietary information highlights the contrast between these two regimes. Clark sought to resign over Richards's push to share all information. Only the personal intervention of OSRD's director, Vannevar Bush, kept Clark at his post. Likewise, Clark refused to be made a government official under a 1944 reorganization, as this would have impaired his ability to deal fairly and to inspire trust. As Clark defended the intellectual property of contributing firms, the antimalarial program expanded in its scope and scale. The proliferation of committees and increasing administrative activities marked a move away from the advisory role of earlier NRC committees. In the end, Bush and Richards took control of the program away from the NRC and vested it fully in the CMR, deploying legalistic assertions of government power. Clark's position as a first among equals was no longer tenable in the new bureaucratic world.

In 1943, the war turned in favor of the Allies. The surrender of the German army at Stalingrad in February and the Allied invasion of Sicily in July were just two turning points. With the growing complexity of wartime research demanding more administration, government functionaries looked to new bureaucratic structures for the management and control of the antimalarial program. They worked changes not just in scale, organization, and methods of drug development, but in the values of science and the scope of government involvement in biomedicine. Growing government bureaucracy impinged on the promises of confidentiality that the NRC had made to commercial firms. It also created a drive for centralization. Personalities, egos, and values had to accommodate themselves to organizational parameters, new power structures, and to the national emergency.

The close of the war saw the advent of a new wonder drug against malaria and reopened the debates about the proper role of government in science, technology, and medicine. Chapter 7, "Chloroquine, Wonder Drug," examines the emergence of chloroquine as a potent and well-tolerated antimalarial. The program tested chloroquine on soldiers, mental patients, and prisoner volunteers. With its promise growing, Rockefeller collaborators took the new drug to Peru for testing in civilian—peasant—populations. Even as the program and its collaborators developed chloroquine for widespread use, CMR was winding down. Discussions of the significance of wartime work and of what should come next began in earnest. At the end of June 1946, the Survey of Antimalarial Drugs was terminated and its many rubber stamps burned. But some antimalarial research was continued under the auspices of NIH's intramural and extramural programs. More broadly, discussions about the role of government in science deployed the antimalarial program as a potential model for postwar research and development. Also discussed in brief are British and German antimalarial research during the war, as well as the significant Australian contribution to the U.S. research program.

The management and administration of science changed during the war, the scale of projects—in dollars, in hours worked, in disciplinary contributions—grew, and proper communication and the distribution of information supported this change in administration and scale. The final form(s) of the antimalarial program did not emerge in a controlled and planned manner but as an evolution in response to military needs and scientific and technological capabilities. The program was a crossroads for essential elements of scientific research traditions and a locus for organizational and pharmacological innovation. Overall, the program was a great success. World War II was the first major U.S. conflict in which fewer U.S. soldiers died of disease than of combat injuries.

The last chapter, chapter 8, "Lessons Learned," sketches the fate of chloroquine and the impact of the wartime program on both antimalarial research and postwar biomedical research. Chloroquine was one of the foundations for the World Health Organization's ill-conceived and ill-fated global malaria-eradication campaign. Though still in use today, chloroquine's efficacy has been severely limited by the rise of drug-resistant strains of malaria. Beyond chloroquine, a number of postwar antimalarials were prefigured or tested in the wartime program. The antimalarial program was a significant reference point for later biomedical initiatives, most notably aspects of the postwar NIH. This book supports accounts of historians and historical actors who felt the wartime work was essential to the future of the NIH. James Shannon—a wartime malaria researcher who went on to become an influential director of the NIH—was but one obvious connection between the wartime regime and subsequent organizations.

Malaria sickens hundreds of millions and kills millions every year. The twentieth century saw little improvement with regard to malaria for the majority of people who live in endemic or hyperendemic areas. With so much still to be done, new structures have begun to emerge: new philanthropic enterprises, new initiatives, and new ways to mobilize capital for the betterment of the poor, programs such as the Bill and Melinda Gates Foundation, WHO's Roll Back Malaria initiative, Medicines for Malaria Venture, GlaxoSmithKline's Malarone donation program, the Malaria Vaccine Initiative, and the Malaria Research Institute. Portions of this discussion resonate with other critical health issues and emerging diseases, such as AIDS, tuberculosis, and West Nile virus. Malaria remains with us all. Both innovation and luck will be needed if the twenty-first century is to have a better record than the twentieth.

But more than just explaining the context and content of the U.S. antimalarial program during World War II, this book is a history of infectious disease and drug development in the first half of the twentieth century. The main narrative ends with the winding down of the wartime program, as malaria research was much less vibrant in the 1950s and 1960s—the heyday of DDT and chloroquine, antimalarial tools developed during the war. For much of the postwar period, malaria research itself was no longer central to infectious disease research or biomedicine. Yet the antimalarial program is critical to an understanding of more recent biomedicine. The history of medicine is moving beyond social history in order to understand twentieth-century, science-based medicine. Part of this has to include research organization. Tools—intellectual and practical—money, and management are all required for modern biomedical research, and this is a story about how such things were mobilized in a time of national emergency and how that mobilization impacted later research.

Chapter 1

Quinine and the Environment of Disease

The malaria parasite is a well organized, highly adapted end-product of thousands of years of biological evolution which would mark it as successful, regardless of the criteria. Species of the genus *Plasmodium* are currently found in every group of strictly terrestrial vertebrates and adaptive capacities have been particularly well demonstrated in birds and primates where the level of speciation is high. When one considers the complexity of the life cycle, including the necessity for adjustment to two decidedly different host environments, the precise combination of temperature and humidity required, plus vector and vertebrate host habits necessary to assure continued transmission of the parasite, its survival in nature alone, is amazing.[1]

Complex, amazing, and highly adapted: This is how a group of researchers at the National Institutes of Health described the parasites that cause malaria. These parasites were not just an admired object of research; they were an enemy to be respected and understood on their own terms. Through the development of synthetic antimalarial drugs in the first half of the twentieth century, malariologists, physicians, and chemists obtained critical knowledge of this successful foe. The scientific, medical, and natural-historical context of these novel pharmaceuticals emerged from earlier understandings of several essential elements: quinine and the cinchona tree from whose bark the drug was derived, the development of synthetic chemicals (drugs) in the fight against disease, the discovery of malaria's causative parasites (several species of the genus *Plasmodium*) and the anopheline mosquitoes that transmit them, and the environmental understanding of malaria.

The embrace of malaria—and medicine more generally—by modern science and technology only added to the disease's many cultural connections. In broader contexts, quinine and malaria played key roles in the birth of the synthetic dye industry, the rise of the pharmaceutical industry, and the development of drugs against infectious disease. These increasingly complex scientific and medical conceptualizations of malaria—and the persistence of the disease—preserved older environmental perspectives on malaria. Of course, germ theory and modern technology brought with them a shift in disease etiology from unhealthy places and bad air to vectors and microbes. These perspectives left behind miasmic theories of disease and took up an ecological approach—a scientific way of treating interconnected networks of living creatures. Ideas about many environments—from the macro scale of rivers and marshes to the micro scale of the blood cell—have thus informed malaria research. Yet even these elements emerged explicitly from older traditions only in the nineteenth century: quinine from a South American bark early in the century and mosquitoes revealed as specific vectors from the wetlands long associated with malaria near century's end. This association of periodic—malarial—fevers with specific "unhealthy" environments goes back thousands of years, and knowledge of an efficacious treatment in the form of cinchona, or Peruvian, bark is now more than four hundred years old. Furthermore, the beginnings of modern chemotherapy and the twin discoveries of the *Plasmodium* parasites and their mosquito vectors were roughly contemporaneous, clustered around the end of the nineteenth century. For malaria researchers in the early twentieth century, quinine, chemotherapy, and mosquitoes were all essential to understanding malaria, as well as its cause, treatment, and control.

Quinine

In addition to being an environmental disease, malaria is unique in being a disease for which a recognized and specific remedy has persisted across several centuries. This specific remedy is today called quinine, an alkaloid drug that was isolated from the bark of the cinchona tree in the early nineteenth century. The use of the bark itself goes back to at least the seventeenth century. With such a long pedigree, quinine's story has almost inevitably incorporated a number of apocryphal episodes.[2] These historical myths were intertwined with changing conceptions of the cause and treatment of malaria and with more general shifts in the cultures of disease intervention. One significant change, a shift toward the chemical, was the creation of quinine itself as a pure salt. Quinine was a purer form of the essential medicinal activity of the crude cinchona bark. It was never an ideal drug, having side effects and often only suppressing infection. Suppression meant that treatment or prevention (prophylaxis) had failed to kill all the parasites, leaving the patient susceptible to relapse. Quinine did not prevent infection but did modify its course such that people could carry on without serious illness. Treatment was further complicated in malaria by recurrence. Even small numbers of surviving parasites could recrudesce and bring on a new attack, and *vivax* malaria could persist in the tissues (liver) for months before renewing its attack upon the host. Quinine and cinchona bark could do nothing to deal with this relapse.

Before quinine, cinchona's history belonged to an older natural-historical and apothecary tradition. It was only during the nineteenth century that the properties of medical substances came to be defined in chemical terms. Therefore, we begin with the bark. For Europeans, the tale of the febrifuge, or fever-reducing, bark of the cinchona tree, often referred to as Jesuits' bark or Peruvian bark, begins on the slopes of the Andes in the late sixteenth century. Sources about the history of quinine are not consistent, particularly with regard to early contacts between the Indians and the Spaniards. While Saul Jarcho's fine book, *Quinine's Predecessor*,[3] debunks many of the earlier accounts, one should not dismiss all these stories entirely as they have been a persistent part of the lore of quinine, a part of its mythology if not its history. An early authority on the history of cinchona is the British geographer Clements R. Markham, who traveled extensively in South America in the 1800s and wrote on the history and natural history of Peru and its environs.[4] In 1862, Markham published an account of his mission to establish cinchona plantations in British India. The British, like the Americans later, were maneuvering to circumvent a Dutch monopoly on quinine, a monopoly that the Dutch had maintained by control of trade since the eighteenth century. Markham's account preserves a mixture of romance, commercialism, and colonialism that is the European, and especially Victorian, inheritance of quinine.

For Markham, cinchona's story began with Spanish colonial expansion in the New World. By 1560, the Spanish military conquest and associated civil wars of Peru were largely over. The early efforts in the collection and shipment of cinchona bark indicate how useful Europeans found the bark to be. There are several reports that by around 1600 some Europeans had been cured of fever by Peruvian bark. While early sources give mixed accounts of whether the local Indians were aware that the bark had fever-reducing qualities, it seems likely that they believed it had some medicinal property. They named the bark *quina-quina*, or "bark-bark," the double name indicating medicinal properties in a plant. The first European purportedly cured of fever by the bark was the countess of Chinchon, wife of the viceroy of Peru. As the story goes, in 1638, the corregidor of Loxa, Don Juan Lopez de Cañizares,[5] on hearing that the countess was in Lima suffering from a tertian fever, sent to her physician—Juan de Vega—a package of the powdered bark, by means of which he effected a complete cure. The countess, greatly pleased by this turn of affairs, purchased a large quantity of the bark and distributed it to the afflicted of the city. On her return to Spain in 1640, she took with her a supply of the bark, introducing it to Europe. After the cure of the countess, the Jesuits were great promoters of the bark in Europe.

Most accounts of the history of cinchona, or of quinine, relate this tale of the countess, if only to dismiss it as apocryphal.[6] In the event, cinchona and quinine retain a fabled past, and use of the bark was well-established in Europe by the middle of the seventeenth century. By the 1670s, the Jesuits were the prime distributors of Peruvian bark, which was sent to Rome by their missionaries.

Through the activities of the Jesuits and others, the bark spread across Europe during the later seventeenth and the eighteenth centuries, although its association with this Catholic order engendered some resistance to its use among Protestants. In 1657, for example, Gabriele Fonseca, papal physician, treated Flavio Cardinal Chigi, nephew of Pope Alexander VII, with the Peruvian bark.[7] Alexander had readmitted the Jesuits to Rome the previous year. In 1678, Louis XIV was building in Versailles and Marly, both malarious places, and Sir Robert Talbor, physician apothecary to Charles II, successfully treated him for obstinate intermittent fever.[8] The next year Louis purchased the secret of preparing quinquina, the extract of the bark in wine, from Sir Robert for a title, a large pension, and two thousand louis-d'ors. Louis's example did much for the reputation of the bark in France. French fabulist Jean La Fontaine wrote an ode, "Poème du Quinquina," in praise of the new medicament.[9] The prevalence of malaria in Europe made the Jesuits' bark a popular and valued import, with local agents gathering the bark in Peruvian forests and selling it to New World middlemen.

This collecting phase continued with taxonomic research in the eighteenth century. In 1735, French naturalist and mathematician Charles de la

Condamine led an astronomy expedition to Peru, with Joseph de Jussieu as physician and naturalist. The French returned with specimens and descriptions of the trees. By 1742, these descriptions and samples were obtained by Linnaeus, who named the genus *Cinchona*, after the countess of Chinchon. Markham insisted on reinstating the first "h" to honor the countess. From the time of Jussieu's and Condamine's reports, around 1740, Europeans attached the febrifuge property not only to the bitter-tasting bark but also to the newly described—and discovered—tree; prior to this, they had known only the bark. Potentially, knowledge of the trees might increase control of the febrifuge property of the bark. A new area of experiment and collection opened to Europeans. In 1760, the Spanish botanist José Mutis described and experimented with several new species; and in 1767–1768 the Spanish government established a cinchona reservation in Peru, near Loxa, for supplying the royal pharmacy.[10] In 1799, Alexander von Humboldt investigated cinchona trees in the Andes of Peru. But it was not until the mid-nineteenth century that the demands of colonial expansion and the capabilities of chemical science gave rise to the cultivation of cinchona—a move away from local gathering and collection and toward colonial plantation agriculture—and this was to happen outside of South America.

In the nineteenth century, cinchona traveled to the laboratory and to the plantation. Experimental science, particularly chemistry, made cinchona and its extracts the subjects of intense investigation. In the laboratory, pharmacists chemically extracted quinine from the bark, purifying and quantifying it. This was a period when the active ingredients of a number of medicinal plants were first extracted. Morphine, strychnine, codeine, caffeine, and other alkaloids were isolated by acid extraction. In Paris in 1820, Pierre-Joseph Pelletier of the École de Pharmacie and Joseph-Bienaimé Caventou of the Saint-Antoine Hospital crystallized quinine salts from cinchona bark extracts.[11]

Meanwhile, synthetic chemistry began to break down the separation between the biological and the chemical. For example, in 1828 Friedrich Wöhler synthesized urea from ammonium chloride and silver cyanate, both considered minerals, and showed that organic compounds might be made from inorganic ones.[12] This process, along with Hermann Kolbe's preparation of acetic acid in 1845, gave hope to some that quinine might soon be artificially—synthetically—formed. In 1854, Adolph Strecker at the University of Christiania (Oslo) determined quinine's empirical formula,[13] a crucial conceptual step in transforming this biological, organic material into a chemical one. In 1856, with this formula in hand, William Henry

Perkin—at the prompting of his teacher August Wilhelm Hofmann—attempted to synthesize quinine ($C_{20}H_{24}N_2O_2$) by oxidizing and condensing allyltoluidine ($C_{10}H_{12}N$). The attempt to synthesize quinine failed, but Perkin serendipitously found that he had created the novel dye mauve.[14] The success of this synthetic dye, in a marketplace that had only known dyes derived from natural materials, launched the fine chemical industry across Europe.[15] The history of dyes and chemistry is intimately bound to the history of infectious disease, particularly through malaria research. The trend toward chemical solutions grew in the nineteenth century, and the medicinal properties of chemicals were extended and refined by researchers such as Paul Ehrlich, a German chemist and immunologist. This work, as we will see, brought new conceptions of disease, its causes, and its cures. Important for quinine was the commercial nature of much of the research: trade in quinine would have consequences not just for South America and Europe but for colonial lands in Africa, India, and Java.

The chemical transformation of cinchona bark into quinine increased the level control of its medicinal properties: the quinine content of bark could be assayed and the purity of its active principle determined. This control of the chemical created new political power and a still greater appetite for the mastery of quinine and cinchona. Once quinine could be extracted and separated from the crude bark, its content could be assayed and the quinine could be purified and measured. Isolated quinine, as opposed to the bark, was more effective, and its effectiveness was further enhanced by using it prophylactically, particularly to secure the health of military and colonial personnel. Access to quinine enabled Europeans to control India and North Africa and to explore and exploit West Africa. Previously, European death rates from malaria had been daunting, and in the case of West Africa, prohibitive. The survival of all the members of Dr. William Baikie's 1854 expedition up the Niger showed that quinine prophylaxis enabled the entry of Europeans into an area where previous death rates among the newly arrived were on the order of 50 percent.[16] Quinine thus augmented colonial military power and reach.

The response among the European powers to the efficacy of quinine was a series of collecting expeditions to South America.[17] Plantation agriculture—the transfer of cinchona to safe, controlled territory—was the ultimate goal of these nineteenth-century expeditions. In 1848, Hugh Algernon Weddell brought from Bolivia to Paris the first cinchona seeds that would be grown in Europe. In 1854, Justus Carl Hasskarl, an employee of the Netherlands East Indian government, brought the first tree to Java; by 1863, the Dutch had more than half a million plants in permanent sites there.[18] And Markham brought the trees to India and Ceylon. As he wrote in 1862, there already existed the danger that "the supplies of bark from South America are not nearly sufficient to meet the demand, and the price is kept so high as to place this inestimable remedy beyond the means of millions of natives of fever-visited regions. For these reasons the incalculable importance of introducing the chinchona plant into other countries adapted for its growth, and thus escaping from entire dependence on the South American forests, has long occupied the attention of scientific men in Europe."[19] Markham was neither the first nor the last to try to circumvent a monopoly supplier of an essential commodity. However, there are many species of *Cinchona*, and the varieties initially cultivated on colonial plantations yielded less than 3 percent quinine sulfate by weight of bark, too little quinine to sustain these enterprises. Luck was against Markham; he would not collect the seeds that would make cinchona plantation agriculture economically viable. That honor was reserved for a more obscure individual, the trader and naturalist Charles Ledger.

British and Dutch plantations in Indian, Ceylon, and Java raced to dominate the cinchona market. Victory came in the 1870s, when the Dutch established a substantial number of *Cinchona ledgeriana* trees in Java. This variety, originally brought out of Bolivia as seeds by Charles Ledger in 1865,[20] had sufficient quinine content, around 10 percent, for commercial exploitation.[21] While the Dutch had previously dominated the market in cinchona bark by controlling shipping and trade, their new success with *Cinchona ledgeriana* extended their dominance by giving them control of production.[22] The British were less fortunate in their attempts to cultivate the tree. The Indian plantations produced a lower-grade mixture of cinchona alkaloids—primarily quinine, cinchonine, and cinchonidine—that was called "quinetum" and later "totaquine." Markham was an early advocate of quinetum use. He believed that the bark grown in India should be processed there for local use. Markham and his collaborators tested the mixed alkaloid preparations and found them to be the most economical product to come from the Indian barks.[23] The British, except in time of emergency, reserved the bulk of this material for Indian use. Markham's protestations notwithstanding, the cinchona plantations of India and Ceylon could not compete with those of Java. Although the League of Nations tested and promoted totaquine in the 1920s and 1930s as a substitute for the more expensive quinine, quinine remained the drug of choice.[24] Meanwhile, using the superior species grown on the Javanese plantations, the Dutch established a quinine monopoly that took its final form as the Kina Bureau in 1910.[25] This type of commodity control, the removal to colonial possessions of a strategic crop, was a typical nineteenth-century stratagem.

In the early decades of the twentieth century, quinine enjoyed a vogue with public health officials. They employed several strategies with mixed results. In the tropics, quinine was primarily reserved for military and colonial elites. These personnel also tried to keep their distance from the native populations who were often viewed as reservoirs of disease. A second approach, typically deployed in the malarial regions of developed countries, such as Italy or the United States, was to use quinine in areas of local outbreaks to prevent further spread of the disease, treating the sick and dosing the healthy prophylactically. Quinine could also be deployed on a mass scale in historically endemic areas without regard to the presence or absence of disease. But overall, quinine was not amenable to these public health uses. It only suppressed infection and could not sterilize the blood. Most importantly from the standpoint of transmission, quinine did not kill the blood-borne gametocyte form of the parasite that infected mosquitoes. Asymptomatic patients could still carry the gametocytes, and, in the case of *vivax* malaria, the hidden, non-blood stage of the parasite could reemerge and trigger a new cycle of infection. Killing the hidden forms and the gametocytes would require new drugs with properties beyond those of quinine.[26]

The rise of science-based industry in the late nineteenth and early twentieth centuries brought a new strategy for commodity control by manufacturing synthetic substitutes, and quinine was no exception.[27] While the Dutch plantations succeeded and the British ones faltered, cinchona continued to follow the changing locations of scientific and technological inquiry—from natural-historical and botanical expeditions in the eighteenth century through the second industrial revolution in the nineteenth. The shift from an agricultural, plantation-based approach to a technoscientific, laboratory-based one placed quinine and malaria control squarely within the mainstream of larger economic and political changes in Europe and the United States. Though this shift continued the chemical trend exemplified by the nineteenth-century French pharmacists, it added a new dimension of industrial scale to the drive for the chemical control of medicinal materials. Industrial nations, such as Germany, the United States, and Britain, would all seek synthetic alternatives to quinine in response to the continued threat of malaria.

Chemists and Chemotherapy

During the period from 1880 to 1939, a number of trends in chemical science and technology began or accelerated. The medical conception of disease, and of malaria in particular, evolved to include germ theory, chemotherapy, and complex environmental vectors like mosquitoes. In the agricultural domain, colonial powers continued to obtain quinine from cinchona trees grown on plantations. New chemical methods and tools transformed the science of natural products and the growth of chemical industry. Large-scale research projects, first developed in the early days of the dye industry, grew and expanded into drugs. Governments, corporations, and foundations established such projects, distributed across specialized institutes, academic departments, and industrial laboratories. Within this framework, the historical trajectory of malaria treatment, based on the use of quinine, accelerated and fragmented. This period was marked by the birth of chemotherapy and the discovery of the microbial origin of malaria.

The transformative belief that health can be enhanced and disease defeated by molecular interventions was part of a broader trend: the increasing conceptualization of biological and environmental materials as being fundamentally chemical in nature. The creative power of twentieth-century synthetic chemistry was the culmination of a century-long project wherein chemists explicitly sought to construct—and later to replace—the products of nature in the laboratory. As the eminent organic chemist, August Wilhelm Hofmann, wrote in the middle of the nineteenth century: "Everybody must admit that the discovery of a simple process for preparing artificially the febrifuge principle of the Cinchona-bark, would confer a real blessing upon humanity. Now we have good grounds for the expectation that constructive Chemistry will not long remain without accomplishing this task. Already . . . numerous substances have been artificially formed, which are in the closest relation to quinine and cinchonine."[28] In the years following Hofmann's pronouncement, chemical results were not quick to appear. Nevertheless, the chemical industry expanded from alkali and acid production into fertilizers and dyes.[29] From dyes, the industry moved into drugs. Changes in industry and science wrought changes in the status and understanding of malaria and quinine.

Although Paul Ehrlich did not coin the term *chemotherapy* until 1907, the final two decades of the nineteenth century were marked by an increasing interest in the chemical control of disease. Today we associate the word chemotherapy almost exclusively with drugs that treat cancer, but historically the word has referred to many chemical interventions in disease. The term often applied to the use of chemicals, or drugs, to treat infection or to selectively kill unwanted cells, whether they were alien organisms invading the body or cancerous cells in revolt from within. For Ehrlich, the term referred specifically to the treatment of infectious disease. For example, his Salvarsan was an arsenic-based chemotherapeutic agent for the treatment of syphilis—a chemical toxic to the spirochetes. From the time of this "magic bullet" against syphilis through World War II, two other noteworthy successes in chemotherapy were the sulfa drugs and penicillin. The sulfas would emerge from synthetic-dye programs in the 1930s as potent antimicrobials, deployed in the chemotherapy of streptococcal and other infections,[30] while the development of penicillin as an antibiotic was one of the great technological success stories of World War II.[31] It should be noted that, institutionally, bacteriology and parasitology were often distinct departments, and that the sulfas and penicillin were active against bacteria, which were smaller, simpler organisms than malaria parasites. Whatever their prey, from the late nineteenth century, microbe hunters had a growing interest in the killing of germs and parasites with specific chemical compounds. The search for these novel therapeutics took place in universities, research institutes, and corporate research laboratories.

Lessons learned in malaria were the foundation for other essential pharmaceutical and institutional developments. By the final decades of the nineteenth century, the synthetic dye industry—inaugurated by Hofmann's British student, William Perkin, mentioned above—was turning its attention to another type of fine chemical, pharmaceuticals. German firms now dominated the industry, and quinine remained a strategic commodity. In this context, chemists made further attempts at the synthesis of quinine and related compounds. Notable among these were Otto Fischer, cousin and collaborator of Emil Fischer, and Ludwig Knorr, then working with Emil Fischer at the University of Erlangen. Emil was a giant in organic chemistry and went on to win the 1902 Nobel Prize in Chemistry. Otto Fischer's synthesis led to kairine, one of the first planned syntheses of a drug. Though kairine showed modest antipyretic activity, it was ineffective against malaria and toxic. In 1883, Knorr produced a less toxic antipyretic, appropriately called antipyrine (see fig. 1.1).[32] In 1888, the dye firm of Meister, Lucius, and Brüning launched antipyrine as one of the first mass-produced pharmaceuticals, alongside Bayer's phenacetin. Salicylates such as aspirin were also found while on the trail of antimalarials and fever-reducing barks, as were later drugs against tuberculosis.[33] Though the novel antipyretics could reduce

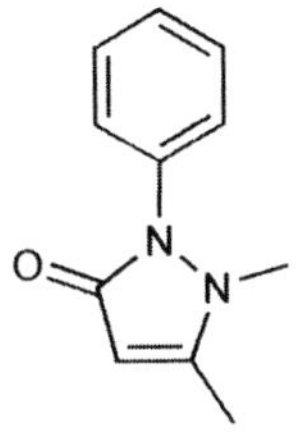

Figure 1.1 Antipyrine

fevers, they were not useful as therapeutics against malaria.[34] The chemotherapy of malaria still had to rely on the natural product quinine.[35]

Paul Ehrlich himself carried forward the chemical assault on malaria. In
1891—the same year that Bayer opened its main scientific laboratory—while
exploring the affinity of dyes for certain tissues, Ehrlich reported weak antimalarial activity for methylene blue, a synthetic dye that selectively stained
malaria parasites in vitro.[36] Methylene blue acted against malaria in the body
as well but caused side effects in patients. The staining of microbes led eventually to rational drug design through the concept of chemical specificity.
Like methylene blue, the later sulfa drugs began as synthetic dyes. Ehrlich's
findings with methylene blue were pioneering in the pharmaceutical field
and constituted the next tentative steps in the search for new drugs intended
to replace or augment quinine.

How such augmentation could be achieved was uncertain. Existing
knowledge suggested connections between immunity and chemotherapy as
related modes in the body's fight against disease. Intellectually, Ehrlich was
the node where these connections came together.[37] Earlier understandings
of chemotherapeutic effects suggest that the body's natural defenses were
augmented by the chemical compounds and that the testing of drugs against
microbes in culture was not well advanced. Ehrlich believed that natural
immunity, the ability of the body to defeat or resist infection—the kind
of immunity observed in vaccination, for example—operated by the same
kind of chemical mechanism as drugs did. The findings of Ehrlich and his
researchers reinforced this concept of drug action.[38] With the chemotherapy
of infectious disease still developing, it was not until the 1920s that one of
Ehrlich's junior collaborators, Wilhelm Roehl, would realize the goal of a synthetic antimalarial.[39]

By the 1920s, mechanisms of action for these chemical compounds
were still not well understood. Wilhelm Roehl—having moved on from
Ehrlich's laboratory to Bayer's chemotherapy institute in Elberfeld—seemed

to associate their activity with that of in vitro antiseptics and not as activators of the immune system.[40] At Bayer, Roehl was testing a promising new drug, plasmochin, against bird malaria in canaries. Roehl compared plasmochin's ability to inhibit the development of parasites "within very wide limits" to the action of mercury bichloride on bacteria.[41] Mercury compounds were topical antiseptics. Roehl's comparison here illustrates that general activity as a germicide was not well distinguished from highly specific antimicrobial effects. So, too, conceptions of drug action remained tangled with the functioning of the immune system. Roehl was puzzled by how plasmochin killed malarial parasites. Did it kill the parasite directly, or did it trigger antibody response, or somehow mobilize the body's cellular immune system? In tests against trypanosomes and the spirochetes of relapsing fever in mice, Roehl showed that plasmochin did *"not* act by producing a general increase in the defensive powers of the body."[42] He proceeded to test the mode of action of plasmochin as an immune activator in his birds. Canaries dosed with plasmochin and challenged with parasite two hours later showed no protection. Roehl concluded that "the assumption of an indirect action" by plasmochin was not confirmed by his experiments.[43] In neither mice nor canaries did Roehl find an immune boost; the activity of plasmochin seemed not to be mediated by the immune system.

In subsequent decades, others continued to pursue the relationship between chemotherapy and immunity in malaria, such as E. M. Lourie,[44] Lucy Graves Taliaferro, and William Taliaferro,[45] all at the University of Chicago Medical School. Lourie established, among other things, that quinine's mechanism of action was not by an increase in immune response.[46] The Taliaferros, too, expanded understandings of drugs and immunity, especially in avian malaria models. The mode of action of antimalarial drugs remained an area of great interest and mystery.

By the 1940s, chemists and immunologists had begun to tease apart the relationship between the body's immune responses and the mechanisms of chemotherapy. With historical and scientific acumen, René J. Dubos, a microbiologist at the Rockefeller Institute for Medical Research in New York, summed up the situation in 1941:

> It is usually considered that chemotherapeutic agents and immune antibodies exert their protective effect against bacterial infections by entirely different mechanisms. Paul Ehrlich, however, believed that the laws of chemotherapeutic action and immunity could be formulated in the same general terms. The living cell was assumed to possess a number

of chemically reactive groups, called "receptors," with which dyes, bactericidal substances, and immune bodies reacted selectively. Ehrlich regarded these "receptors" as definite chemical entities, capable of entering into union with dyes, antiseptics, and antibodies. Characteristic staining reactions, differential susceptibilities to toxic substances, and specific reactions with immune bodies could all be explained by postulating the existence of a sufficient number of "receptors" in the bacterial cell. . . . Unfortunately, neither Ehrlich nor his immediate followers succeeded in identifying the chemical nature of these "receptors," or even in demonstrating their existence as well-defined entities; the receptor theory therefore fell into disrepute and was often considered an attempt to mask ignorance under a covering of words. During the past two decades, however, immunochemistry has in several cases given reality and chemical definition to the "receptors" postulated by Ehrlich.[47]

For Dubos, the interactions of cells—living entities—with their environment was chemically mediated. As he was a key connection between the realm of chemotherapy and the environmental movement later in the century, Dubos's words merit close attention.[48] With the function of the immune system separated from the function of drugs, Dubos still saw much that needed explication with regard to drug action:

> There are of course many ways in which it is possible to interfere with the parasitic career of a virulent organism, and it would be futile to try to force the mechanism of action of the different therapeutic agents into one and the same pattern. But in any case it appears justified to claim that the rational development of antisepsis and chemotherapy has much to gain from a better knowledge of the chemical architecture of the bacterial cell for, in Paul Ehrlich's words, "only such substances can be anchored at any particular part of the organism which fit into the molecule of the recipient combination as a piece of a mosaic fits into a certain pattern."[49]

Ehrlich and others transformed the understanding of drugs and immunity and made all these interactions *chemical* in a profound and fundamental way. These chemical understandings of pharmacology and biology would transform biomedicine.[50]

Malaria and Mosquitoes

For nearly all of its recorded history, malaria has been a disease of place. The name we give malaria in English today was derived from the Italian for "bad air," and malarial fevers were often associated with the bad or corrupt air of swamps and marshes—miasmas, as these foul and pernicious effluvia were often termed. Since ancient times, malaria in Europe was documented in wetlands, such as the famously deadly Roman Campagna surrounding the Italian capital. Tales of intermittent fevers abound, invoked in such historically significant deaths as that of Alexander the Great and Alaric, king of the Visigoths, who sacked Rome in 410 C.E.[51] As diseases of place, these fevers could be controlled by drainage and engineering, an early example being that of Selinunte. This city in Sicily was relieved of its burden of fever by the Greek philosopher-physician Empedocles who, in the fifth century B.C.E., altered the course of a local river and made Selinunte's environs more salubrious.

Environmental variables continued to be suspect in the coming millennia. At the end of the nineteenth century, noted Italian malariologist Angelo Celli listed soil, water, and air as the "three principle factors" contributing to "local or physical causes of predisposition or of immunity" to malaria. Celli asserted these factors just at the historic moment when mosquitoes were revealed as the vectors of malaria. He acknowledged this new fact but knew that location remained a critical variable in the disease. "Up till a few months ago this was believed [by Italian malariologists] to be one of the most typical soil diseases, like tetanus and anthrax. This can no longer be maintained *sic et simpliciter*; but, on the other hand, it is undoubtedly, as we have said, a typical local or autochthonic epidemy. It is interesting, therefore, to study the local causes which favour or do not favour its production."[52] In the nineteenth and twentieth century, the Italians, like the Greeks before them, continued to employ engineering projects and land reclamation as part of a program to eliminate malaria from the country. The Italians referred to these efforts collectively as "bonification," a process of transforming disease-ridden places into good productive land. For example, between World War I and World War II, 200,000 acres of the infamously deadly Pontine marshes were reclaimed.[53] These environmental interventions to alter places and geography in order to control intermittent fevers are as ancient as malaria's written history.

Late in the nineteenth century, malariologists transformed malaria biologically. The basis of this transformation was the visualization of the malarial parasites in blood and the unraveling of their transmission via mosquitoes. Mosquitoes, it turned out, were what made wetlands unhealthy. Place remained an essential part of malaria's culture, but by the end of the nineteenth century, this connection was no longer mediated by miasmas or corrupt air, but by arthropod vectors: *Anopheles* mosquitoes carried malaria from person to person. Three names are famously associated with these transformations: Alphonse Laveran, Ronald Ross, and to a lesser extent Giovanni Battista Grassi. In 1880, Laveran (who won the Nobel Prize in Physiology or Medicine in 1907), a French army doctor working in Algeria, discovered the malarial parasite in human blood cells. Within a decade, his findings gained wide acceptance. In 1897, Ross (who won the Nobel in 1902), an officer in the Indian Medical Service, discovered the human malarial parasite in *Anopheles* mosquitoes.[54] The scientific study of malaria mosquitoes and their ecology would take its first form when Ross, following up on his *Anopheles* research, traced the full life cycle of the avian parasite in its mosquito vector in 1898. In the fall of 1898, Italian doctor Grassi, along with Giuseppe Bastianelli and Amico Bignami, demonstrated the life cycle of *Plasmodium falciparum* (aestivo-autumnal fever) in humans and *A. claviger* mosquitoes. The Italians had done likewise for the other human malarias of Europe, *P. vivax* and *P. malariae*, by the end of 1899. The priority claims of Ross and Grassi became the source of one of the early twentieth century's bitterest and longest scientific feuds, and I will not dwell on them here.[55] It is sufficient to note that, by the beginning of the twentieth century, malaria joined yellow fever and filariasis as a disease transmitted by mosquitoes.

The discovery of mosquito transmission broadened the scope of prevention beyond measures such as the drainage of wetlands and the use of quinine to secure the health of colonial personnel. In the early days of the twentieth century, prevention took a number of forms, most notably drug prophylaxis and the elimination of mosquitoes. Mosquitoes could be killed, their habitat destroyed or disrupted, or they could be kept at bay with screens and nets. Prevention in these terms brings to mind concepts of separation or protected interfaces: Keeping mosquitoes away from one's skin could prevent the transmission of the disease. For example, this interface between mosquito and human could be physically obstructed with a window screen or a bed net. The propagation of malaria requires many interfaces to function without disruption. The parasite must cross many cell membranes in the human host and traverse an entire mosquito in a number of forms to successfully complete its life cycle. Each of these interfaces is a possible point of attack in the battle against malaria. The choice of attacking malaria medically with drugs or environmentally by going after mosquito vectors became one of the great philosophical divides in public health. After his discovery of the mosquito as vector, Ronald Ross became the great proponent of mosquitoes as the crucial variable in malaria transmission, while famed German microbe hunter Robert Koch championed medical intervention.[56]

Many joined this battle. The Rockefeller Foundation, from its inception in 1913, sought to eliminate malaria both by the control of mosquitoes and the study and distribution of antimalarial compounds. The foundation had many collaborators in its campaigns against malaria. In 1921, while working for the U.S. Public Health Service, Marshall A. Barber—along with his assistant Theodore Brevard Hayne and the entomologist William Komp—developed Paris green, a poison that mosquito larvae would eat when it was scattered on water.[57] Barber was at this time a once-and-future Rockefeller employee. He worked for the International Health Board from 1915 to 1917, the Rockefeller Institute from 1918 to 1919, and the International Health Division (IHD) from 1929 to 1939. For two decades, the Paris green larvicide was an essential component of malaria control projects around the world. In Italy, governmental and private institutions deployed land reclamation, mosquito control, and quinine against the disease. At the beginning of the twentieth century, Italian malariologist Angelo Celli chronicled the long history of malaria and malaria control in the Roman Campagna. Celli's editor (and daughter) brought the story forward into the twentieth century in her epilogue, noting that during the period from 1862 to 1912, the Italians spent $62.4 million on land reclamation, or bonification, projects: "But in spite of all the years and all the millions spent for hydraulic reclamation only a minimum success in sanitation was obtained as compared with that which during the short period of 10 years has been obtained by the use of State quinine, and that, too, with a large profit."[58] Now that the role of mosquitoes was visible, this difference in success was now comprehensible: "We can easily understand to-day the reason for the limited advantages which were obtained through hydraulic reclamation, since that very seldom eliminates the anopheles."[59] In places where vector mosquitoes continued to breed, drugs might work better than drainage. Most famously, DDT—the insecticide developed during World War II and deployed around the globe in subsequent years—exemplified a new type of intervention made possible by the discovery of mosquito vectors.[60]

Mosquitoes anchored malaria to the watery places where they bred, cementing the association of malaria to specific locations even while they made malaria control more complex. Pre–World War II antimalarial campaigns in the United States reveal this complexity, as the government made substantial efforts to intervene in malaria in the South using drainage and engineering. These federal efforts coincided with the decline of malaria, but whether they were causal is a matter of much contemporary and historical debate.[61] As malariologist Marshall Barber wrote, "In comparing the factors which contributed to the decline of malaria in the United States, we find it difficult to say which is of most weight; for they vary greatly according to time and locality." Barber had pointed out that land use and water could help or hinder the disease: "In one region malaria diminished when the land was drained, in another when it was flooded and devoted to rice cultivation; in a third when the woodlands were cleared, and in a fourth when an almost treeless prairie was cultivated." At the same time, people had more access to health care, better housing, and improving diets. Barber, having considered "the great bulk of the decrease in malaria which has been noted all over the country, from the Great Lakes to Texas and through many years," gave "the greater credit to screens, quinine, and improved medical treatment."[62] Wherever one might give the credit, each malarial locality had to be assessed and surveyed to understand how the disease and vectors operated.

Environment and Ecology

The ecology of mosquitoes provided another reason for scientists to view malaria from an environmental perspective. The insects further complicated an already complex disease. Malarial parasites did not just reside in the human body, and they could not be transmitted between human hosts by most normal contact.[63] Malaria parasites were large (compared to bacteria) multistaged creatures that depended on two distinctive hosts. For both these reasons, place and complexity, malaria workers were predisposed for seeing the disease from an environmental perspective.[64] Although most of this book focuses on the laboratory and clinic, we must remember the environmental context of malaria as a disease. This understanding of malaria has a long history and was certainly in the minds of scientists and physicians as they captured parts of this broader environment within their labs. A view of malaria in the context of its hosts and its environment might be termed an ecological or natural-historical perspective. Ecology is the scientific study of living things in their environment and often carries antireductionist overtones.[65] In the twentieth century, the use of the term natural history—a field more associated with an earlier period—signals a similar, more descriptive, holistic view of the natural world. As Marshall Barber, late of Rockefeller's IHD, wrote in 1946, "I have given considerable space to the natural history of mosquito vectors, a knowledge of which, I trust, will aid in understanding the methods of preventing the disease."[66]

Another promoter of natural history in the twentieth century was Marston Bates, a Rockefeller researcher and entomologist who spent much of his career working with mosquitoes. Bates had an inclusive meaning for the term natural history, "so that it would cover both the field and laboratory study of living organisms, because both types of study are intimately related."[67] In his 1949 book, *The Natural History of Mosquitoes*, he promoted this natural-historical perspective. Bates was opposed to compartmentalization and the closure of disciplinary boundaries: "The use of a term like 'natural history' in itself symbolizes a rebellion against the endless compartmentation of the biological sciences into specialized and mutually exclusive 'ologies,' but it is not intended as a substitute label for the entire field of biology." For Bates, biology remained an "ology" and therefore potentially too analytic or reductionist. "Biology necessarily covers all aspects of the study of organisms and living processes without stressing one particular point of view more than another, while natural history would levy contributions from the various specialties only in so far as their material would directly help the understanding of the living, functioning, whole organism."[68] Bates's twentieth-century natural history would take advantage of modern science but not lose sight of the intact organism. For Bates, natural history would include elements drawn from "ologies" such as morphology and physiology. This approach was of great value to those who studied malaria and mosquitoes because it would keep them aware of the bigger picture and the subtleties and complexities of the disease and its hosts.

Such a holistic view is also essential to the historian of a disease as complex as malaria. The interaction of many scientists, patients, organisms, and ecosystems is the historical object we are exploring, not the isolated results of one study or technological intervention. History writing aside, the necessity of taking environment into account was a persistent theme in malaria research. The natural-historical—or ecological—perspective produced a number of larger-scale environmental models used by other Rockefeller workers, such as Paul Russell, Wilbur Sawyer, and Lewis Hackett. Hackett's *Malaria in Europe: An Ecological Study* had, as the subtitle suggests, an environmental approach to the problem of malaria in its European context.[69] Hackett emphasized the complex—often confounding—interaction of climate, geography, technology, and immunology with humans, mosquitoes, and parasites. Hackett, like Sawyer and Russell, was associated with Rockefeller's IHD.

With regard to tropical medicine in general, Wilbur Sawyer, director of IHD, emphasized the importance of the environment in his 1937 presidential address to the American Academy of Tropical Medicine. North American investigators could not expect to reap the benefits of their expenses and sacrifice "without study of disease in its natural surroundings." [70] For Sawyer, "The natural tropical environment is not definable in terms of heat and humidity." It was "a thousand different and complex environments," involving local climatic, social, and economic conditions as well as race, nutrition, and "especially arthropod vectors of disease and animal hosts" (11). In Sawyer's framing of tropical diseases, the most important one, transcending all others, was malaria. Making the case for the cross-fertilization of laboratory and field—between "the field" and "centers of learning"—Sawyer asserted that malaria was actually not a single disease: "A superficial knowledge of malaria may be gained from lectures, books, prepared specimens, and observation of the occasional patient who enters our northern teaching clinics. A real understanding of malaria, however, requires observation and experience in several environments, for this disease varies from place to place in the species of plasmodium, the clinical picture, the species and race of the anopheline vector, and the local conditions favoring transmission" (14). [71] However, the tropical field worker or clinician might lack for other malaria essentials, such as scientific exchange, current journals, and "elaborate laboratory apparatus and special experimental animals" (16). Beyond the natural environment of the disease, it was these appurtenances that formed another essential medical/scientific environment. As Sawyer said, "There is another environment, broadly speaking, which is indispensable to study and research in tropical medicine. It is the academic environment consisting of library, laboratory, and association with other scientists" (15). Sawyer proceeded to acknowledge that such environments were more numerous in the temperate regions than in the tropics and that they were "built up slowly." In Sawyer's construction, those who studied and treated disease had to be understood in the context of their own environments.

Almost two years before Sawyer made his case before his peers, Paul Russell of Rockefeller's IHD addressed the third-year class of the Harvard Medical School. Russell, too, sought to emphasize biological interactions and the environment with his topic: "Preventive Medicine as Exemplified by Malaria." Russell employed the agricultural analogy of seed, sower, and soil, where the seed was an infected and infectious individual carrying the gametocytes, the sower was the *Anopheles* mosquito, and the soil was the individual whose blood was accessible to the mosquito and susceptible to infection. [72] From a preventive medicine or public health standpoint, Russell said that the factors contributing to endemic and epidemic malaria might be grouped in three categories: "the *human host* as seed or soil, the *insect* as sower, or the *environment* which is influential as regards both man and insect" (emphasis in the original).[73] Following a discussion of host susceptibility featuring William Taliaferro's immunological work in birds and monkeys, Russell moved on to "man's ability to modify malaria by manipulation of environment" (14). He cited "slovenly methods of agriculture," "grossly defective hygiene," and lastly "engineer-made malaria" as negative human impacts on the malaria environment, before moving on to the subtleties of proper malaria control through environmental interventions, with all their "technical, social, legal, and economic implications" (15–23). In Russell's view, all this was in aid of species control as the most feasible approach to malaria control (25–26). Species control was a measured approach to going after the malaria vectors, attacking only those species of *Anopheles* mosquitoes that were responsible for malaria transmission in a given area. Though Russell had a specific agenda to press, it nevertheless required him to frame the disease problem in broad environmental terms.

These environmental terms were not limited to those who worked in the field or oversaw large-scale antimalaria campaigns, such as the Rockefeller officers cited above. Another researcher who kept environmental factors in mind, although his research was largely confined to the laboratory, was Robert Hegner. Hegner had founded the program in medical zoology at the Johns Hopkins School of Hygiene and Public Health. Hegner and his colleagues were keenly interested in the impact of environment on parasite development, especially avian malaria. As outgoing president of the American Society of Parasitologists, Hegner said in 1936, "For the most part investigators have devoted their time and efforts to attempts to eradicate parasitic organisms, and comparatively few have endeavored *to improve the environment in the host in favor of the parasite.* No one knows what factors prevent a certain species of parasite from living in a given species of host, but it might be possible to modify the host in some very simple way that might even occur in nature so as to render it susceptible to infection."[74] This experimentally produced susceptibility might reveal why hosts were susceptible or open up new model organisms to infection, expanding the possibilities for research. Choosing an example from bird malaria, Hegner posed questions regarding the chain of causality that led to patterns of development in the parasites. As in humans, certain bird malarias reproduced synchronously in the blood. Hegner postulated that the timing of this asexual cycle could be controlled in one of two ways: It might be governed by the parasite's genes and be impacted only temporarily by environment, or it might be "forced on the parasites by the activities of the bird or the diurnal variations in the environment" (11). In summarizing, Hegner related the world of the laboratory to the world of nature: "Our plan has been to note the reactions of natural and foreign parasites to modifications in the host. In every case the modifications were brought about by changes in the environment of the host that might easily occur in nature" (11). Hegner sought to understand nature by capturing parts of it in the controlled environment of the laboratory and modifying variables, such as light and temperature, to observe behavior that might have occurred in nature.

Though Hegner passed away in 1942, this environmental understanding persisted in his department and in the U.S. wartime antimalarial program. One of Hegner's last students, Myron Simpson, examined periodic behavior in avian malaria reproduction in ducks. These "rhythms" were part of the interplay of intrinsic properties of the several organisms and their environment, conceived as both the external world and the biological space within the hosts. Grasping and understanding the complexity of the living systems was an essential first step to malaria research: "The complex animal body, when considered in relation to its own tissues or its parasites, becomes an intricate environment more or less complete within itself. Hence, in studying the tissues of an organism or the species living within it, one must consider the inherent potentialities of cell or parasite as they are allowed expression by the regulated physiological processes of the organism itself."[75] Simpson's interest was in the parasites' periodic behavior and environmental conditions such as host age and day-night cycles. He explored the interaction of biological function and environment. These were his essential variables in his biological models. Complexity, environmental contexts, and interaction between parasite and host were central concerns of researchers like Simpson and Hegner. We will revisit this in discussions of animal models in the following chapter.

Even newcomers to malaria research were keenly aware of location and environment. Eli K. Marshall Jr. was a Hopkins pharmacologist and chemist well known for his pioneering work on the sulfa drugs—antimicrobials that had emerged in the 1930s and 1940s. With the outbreak of World War II, however, Marshall worked more and more with malaria chemotherapy, contributing greatly to the antimalarial program. In 1944, when Simpson was writing about microenvironments in his thesis, Marshall was raising concerns about the use of avian models of malaria and with the microenvironments seen by malaria parasites in birds. At a conference on malaria on 29 March 1944, Marshall expressed these concerns to his colleagues. "Unlike the work with the sulfonamides where one is dealing with only one stage of the infecting organism and where there is good comparison between mouse and man as regards the absorption, degradation, and excretion of the sulfonamide, in malaria the life cycle of the parasite is not even known, and it is possible that one may be dealing with five different forms." At that time, these five were the sporozoites, the cryptozoites (as the yet-to-be-revealed liver stage was known), an exo-erythrocytic form (now called the merozoites), the trophozoites, and the gametocytes. Marshall pointed out that each "of these forms may be in different environments" and that it was "essential to know whether the action of drugs on the various stages of parasite are qualitatively or quantitatively different."[76] As he traced the subtleties of actions of drugs through the complex environments of various hosts, Marshall's wartime malaria work would expand the field and contribute the twentieth-century revolution in pharmacology.

Like Hegner's, Marshall's malaria models were generally not mammals but birds. With different parasites, different life stages, and different hosts, one had to account for many microenvironments. In the face of these complexities, malaria researchers from Laveran to Hegner to Marshall would again and again return to birds and their malarias while looking for new therapies and new insights into human malaria biology. Always in the background was the question of how similar were these bird diseases to the human malarias—would the research be relevant to human treatments? These malarial birds were central to the development of antimalarial drugs, and they are our next stop in this history.

Chapter 2

Avian Malaria

The period between World War I and World War II was a productive one for antimalarial research. The first successful environmental insecticide, Paris green, was developed against mosquitoes. And on the drug front, new methods for testing antimalarials in animals—in birds, in fact—would emerge in the Bayer laboratories. These methods would persist as the backbone of antimalarial drug screening throughout the war and into the late 1940s. To appreciate the work done by the U.S. wartime antimalarial program, we need to understand the research tools available to it. What were the shapes and capabilities of model systems for malaria research? To understand the development of drugs in the first half of the twentieth century, we need to know how Bayer's innovations with animals came to be. How did canaries with malaria become a transformative technology for pharmaceutical innovation?

The use of bird parasites as research tools and models of human disease began simply. Malariologists brought small, wild-caught birds into the laboratory and passed their parasites on to other local birds or canaries from the neighborhood pet store. The wider research community evinced little resistance to the idea that sparrows or canaries might be suitable for medical research. Indeed, Alphonse Laveran seems to have met less resistance to his suggestion that physicians should study malaria in birds than to his initial discovery of malaria's causative parasites in human blood. And Ronald Ross's widely accepted priority claim to the discovery of mosquito transmission rested largely on his own work with birds and their vector mosquitoes. From these foundations, the complexity of avian model systems would grow as researchers discovered new varieties of malaria, paired them with new mosquitoes, and asked new questions. With regard to chemotherapy, the additional host preferences expanded potential laboratory subjects from canaries to chickens and ducks: commercially available birds that would soon allow rapid expansion of research in a time of national emergency. For malaria before 1950, it was birds and their malarial parasites that were key to research, not the rodents that one typically envisions in a biomedical laboratory.[1] This story of avian malaria has its beginnings in the late nineteenth century, but its key innovator was Paul Ehrlich's chemotherapy pioneer, Wilhelm Roehl.

Little known today, Roehl was one the pioneers of modern drug discovery, having trained with Paul Ehrlich. Roehl worked in Ehrlich's laboratories on two occasions, first in 1905–1906 and again from 1907 to 1909. It was during these crucial years that Ehrlich's group discovered Salvarsan, the revolutionary chemotherapeutic agent against syphilis.[2] Roehl's work on trypanosomes (the parasites associated with sleeping sickness) helped refine Ehrlich's thinking with regard to chemotherapy, drug resistance, and receptor theory—as Ehrlich acknowledged in his Nobel lecture in 1908.[3] Roehl did the bulk of his trypanosome work in mice, using more than one thousand white mice and treating them with various active arsenic compounds and dyes. He also ran comparative tests in two other standard lab animals, the rabbit and the guinea pig.[4] Speaking about the methods of chemotherapy in 1907, Ehrlich said that hundreds or even thousands of compounds had to be tested in animals before even a few therapeutic chemicals could be identified. From the effects of these chemical compounds on animals, Ehrlich and his collaborators were able to obtain hints "as to what to avoid, and in what direction therapeutics should proceed."[5] This use of laboratory animals as models of human disease was at the center of the new chemotherapy and of Roehl's contributions to drug discovery.

Beyond the routine utility of animal testing in chemotherapy, the inability of researchers to infect animals with human malaria or to grow these parasites in test tubes or on plates (in vitro cultures) increased the need for animal models. In vitro systems in bacteriology, for example, had allowed many germs to be cultured in dishes with no other organisms needed to maintain the disease agents in the lab. In relation to other diseases, malaria's lack of such simple systems was a persistent hindrance to research. In his 1967 presidential address to the Royal Society of Tropical Medicine and Hygiene, the eminent malariologist Percy C. C. Garnham discussed the historical significance of Koch's three postulates for proof of the cause of disease: "the presence of the parasite in all the lesions, its isolation in pure culture, and its ability to reproduce the disease in laboratory animals." Garnham mused about the unfortunate status of malaria: "Incidentally, the second and third of these postulates can scarcely be said to have been fulfilled for the malaria parasites: the latter can hardly be maintained in pure culture and they will only infect splenectomized marmosets, gibbons or chimpanzees—which are not exactly laboratory animals."[6] Garnham's concern was historically common among malariologists. Researchers regularly cited the difficulties of working with malaria in the lab. Robert W. Hegner and his coworkers at the Johns Hopkins School of Hygiene and Public Health echoed Ehrlich in valuing animal research: "Animal experimentation is essential in the trial of any new therapeutic agent. . . . Fortunately this can be done with most of the important parasitic diseases of man." But for malaria, however, the Hopkins workers shared Garnham's later lament, as "malaria offers an exception and it has therefore been necessary to utilize the similar diseases of birds."[7] Roehl's innovations would fill a critical need in the chemotherapy of malaria.

From the 1890s to the 1940s, avian malarias were the dominant research tool in chemotherapeutic research, in the immunology of malaria, and in the biology of the malarial organism. Their dominance would only gradually diminish. Paul Russell, of the International Health Division of the Rockefeller Foundation whom we last encountered presenting his environmental model of malaria to the medical students at Harvard, was a promoter of avian malaria models, commenting in 1931, "The longer I work with bird malaria the more firmly I am convinced that it is a reliable indicator for human malaria."[8] In the early days of parasite research, the ready availability of bird malarias played a role in their selection as research models. "Infected birds may be secured almost anywhere," wrote Reginald Manwell in 1934.[9] Manwell had trained at Johns Hopkins, earning his DSc there in 1928. Manwell favored English sparrows as sources of parasites. Change would only come after World War II, when the rodent malaria *Plasmodium berghei*, discovered in 1948, became one of the most productive models in malaria research.[10] And it was not until the 1970s that William Trager and James B. Jensen would successfully culture *Plasmodium falciparum* in vitro through a portion of its life cycle in human blood.[11] Before the development of rodent models and this breakthrough in culturing, bird malaria was the best model and often the only hope of researchers seeking new insights and new tools.

Avian Malaria before Roehl

By the 1920s, when Roehl took them up, avian malarias were already well established as general tools for malaria research, particularly with regard to the biology of the parasites. No less an authority than Alphonse Laveran—the discoverer of malarial parasites in human blood—had exhorted his fellow physicians and malariologists to study the blood parasites of birds to learn more about human malaria. As he wrote in 1891,

> Direct observation of the parasites of human malaria appears today to have yielded all that it can, and I believe that to solve the still obscure questions relating to the development of this parasite, it is necessary to follow a slightly divergent path and study the analogous parasites that exist in diverse animals. The blood-borne parasites of birds described by [Vasilii] Danilewsky are of particular interest from this perspective, on account of their great resemblance to human malaria parasites; thus are physicians led to encroach upon the domain of the naturalists and attend to these avian parasites.[12]

Many heeded this exhortation. Within a decade of Danilewsky's 1885 observations of avian parasites[13] and the general acceptance of Laveran's claims about the protozoan etiology of human malaria, bird malaria was intimately associated with its human cousins. For example, in their seminal paper on human malaria, William Sydney Thayer and John Hewetson passed over the blood-borne parasites of most other animals to provide a brief but thorough review of avian malaria in 1895.[14] As these two Hopkins doctors wrote, "It has been clearly shown that birds may suffer from a malarial infection very similar to that in man." The most famous physician to take up the study of avian malaria was Ronald Ross—whom we also met in chapter 1—whose studies of bird malaria in 1897–1898 established mosquitoes as the vectors for malaria. From Laveran's investigations through World War II, avian malarias were central to understandings of the biology and control of the human disease.

Others shared Laveran's and Ross's enthusiasm for birds. Following on Laveran's discovery, William G. MacCallum of Johns Hopkins made the next major contribution to the understanding of human malaria. MacCallum—who is still well-known among malariologists—used the blood of both crows and people to give meaning to the observed motion of the parasites in freshly drawn blood. It was this motion, seen through the microscope, that had led Laveran to his initial observation of the parasites. In the summer of 1897, MacCallum, back home from his medical studies at Hopkins, drew blood from sick crows in Dunnville, Ontario. In this blood, he saw parasites of the genus *Halteridium*, distinguishing two forms of the parasite: a granular form that emerged from the corpuscle and was quiescent, and a transparent, homogenous form that erupted from the blood cell with great activity and "threw out active flagella." Although many had described the flagellation, or exflagellation, of the parasites—a process wherein the parasites burst forth from the red blood cells and formed motile, elongate bodies, or *flagella*—it was MacCallum who observed the two forms in the same microscopic field and gave lasting interpretation to this behavior. Often quoted by malariologists, this passage contains MacCallum's key observations:

> Then came the acme of the process. One of the four flagella passed out of the field, but the remaining three proceeded directly toward the granular form, lying quietly across the field, and surrounded it, wriggling about actively. *One of the flagella, concentrating its protoplasm at one end, dashed into the granular sphere, which seemed to put out a process to meet it, and buried its head, finally wriggling its whole body into the organism, which again became perfectly round.* The remaining flagella, seeking to repeat this process, were evidently repulsed, and soon became inactive and degenerated. . . . Soon all became quiet again . . . what now had become an elongated fusiform body, which soon swam away with a gliding motion. [emphasis in original]

MacCallum's conclusion: "Have we not here, without much doubt, a sexual process in the organisms the result of which is the motile vermiculus?"[15] The parasites were reproducing sexually in the cooling blood.

MacCallum was able to garner his critical insight because his avian parasites and their highly susceptible hosts had a distinct advantage over the malaria he observed in the clinic. Unlike infected human blood, which showed him few sexual forms in any given microscopic field, his crow blood gave him a high enough density of parasites to find this key observation. In spite of differences between the crow disease and human malaria, MacCallum was confident that he could confirm his findings in the human case. Indeed, activated by his avian observations, MacCallum soon found sexual reproduction in the human parasites, complete with passive and active forms.[16] MacCallum used an avian model of the disease for insight into the biology of the human parasite. This mapping of findings in birds to those in humans was a persistent method in malaria research throughout the first half of the twentieth century. Its continued productivity required a rich array of avian model systems and the movement of people and materials between field, laboratory, and clinic—much as MacCallum moved from the meadows of Ontario to the clinics of the Johns Hopkins Hospital.

MacCallum's *Halteridium* was only one bird parasite employed as a malaria research tool. Numerous others, mostly of the genus *Plasmodium*, were isolated and developed. Four *Plasmodium* bird-malaria models provided the resources for the U.S. antimalarial project conducted during World War II. These four avian species—which emerged as distinct and stable entities from the 1920s to the 1940s—were *P. relictum*, *P. cathemerium*, *P. gallinaceum*, and *P. lophurae*. Though I will not dwell on it here, most *Plasmodium* species required some negotiation before nomenclature, host specificity, and morphology could be established.[17] Each merits attention to its identification and its place in the laboratory and field.

In the first years of avian malaria research, *P. relictum* was the predominant species. Although it was one of the earliest of the parasites identified, *P. relictum*'s name and identity took the longest to stabilize. Later writers frequently attribute the species' first description to Vasilii Danilewsky.[18] However, his belief in the unitary nature of malaria—that all malaria parasites in humans and animals shared a single causative agent whose appearance and development varied from host to host—makes his early association with *P. relictum* difficult to confirm. *P. relictum*'s promiscuous host choice among many kinds of birds—one of the largest range of natural host species of any malaria parasite—no doubt contributed to some confusion about its naming and nature. More certain identification occurred in Sicily by Giovanni Battista Grassi and Raimondo Feletti in 1892.[19] Unlike the parasites of humans, *P. relictum* was transmitted primarily by mosquitoes of the genus *Culex*,[20] and it was in this connection that *P. relictum* made its first major contribution to medicine. Ronald Ross made his discovery of the mosquito transmission of malaria using *P. relictum* and *Culex*—most likely *Culex pipiens fatigans*. Ross was not an expert entomologist, identifying these mosquitoes as "gray." Indeed, his early failure to distinguish the gray mosquitoes (*Culex*) from their "dapple-winged" (*Anopheles*) relatives may have been responsible for his first charting the development of an avian parasite rather than a human one. Well aware of MacCallum's observations on the sexual reproduction of the parasites, Ross completed this avian work—conducted largely with wild-caught larks and sparrows—in July 1898. But the story of *P. relictum* does not end with Ross.

Plasmodium relictum is capable of infecting domestic as well as wild perching birds. Among its susceptible hosts is the canary (*Serinus canarius*).[21] While

Roehl was preparing his early projects at Bayer, another worker in Germany was taking the first steps to bend avian malaria to the purposes of chemotherapeutic research. Working at the Institute for Tropical Medicine in Hamburg, Phokion Kopanaris noted the great similarity between avian malarial parasites and those of humans. In 1911, Kopanaris described his experiments testing quinine and Salvarsan against bird malaria. (Salvarsan, Ehrlich's anti-syphilis drug, had previously shown some activity against human malaria.) Kopanaris used canaries artificially infected with *P. relictum* as his research materials. He tested known human drugs against the animal parasites and demonstrated that what worked in humans could also be efficacious in bird disease.[22] A decade later, Wilhelm Roehl, working for Bayer at Elberfeld, adopted and adapted this model system of canaries.

Roehl and His Canaries

As a nation, Germany had a number of good reasons for working on synthetic antimalarials. In World War I, its troops in East Africa had suffered greatly from a shortage of quinine. The shortage also hampered the German army in the Balkans and Turkey. While having little colonial access to quinine, Germany had unmatched resources in the synthetic dye industry and Ehrlich's research in chemotherapy. As a company, Bayer had a profit motive for pursuing quinine substitutes. Yet as we saw in chapter 1, many had tried and failed to replace natural quinine. Achieving this long-desired end would require something more than motivation. Wilhelm Roehl would provide the necessary tools for success.

Roehl was born in Berlin in 1881 into a family of mathematicians and theologians. From a very young age, he was interested in biology and animals, enlisting his mother in projects that involved boiling down the skeletons of the occasional owl or hedgehog.[23] After attending gymnasium in Naumburg and Halberstadt, Roehl studied medicine at the Universities of Halle and Heidelberg, passing his state exam in the fall of 1903 and receiving his medical doctorate *summa cum laude*. Roehl worked at research institutes in Heidelberg and elsewhere before coming to Ehrlich's Institute for Experimental Therapy in Frankfurt in 1905. Frankfurt would prove to be an important locale for Roehl. In September 1909 came a moment crucial to Roehl's future: he met Carl Duisberg at a lecture in Frankfurt by Paul Ehrlich on the fundamentals of chemotherapy.[24] Duisberg was a member of the board of management at the chemical and dye company Bayer, and shortly thereafter he sought out Roehl to bring this new expertise in chemotherapy to Bayer.

After a brief stay in Giessen, Roehl was persuaded to work for Bayer, who sent him to Vienna for further training in pharmacology with Hans Horst Meyer. In the spring of 1911, Roehl came back to Germany and fitted out a small chemotherapy laboratory in Elberfeld. Except for his military service during World War I, Roehl would work for Bayer until his death in 1929 at the age of forty-seven. In his time at Bayer, Roehl worked on a range of medical problems, including sleeping sickness and malaria. Where his earlier work had involved mice and trypanosomes, his animal model for malaria would employ birds and bird malaria.

Roehl, like others, believed that malaria research was hindered by the lack of good model systems for research. He found it remarkable that—despite a number of possible leads, all of which had been around for years—the new chemotherapy had turned up no new chemical compounds active against malaria. The only materials to show any significant activity remained quinine (and the other cinchona alkaloids), arsenicals like Salvarsan, and the methylene blue dyes. Why had no new antimalarials been forthcoming? Clearly, in Roehl's opinion, it was the lack of good methods of animal testing. A tractable, scalable, and quantifiable animal system was lacking. Roehl further noted that while drugs with activity against human malaria had been shown by Kopanaris and others to be active against avian malaria, no one had done the reverse: discovered "an effective substance against malaria in birds which later proved effective against human malaria."[25] Kopanaris had treated bird malaria with drugs already known to be active against human disease. To impact human health, the epistemological arrow would have to be reversed.

In addition, Roehl identified a critical quantitative problem with previous chemotherapeutic work on avian malaria. This was what one might term today a drug-delivery problem, particularly with bitter-tasting, potentially toxic alkaloids such as quinine. Other researchers had delivered their drug compounds to the birds by intramuscular or subcutaneous injection. Such injections of natural alkaloids produced almost immediate toxic and inflammatory effects, forcing researchers to limit themselves to testing only very low dosages. But these low doses made any antimalarial activity easy to overlook. These difficulties could be overcome by adding the candidate drugs to the birds' food, potentially allowing for continuous administration with the food. This method, too, had drawbacks. Roehl observed that some of his canaries "would rather starve than to swallow the bitter drug."[26] And this method demanded larger quantities of the chemical compounds and prevented precise measurement of dosages. For proper chemotherapy research, a new method of delivery would be required.

For Roehl, quantitation was key to drug screening. He therefore borrowed a technique previously used on mice. He administered the drugs in solution by means of an esophageal tube, employing a fine catheter attached to a syringe. With this setup, Roehl could gradually deliver a carefully measured dose—say one milliliter—to a canary weighing only twenty grams. The birds might occasionally regurgitate the solution, but Roehl was nonetheless able to quantitatively demonstrate the efficacy of a number alkaloids. Roehl's first tests were made with quinine, using canaries infected by intramuscular injection of diseased blood. Normally parasites would appear in the birds' blood after four or five days, but Roehl could suppress the appearance of the parasites for ten days or longer if he treated the canaries daily for five days after inoculation with sufficiently strong solutions of quinine. Roehl employed untreated controls in each series of infected birds to forestall false conclusions. He assigned primary importance to the observation of parasites, noting whether their appearance in the blood was delayed relative to controls.[27] Roehl took Kopanaris's canaries and *P. relictum* and made them a tool for quantifying the efficacy of antimalarial drugs. Roehl then went one step further and related efficacy to toxicity. By his new method, he determined both the effective dosages (concentrations) and the maximum tolerated doses.

Of course, the most important step for Roehl was to move beyond quinine and search for new drugs. To do this, he took his avian system—and his observation of parasite suppression in the blood—and screened synthetic compounds. Over the course of three years, the Bayer group screened several hundred compounds. Bayer's chemists, and their store of knowledge and materials from decades in the dye industry, provided Roehl with these substances. He was able to identify the first synthetic antimalarial to rival the natural compound, quinine. One can hear the pride, teamwork, and triumph in Roehl's words: "Only after my quantitative method had been elaborated was it possible to test the substances chemotherapeutically in animal experiments. Further collaboration with chemotherapists and chemists then led rapidly to the discovery of the active series, the systematic elaboration of which finally yielded Plasmochin."[28] Plasmochin—also called plasmoquine or pamaquine—was the first commercial synthetic antimalarial. We will revisit plasmochin in its chemical and clinical context in the next chapter.

To prove his new drug and his new method, Roehl tested plasmochin against the benchmark antimalarial, quinine. In Roehl's tests, quinine was effective only at a dilution of 1 to 800, but plasmochin was active against the avian malaria even at a dilution of 1 to 50,000, more than a sixty-fold increase in potency. In addition, Roehl found plasmochin in birds to have much greater spread between its minimum effective dose and its maximum tolerated dose—its therapeutic ratio. Plasmochin gave a therapeutic ratio of 1 to 30, compared to quinine's 1 to 4.[29] In birds, Roehl had a synthetic drug more potent than the long-serving natural compound. For Roehl, this was just the beginning: "For the first time this inferential transfer of results from canary to man has been justified by Plasmochin. For the first time a synthetic alkaloid has been discovered which has proved efficient in bird malaria and thereafter also in human malaria. I am convinced that this path can be successfully followed again and that we have reached the first stage in a great development of chemotherapy."[30] Roehl had successfully extended his findings from the bird model to human malarias.

Bird Malaria after Roehl

After Roehl's death in March 1929, Walter Kikuth, fifteen years his junior, took his place in Elberfeld. Kikuth, a physician, had trained at the Institute for Tropical Medicine in Hamburg. With Kikuth in place, the chemotherapy program at Bayer was in full swing. He and others at Bayer sought to refine their model systems ("Modellversuch").[31] A British malaria worker and Rockefeller collaborator, S. P. James, got a glimpse of this operation during a visit to Bayer's Elberfeld Institute in the fall of 1931—paid for by the Rockefeller Foundation and at the invitation of Werner Schulemann,[32] the leader of the Bayer team. James noted the centrality of animal models to the research. Indeed, he was astounded by the quantities of birds and other animals that Bayer employed in its research.[33] James noted that, following Roehl, the Germans had used blood inoculation as a means of transferring infection from canary to canary, but that some six weeks prior to his visit they had instituted some new procedures. Following James's own work, Kikuth's group had added mosquitoes as natural vectors to their model systems.[34] By the time of James's visit, Bayer's mosquito facilities were operational. James's description of the Bayer program reveals something of his own pride as an innovator in prophylactic research as well as his desire to further his own research agenda:

> They showed me these arrangements which consist essentially in the provision of a room which is kept . . . at a constant temperature of 25º C and with a saturated atmosphere. The mosquitoes (*Culex pipiens*) are reared from the egg and larvae in this room and are infected by being

allowed to feed on malaria-carrying canaries and by being kept in the room for the requisite number of days. They are then used for infecting other canaries by their bites. . . . The arrangements left little or nothing to be desired and there is no doubt that in a short time "prophylactic tests" on bird malaria similar to those conducted on human malaria at Horton [James's malaria prophylaxis lab in Epsom] will be part of the routine of the department. The work was in the hands of a senior female assistant, well educated but not a graduate in science or medicine.[35]

James's praise of this system was, in part, a plea to his Rockefeller colleagues to fund the establishment and staffing of similar state-of-the-art facilities in Great Britain. Kikuth and Schulemann not only adopted James's innovation, they used Bayer's capital resources to create an industrialized mosquito facility.

Central to James's innovation was his belief that a successful prophylactic drug had to be active against the malarial stage (sporozoites) first injected by the mosquito rather than against the parasite in its latent phase or the subsequent blood stages. Mosquito bites were only one of three ways to transfer infection in the laboratory. One was injection with infected blood that challenged the new host with the blood stages of the parasite, the method originally employed by Roehl. The two other modes that challenged the new host with infectious sporozoites were the injection of ground-up infectious mosquitoes or the natural way, in which the mosquitoes did the injecting.[36] James advocated the more complex model involving live mosquitoes as better suited to the study of prophylaxis.[37] For James, sporozoites were essential for the testing of prophylactics. He had shown in humans that standard doses of quinine before and after blood inoculation could halt transmission, but that sporozoite (mosquito) transmission was much more virulent.[38] He found Bayer's efforts much improved by the addition of mosquitoes.

James's was certainly not the last word on avian malaria research or mosquitoes. But for a time at least, canaries alone would no longer be sufficient, and Bayer had added mosquitoes to the mix. Some, such as Paul Russell of Rockefeller's IHD, had their doubts about the usefulness of the added complexity. Russell was not certain that mosquitoes were necessary: "And while there is unquestionably a difference between mosquito and needle inoculated avian malaria this difference is not so wide as might be thought."[39] James came from a more academic world than Bayer's industrial realm. And his work had challenged the adequacy of Bayer's productive, but mosquito-free, model system. Plasmochin, the first successful synthetic antimalarial, had emerged from the mosquito-free, chemically oriented research program. Bayer then specifically moved to address the *prevention* of malaria as distinct from the *treatment* of malaria. In the preexisting system, patients in the clinic—already infected—could be modeled without mosquitoes. James's work suggested that true prophylactics—preventatives—needed a model of uninfected hosts subjected to sporozoites from infected mosquito. Therefore malaria research might require both a vertebrate host (bird; intermediate host) standing in for a human and an arthropod host (mosquito; definitive host) brought into the laboratory from the field. Though Bayer might add other organisms to their model systems, with regard to parasites, *P. relictum* continued largely to satisfy Bayer's research needs.[40] Other programs, with less concern about chemotherapy and the needs of the marketplace, made avian malarias themselves the object of scrutiny. For example, in universities departments, the search for new experimental results led to the introduction of novel avian parasites as research models.

At Johns Hopkins in Baltimore, interest focused on the biology of avian parasites including the delineation of new and known species. Writing about avian malarias in 1926, Robert Hegner said his department of medical zoology had been conducting research on bird malaria since the Hopkins School of Hygiene and Public Health had been organized a decade earlier. In the 1920s, Hegner's people employed two strains of avian parasite: one from New York sparrows—possibly *P. relictum*—and the other isolated from Baltimore sparrows. For hosts, malaria researchers at Hopkins regularly used female canaries purchased from Baltimore pet dealers, as male canaries—more brightly colored and more likely to sing—were preferred in the pet trade. Though Hegner was careful to cite therapeutic studies, the major focus at the Hopkins School of Hygiene and Public Health was biological. A number of Hopkins's researchers built the malaria program. In chronological order, they were Eugene R. Whitmore, Shulamite Ben-Harel, George H. Boyd, Lucy Graves Taliaferro, Kosta S. Drensky, R. F. Feemster, C. F. Scudder, Edwin H. Shaw, and Ernest Hartman.[41] The last of these, Hartman, characterized a novel species of avian parasite, *P. cathemerium*.[42] Hartman, born in 1896, received his DSc from Hopkins in 1926 while employed in the department.

Over the course of several decades, Hopkins researchers developed and studied *P. cathemerium*. Working at the Johns Hopkins School of Hygiene and Public Health at roughly the same time that Roehl was developing his canary/*relictum* model, Hartman isolated his parasite from a house or English sparrow in Baltimore in October 1924. In the following years, Hartman refined knowledge of *P. cathemerium*, determining its host requirements and showing that its morphology and life cycle were preserved during passage from one host species to another. After transferring the new parasite from his original sparrow into canaries, he infected other passerine hosts (perching birds), first the European siskin (*Spinus spinus*) early in 1926, then from canary to both cowbird (*Molothrus ater*) and red-winged blackbird (*Agelaius phoeniceus*) that summer, and finally, some seven months later, back into canaries. Coupled to canaries, the new *P. cathemerium* was a fruitful system for Hopkins researchers right through World War II. A number of significant examples may be cited. Lucy Graves Taliaferro showed periodicity for a nonhuman malarial parasite, Clay Huff studied the problem of immunity in mosquitoes, Reginald Manwell studied relapse in bird malaria, Khwaja Samad Shah studied the development of the parasite's sexual stages, Redginal I. Hewitt examined the dependency of infection on the age of the red blood cells, and Robert Rendtorff examined the early development of the parasite.[43] Each of their avian investigations was intended to illuminate the life cycle and preferences of comparable human parasites. All these researchers would go on to successful careers in parasitology.

Throughout the interwar period, the rationale for working with *P. cathemerium* and other avian malarias remained consistent with Laveran's nineteenth-century declarations, though the scale of modeling grew beyond the direct comparison of the parasite development into subtler biological questions and the wider ramifications of diversity among *Plasmodium* species. As Laveran suggested, "To solve the still obscure questions relating to the development of this [human] parasite, it is necessary to . . . study the analogous parasites that exist in diverse animals."[44] *P. cathemerium* displayed a wide variety of behavior analogous to the human parasites. With the outbreak of World War II, *P. cathemerium* research continued at Hopkins, and the frame for avian malaria continued to expand.

Two wartime dissertations illustrate the increasing range of questions addressed with avian malarias: host requirements and basic parasite biology, problems not directly applicable to military needs. One of Hegner's last graduate students was Marion M. Brooke, who completed his dissertation in May 1942. His thesis dealt with the link between malnutrition and malaria in many regions of world. As a preamble to the need for more experimental data, Brooke cited much of the epidemiological evidence for the positive correlation between malnutrition and malaria. His first and nearest example was the "malarious South" which was the "most poorly nourished region of the United States." After a number of such examples, Brooke concluded that although there was "generally accepted belief that malnutrition must predispose a population to more severe malaria," there was surprisingly little research "even remotely bearing on this relationship."[45] To fill this lacuna, Brooke examined the effect of reduced or deficient diets on several species of malaria parasites using several avian hosts: canaries, pigeons, and ducks. Brooke reasoned, "Many phenomena concerning malaria have been found to be similar, if not identical, in both bird and man in spite of their phylogenetic differences. Therefore, it seemed possible that facts gathered on the effect of malnutrition upon avian malaria might throw light on the human situation."[46] Brooke looked to avian malarias for answers regarding human epidemiology. Clearly, the mapping of avian disease onto the human condition was becoming more complex and sophisticated.

Myron Simpson also worked on the broader implications of these avian models. Writing in 1944 on his *P. cathemerium* work, Simpson related how the stimulus of war increased the volume and pace of malaria research, especially chemotherapy, and how this in turn had brought the realization that much remained unknown with regard to the biology of the parasite. The wartime therapeutic agenda was the rationale for the pursuit of parasite biology in model systems. And bird malaria was one place wherein to seek this knowledge. Findings in birds were frequently translatable into data about the human disease, "or if not immediately applicable, at least tend to indicate directions in which human malaria research may well proceed with hopes of eventual success."[47] Simpson was examining the periodic behavior in the parasites' reproduction in ducks. These "rhythms" were part of the interplay of intrinsic properties of the organisms—intermediate and definitive hosts and the parasites—and the environment, conceived as both the external world and the biological space within the hosts. Grasping and understanding the complexity of the living systems was an essential first step to malaria research: "The complex animal body, when considered in relation to its own tissues or its parasites, becomes an intricate environment more or less complete within itself."[48] Simpson's primary interest was in the parasites' periodic behavior—specifically synchronicity, periodicity, and length of the asexual cycle—and environmental conditions such as host age and day-night cycles. These were his essential variables and increased the reach and breadth of these biological models.

For new research niches such as these, *P. cathemerium* was one of the most productive malaria models from mid-1920 through the early 1940s. Similarly productive of new data was *P. gallinaceum*, first isolated and characterized in 1935.[49]

Bayer's launch of its second synthetic antimalarial, atabrine, in 1932 had further enhanced the status of Roehl's model, and the search for new avian malarias had continued apace. As Émile Brumpt wrote from Paris in 1935: "The practical importance of these avian *Plasmodium* is very great for studying the treatment of human malaria. Indeed, since 1926, studies of the action of drugs on avian parasites have yielded many synthetic products (plasmochin, atabrine, etc.)—substitutes for quinine, of use in human pathology."[50] Brumpt was promoting his newly characterized avian parasite, *P. gallinaceum*. While *P. relictum* and *P. cathemerium* were largely parasites of the passerine (perching) birds, *P. gallinaceum* was a parasite of chickens and other fowl. According to Brumpt, *P. gallinaceum* was first observed by one of his former students in the city of Nhatrang in French Indochina (Vietnam) in 1910. This student demonstrated the blood inoculation from one hen to another and, on his return to Paris, brought beautiful smears of the parasite to Brumpt. These slides rested comfortably in the collections of the parasitology laboratory for more than two decades. Then, in 1935, prompted by reports coming out of Ceylon of imported birds dying of a *P. relictum*-like infection, Brumpt returned to the old smears and published descriptions of the parasite, which he named *P. gallinaceum* after its chicken host, *Gallus gallus*. Brumpt also toured the Far East in search of live parasites, finally acquiring some of the survivors of the Ceylon outbreaks and returning with them to Paris, where he established the strain in new hosts.[51]

Plasmodium gallinaceum, promoted by Brumpt, was a very productive model organism. As malariologist P.C.C. Garnham wrote in 1966, "Brumpt, with characteristic generosity, immediately distributed the parasite to everyone who wanted it, thereby . . . opening the floodgates to a tide of scientific papers which now number a thousand or more."[52] Brumpt himself was quick to suggest that while the parasites of the smaller passerine birds had been invaluable in the study of human malaria, a species capable of infecting larger domestic fowl would be still more precious.[53] Brumpt also saw value in *P. gallinaceum* for chemotherapeutic studies.[54] *P. gallinaceum* was an excellent model system because of the size and availability of its host and because of its adaptability to many hosts. While the natural host of *P. gallinaceum* was the jungle fowl, it was found in the laboratory to infect not just all European breeds of domesticated chickens but also geese, pheasants, partridges, and even peacocks, and it was transmitted by a very large number of mosquito species, being one of the most oligoxenous malaria parasites known.[55] The availability of a parasite for use with cheaply and readily obtainable chicks was crucial to opening the floodgates to thousands of publications. Prior to Brumpt's discovery, no species of malaria was known to infect chickens. The ease of use of *P. gallinaceum*'s host, the chicken, was key to its widespread adoption as a model integrable into a range of research programs.

Brumpt's *P. gallinaceum* prompted others to look for new parasite species in exotic fowl. The next major isolation was of *P. lophurae*. Though *P. lophurae*, like *P. gallinaceum*, originated in the distant east, Lowell Coggeshall of Rockefeller's IHD did not have to travel far to collect it: he had only to go from Manhattan to the Bronx.[56] As Coggeshall described his own motivation, "Since Brumpt showed that a variety of birds are susceptible to [*P. gallinaceum*], and since he also suggested the natural host was a wild bird, it seemed possible that birds imported into this country from tropical Asia might harbor a similar parasite." Coggeshall, in cooperation with an ornithologist and a pathologist at the New York Zoological Park, examined the blood of birds at the Bronx Zoo—birds that had originated in Borneo and Ceylon—and injected the exotic blood into day-old chickens. Then in June of 1937, one bird yielded exciting results: A fireback pheasant from Borneo (*Lophura igniti igniti*) showed a novel plasmodium infection that was readily transmissible to the chicks.[57] Coggeshall named the new parasite for its pheasant host: *Plasmodium lophurae*. The new parasite was infectious in chickens, but, unlike Brumpt's parasite, it was not invariably fatal to young chicks, producing "only a moderately severe disease." Such distinguishing properties allowed new model organisms to complement existing ones.

To complete the disease model Coggeshall needed a competent vector, and for these experiments he turned to his colleagues Carl Ten Broeck and William Trager at the Rockefeller Institute for Medical Research in Princeton. They demonstrated infectivity in the *Aedes aegypti* mosquito, better known for its role as a vector for yellow fever. However, this vector and this parasite were not as tractable as at first seemed the case. As Trager observed, he, Coggeshall, and Clay Huff all found that the same strain of *Aedes aegypti* yielded an infection rate much below Coggeshall's initially reported 60 percent.[58] It took Trager and others several years to develop and disseminate a suitably susceptible strain of the *A. aegypti* for use with *P. lophurae*.[59]

On the vertebrate side, *P. lophurae* found an excellent experimental host in the Peking duck. Very young ducklings, between a few days and few weeks old, were highly susceptible to the parasite. Henry A. Walker and Harry Benjamin van Dyke of the Squibb Institute for Medical Research got their start using *P. lophurae* in ducks with the help of Robert Hegner and Evaline West at Johns Hopkins. Hegner and West supplied them with ducks infected with the "Coggeshall strain" of *P. lophurae* and provided them with information on the laboratory handling of the parasite. For their work on sulfonamides as antimalarials, the Squibb workers found this model system invaluable: "The course of infection by the Coggeshall strain of *P. lophurae* in the duck is particularly suitable for chemotherapeutic study because the number of parasites in the blood usually grows rapidly until death occurs."[60] In this Hopkins model, the ducklings were inoculated intravenously with citrated blood from an infected duck. A parasite as virulent as *P. lophurae* might not be able to propagate in natural populations because of its rapid lethality—untreated ducklings usually died in five to sixteen days[61]—but with proper handling in the lab, it was an excellent screen for potential antimalarials. Compared with other avian parasites, it was particularly useful to the workers at Squibb: Alone among their experimental infections, *P. lophurae* was sensitive to sulfonamides, making it a good model system for drug screening.[62]

The late 1930s saw not just the spread of new model systems based on *P. gallinaceum* and *P. lophurae* but increased attention to chemotherapy brought on by the growing threat of war. Malaria has, throughout history, thrived in conflict, especially in the ranks of nonimmune soldiers transported to endemic areas. Interest in this more pressing and practical agenda, that of keeping troops in the field, made attention to transmission and mosquitoes essential.

In addition to identifying the parasite, it was necessary to identify specific vectors for *Plasmodium* model species. Discovery of a new avian malaria led to a search for a mosquito capable of transmitting that particular strain or species from one host to another. Model systems often required entomological inputs. For example, following Lowell T. Coggeshall's 1940 solicitation on behalf of the Rockefeller's IHD to join in a "unified attack upon malaria," Harry Beckman of the Marquette University School of Medicine in Milwaukee wrote back to describe his program and his models. Beckman was primarily interested in malaria prophylaxis. His group therefore occupied themselves as much with mosquitoes as with parasites. Indeed, Beckman had established their mosquito colony (*Culex pipiens*) several years earlier. These insects allowed them to transmit *P. cathemerium* "exclusively through the injection of sporozoites," without recourse to the injection of infected blood. This in turn allowed Beckman to study experimental infections that more closely resembled "naturally-acquired malaria." To maintain all this, the mosquitoes and the infected birds were kept in a room much like that at Bayer. Temperature, humidity, and light had all to be carefully and continuously controlled.[63] Beckman had within his lab an automatically controlled ecosystem for the preservation and propagation of his avian disease and both of its hosts.

The continued expansion of model systems to capture more and more of the field in the laboratory was a common element of avian malaria research during the 1930s. A Rockefeller-funded industrial-academic collaboration provides a fine example to illustrate how avian model systems had matured since Roehl's initial feeding tubes and blood injections. On the eve of U.S. entry into World War II, a typical chemotherapeutic problem—in this instance inquiry into the activity of sulfanilamide as a prophylactic—might take this form:

> In the past, investigation of the prophylactic effect of sulfanilamide derivatives against sporozoites has not been possible. Technical difficulties in the administration of sulfanilamide derivates to canaries in such a way as to maintain adequate blood concentrations have prevented the use of P. cathemerium for this type of work. These difficulties do not apply in the case of ducks; however, no satisfactory vector has yet been found for P. lophurae. Research into the prophylactic effect of drugs will now be carried on in this laboratory [IHD, NYC], since blood concentrations of sulfanilamide derivatives are easily maintained in chicks, and an efficient vector for P. gallinaceum in Aedes aegypti should furnish the necessary sporozoites.[64]

These model choices and decision points merit a quick review. The chemical, or biochemical, properties of the drugs to be tested, sulfanilamides, did not allow the researchers to use canaries as hosts. Ducks, in contrast, would maintain suitable levels of the drugs, but their parasites, P. lophurae, could not be delivered by mosquitoes. Researchers' interest in prophylactic drug studies meant that the chemical compounds must be tested against sporozoites, the form of the parasite that entered the bloodstream in the saliva of infected mosquitoes. With these constraints and with the extant resources, the researchers employed a model system consisting of young chickens, P. gallinaceum, and A. aegypti as mosquito vectors. For their investigations, they needed the drug, the vertebrate and arthropod hosts, and the parasite all functioning as a single, competent chemical and biological system. This use of these avian models in chemotherapy required that Eli K. Marshall, at

Hopkins, study other drug properties in other systems. Marshall investigated the "absorption, excretion, distribution, and toxicity of sulfanilamide derivatives" in canaries and ducks, as nothing was known about these compounds in birds. These extended systems of screening for activity, metabolism, and toxicity were subsequently mobilized for war work.

At any time, malaria researchers required models—biological systems in the laboratory and the field. The avian malarias served this purpose. Avian malaria systems consisted of outbred, market, or wild birds; mosquitoes naturalized to the laboratory; and strains and species of parasites isolated in the wild (often from multiple sources), passed through laboratory animals for stabilization, and then exchanged among researchers. The nearness of these animals to the pet shop, the farm, and the field made them far from genetically uniform while their distance from human malaria often rendered their correlation with human disease inexact. The avian parasites did not appear identical to human parasites under the microscope, the vector genera varied, and even avian blood cells were distinct, being nucleated, unlike the cells of mammalian blood, for example. Even the human disease against which any model must be mapped was not a singular entity but was comprised of several species of parasites with distinctive life stages, symptoms, responses to therapeutics, and dozens of localized vectors. If distinct in morphological and phylogenetic detail with regard to host, parasite, and vector, the avian malarias could be viewed as congruent if viewed over the whole life cycle of the organism, its many stages and forms, and in many locations and transformations, including at times the role of vectors and response to drugs. The capture of more of the parasites' wild ecology within the confines of the laboratory facilitated the mapping of findings in birds to findings in humans, the epistemological arrow whose direction Roehl had first reversed.

Complexity became a virtue in many malaria systems. Thus, even the laboratory research on malaria required an environmentally large frame for the disease, and the early researchers—such as Ross, MacCallum, and Hartman—who collected vectors, hosts, and parasites needed this ecological perspective. To map the avian disease onto the human disease, malariologists had to see the disease in a larger, environmental context rather than as a singular isolate that caused infection in animal and human alike. This environmental frame might be the blood of a canary, the gut of a mosquito, the temperature-controlled insectarium, or all of these and more, depending on the individual research agenda. The difficulty of conducting infectious disease research with human subjects made these bird systems essential to many kinds of malaria work during this period. From canaries to chickens and beyond, subsequent expansion of model systems encompassed more of malaria as a disease in the field and in the clinic.

The canary model of Kopanaris and Roehl was successful well into the 1930s, as suggested by the Hopkins-trained Reginald D. Manwell in 1934: "For the study of the course and pathology of a malarial infection canaries are very suitable, since they are virtually always free from such infection to begin with. The effect of quinine and plasmochin treatment is also interesting to follow. . . . In all these respects malarial infection in birds closely resembles that in man." [65] The workers at Bayer used the canary model to develop a second—and less toxic—synthetic antimalarial in the 1930s, atabrine. We will see more of atabrine and plasmochin in the next chapter where we look at the chemical and clinical aspects of chemotherapeutic research. A focus on the chemical will bring us back to Germany and Bayer, a company whose major resources lay in their synthetic chemistry expertise and in their large collection of existing chemicals, synthesized both for dye research and for pharmaceutical and antiseptic programs.

Chapter 3

New Drugs

Quinine—how to use it, make it, and especially replace it—remained a subject of much interest in the first half of the twentieth century. And with good reason. Although precise numbers on disease and disability were (and are) notoriously difficult to collect, especially for diseases like malaria that are at their worst among the world's poorest, in 1926, the League of Nations estimated two million deaths per year from malaria. Since the death rate was three to four per 1,000 cases, this meant an estimated 650 million cases of malaria, or roughly one-third of the human race.[1] During the 1930s, estimates of the total number of malaria cases worldwide varied from 300 to 800 million.[2] In Europe and North America, the quinine question involved public health, philanthropy, and national security.

Nations employed two strategies for medical intervention in malaria. Some, especially the Dutch, continued to obtain quinine from cinchona trees grown on plantations. For others, the solution was a synthetic substitute for natural quinine. Overall, companies, foundations, and nations turned more and more toward chemistry as a way of coping with malaria. As we saw in the previous chapter, a program of testing chemical agents against avian malaria was initiated by Bayer in Germany in the 1920s. In the years between the two world wars, efforts to replace quinine moved through the laboratory, the clinic, and marketplace.

First-Generation Synthetics

The Germans had good reasons for seeking synthetic antimalarials. A number of local pressures fueled their efforts. In World War I, German troops in

East Africa, the Balkans, and Turkey suffered greatly from a shortage of quinine. While having no colonial access to quinine, Germany had unmatched resources in the synthetic dye industry and chemotherapy. The major German effort in malaria chemotherapy followed the development of Roehl's avian model for malaria. The antimalarial project begun by Bayer (a division of I. G. Farben from 1925 until 1945) and their collaborators in the 1920s would prove to be one of the largest and most successful research efforts of its kind.[3] For a chemical and pharmaceutical company like Bayer—and its U.S. corporate partner, the Winthrop Chemical Company, Inc.—synthesizing active compounds and marketing them as drugs were the two critical activities.[4] The chemical problems, though complex, were often less difficult than market competition and consumer perceptions. We turn first to the chemical challenge of finding a synthetic replacement for quinine.

As discussed in chapter 1, the mode of action of antimalarial drugs was not well understood in the first half of the twentieth century. But the chemical shapes and structures of these drugs, both natural and synthetic, were knowable,[5] as were their activities against parasites. Chemists' structural drawings, like the ones that appear in this chapter, were a shorthand for the chemical, physical, and biological properties of chemical compounds.[6] The chemists and their collaborators could establish structure-activity relationships and used chemical structures as models for biological activity: add a carbon atom here and toxicity goes down, add a nitrogen there and activity goes up. Wilhelm Roehl and his collaborators could map chemical composition and shape against the activity of potential drugs in birds and humans. Scientists at Bayer in Elberfeld were able to screen thousands of compounds using Roehl's system of canaries infected with an avian malaria, *Plasmodium relictum*. Roehl had tested an extensive series compounds of the quinine and quinoline types, "as well as basic substances of dye stuffs and other origin," since his arrival at Bayer in 1911. These came to his group from chemists working the "Farbenfabriken"—the dye factories and labs. Roehl first tested these on trypanosomes, the organisms associated with sleeping sickness, that he had worked on previously at Ehrlich's institute. Later he screened them against his avian malaria in canaries, "unfortunately always without success."[7] Thus, the work at Elberfeld involved not just the random screening of compounds but the development of a series of structure-activity relationships.

For work on antimalarials, quinine was the obvious chemical starting point. Using quinine as a lead compound, several workers sought to chemically modify the quinine nucleus and to synthesize various quinoline compounds.[8]

A *lead* compound is one that provides a starting point from which to explore chemical and biological space.[9] It is the first structural model for a possible drug and generally shows some desired property or properties. This compound, like a clue in an investigation, could lead chemists to compounds, perhaps in its family of related compounds, whose properties more and more closely match those they were seeking. In the case of quinine and Bayer, the desired property was antimalarial activity. Along the path to new compounds with this property might be compounds with additional desirable properties, such as low toxicity, ready availability from simple starting materials (cheapness), or the ability to kill multiple life stages of the parasite. Bayer began with research on quinine, making "chemical attacks on the positions indicated by arrows," as in figure 3.1.[10]

The Bayer researchers initially assumed that any compound active against malaria must retain certain of quinine's chemical substructures. Its quinoline nucleus should be maintained, as well as the basic (salt-forming) nitrogen (N) attached by a carbon chain to the 4-position of the nucleus. Under these assumptions, quinine was the lead compound, and Bayer's researchers began by chemically altering quinine itself. The natural product proved a poor model, as one of the scientists heading the project, the physician and chemist Werner Schulemann, said: "In spite of much excellent synthesis, however, the desired goal was not reached."[11] The investigations into quinine and closely related compounds did not result in compounds with significant, or enhanced, antimalarial activity.[12] Although Schulemann and his colleagues moved on from quinine as a lead compound, they would return to

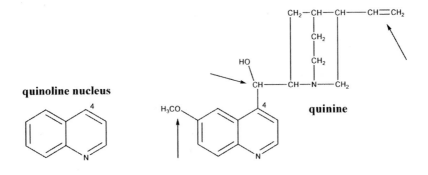

Figure 3.1   Quinoline nucleus and quinine structure with points of modification

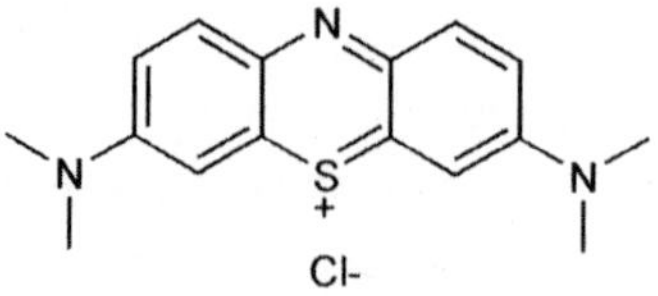

Figure 3.2   Methylene blue

its quinoline nucleus.[13] These concerns with chemical structure and shape were part of a broader shift toward a molecular understanding of medicine.

Schulemann—and his colleagues Fritz Schönhöfer and August Wingler—also pursued a structural line of inquiry starting with Ehrlich's methylene blue work and again using the Roehl avian model as an assay. Ehrlich had demonstrated that methylene blue, which stained malaria parasites in vitro, also had antimalarial activity.[14] Compounds that were structurally similar to methylene blue were synthesized at Bayer to follow up on this lead.[15] Notice in figures 3.2 and 3.3 how each of the series was made by adding carbon chains (the zigzag lines) and more to methylene blue's nitrogens (N). Compounds I and II, where the dimethyl side chains of methylene blue (the single lines attached to the nitrogens on the left and right of the molecule) had been modified, were found to be slightly more effective than the parent compound: the structural changes increased their antimalarial properties relative to methylene blue. However, their "therapeutic index"—that is, the ratio

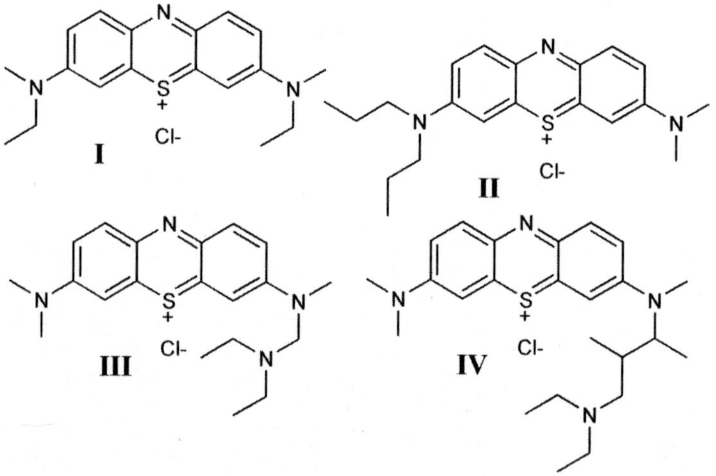

Figure 3.3   Compounds from the methylene blue series (Cl- indicating the compounds were isolated as chloride salts)

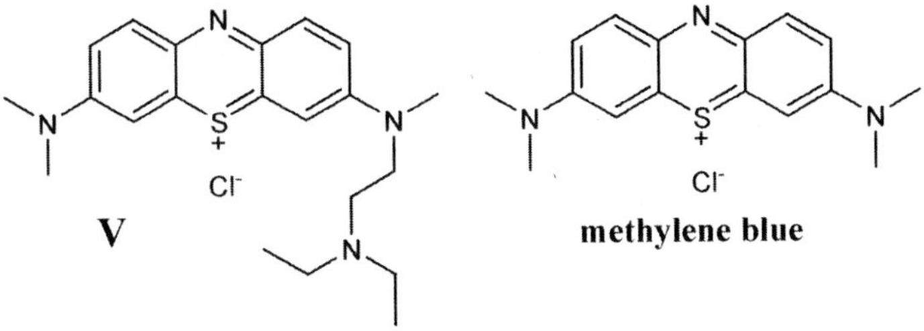

Figure 3.4 Compound V

of the effective dose to the tolerable dose—was still very low, around 1 to 1. Bayer's chemists found that they could improve this ratio by adding basic groups—in the sense of "opposite of acid"—to the amino side chains, as in compounds III and IV. The amino groups on the side chains were those with the nitrogen (N) in them. The chemists found another promising side chain with compound V (see fig. 3.4). With these findings, they extended to other classes of compounds the principle that effectiveness could be enhanced and toxicity reduced by the addition of basic alkyl groups (nitrogen-containing side chains). The other compounds were built primarily around the ring structures of other synthetic dyes, such as triphenylmethanes, azines, and oxazines. It was in the quinoline series, however, that success came first.

Having established in the methylene blue series the hypothesis that certain nitrogen-containing side chains increased antimalarial activity and decreased toxicity of a given chemical structure, Schulemann and the Bayer chemists started over with a simpler structure, the bare quinoline nucleus found at quinine's heart, and added their new active side chains.[16] Using the quinoline nucleus as a starting point vastly simplified the chemical exploration of the quinoline compounds by disposing of the structural and stereochemical complexity of quinine itself. Fritz Schönhöfer produced a series of quinoline compounds. He originally added the amino group to the quinoline nucleus at the 6-position, but these attempts yielded only tarry messes. Then the chemists moved on to the 8-position, and these compounds proved promising.[17] Even Schönhöfer's first simple 8-aminoquinoline, compound VI, proved active, showing several times the activity of quinine in the Roehl canary test (fig. 3.5).

Schulemann and his group pursued both variation and stability in developing their several series of compounds. They constructed each series around a different central structure, or nucleus, but with similar side-

quinoline   VI

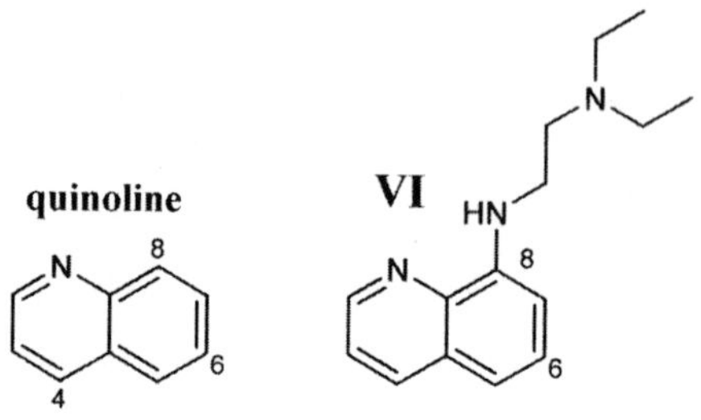

Figure 3.5 Quinoline and Fritz Schönhöfer's first simple 8-amino-quinoline

chain modifications, and they varied the side chains attached to the central structures while keeping a stable eye on the lead compounds that showed the best activity, such as quinine and methylene blue. Schulemann constructed a side chain diagram, giving a sample of the many side chains that the chemists synthesized, each of which was attached at the 8-position to yield a potential antimalarial compound (fig. 3.6).[18] The shape and chemical composition of each of these side chains allowed Bayer to predict antimalarial action of the structures and further refine requirements.

With the 8-amino series showing promise, Werner Schulemann pointed out that quinine had a methoxy group ($-OCH_3$) that was essential for activity, so Schönhöfer added one at the 6-position, producing a compound that Roehl "baptized" A-prochin. Schönhöfer then produced a whole series of compounds—A-prochin, Be-prochin, Ce-prochin, and so on—with slight variations. Beprochin (as it was written in later publications) turned out to be the star of the series. Produced in 1924, Roehl found this compound to be well-tolerated by the canaries and very active—more than thirty times more active—than other compounds in the series. It was subsequently named pamaquine and later marketed as plasmochin or plasmoquine (fig. 3.7). With a therapeutic index of 1 to 30, plasmochin was the first successful synthetic antimalarial.[19]

From Bird to Man

Once plasmochin had been synthesized, Bayer still had much work to do. Drugs had to pass clinical tests in humans, chemists had to scale up synthesis processes—to large volumes in the case of successful drugs—and agents and detail men had to market the new drugs to doctors and patients. For plasmochin, human tests began with Dr. Franz E. Sioli, director of the regional asylum in Düsseldorf (Provinzial-Heil und Pflegeanstalt). Sioli—

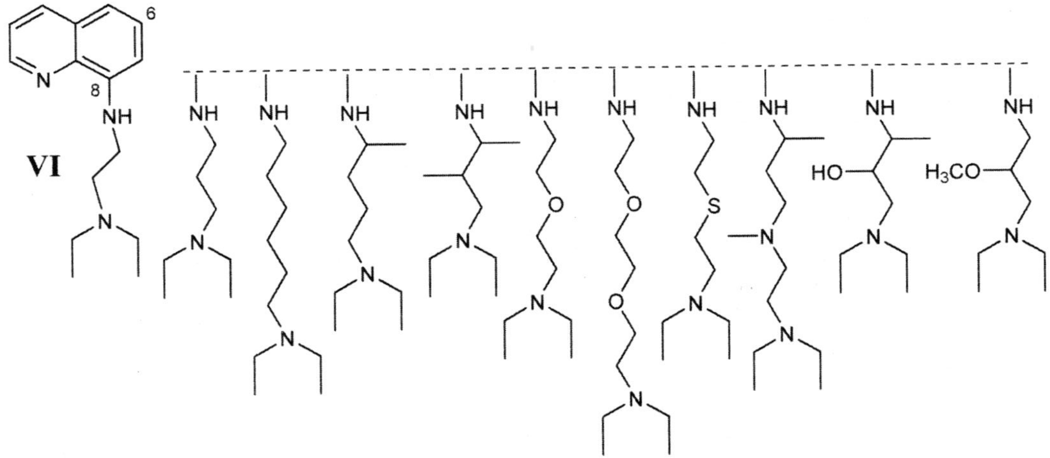

Figure 3.6 Schulemann's side chain diagram

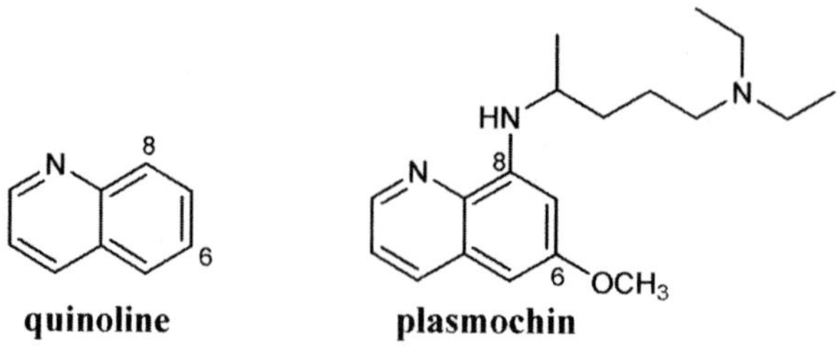

quinoline   plasmochin

Figure 3.7   Plasmochine or plasmoquine

like S. P. James in England and others elsewhere—employed malaria therapy to treat syphilis.[20]

In the 1910s, the Austrian doctor Julius Wagner von Jauregg had developed this treatment of general paresis due to syphilis. His approach showed
such apparent success (today there is some argument about whether the therapy did work) in mitigating this intractable and devastating disease that Von
Jauregg won the 1927 Nobel Prize in physiology or medicine for this work.
Malaria therapy was a significant clinical advance: At the time, approximately 15 percent of patient populations in mental hospitals were paretics,
and late-stage syphilis of the brain (neurosyphilis) did not respond well to
Ehrlich's drug Salvarsan.[21] The use of high-grade, malaria-induced fevers in
the controlled environment of hospital wards gave malaria researchers a fer-
tile, if ethically fraught, new domain for experiment. In the normal course
of malaria therapy, doctors often terminated the malaria with quinine after
a series of fever spikes occurred. To test new drugs, researchers could substitute the new compounds in place of quinine. Thus, in March 1925, the Bayer
team sent their new beprochin (plasmochin) to Sioli.

Before developing a treatment regimen, Sioli undertook a crude investigation into the human toxicity of plasmochin. He treated three mental patients
with gradually increasing daily dosages—to a maximum of 5 x 0.05 grams
over the course of one day—in order to find the tolerable dose: 3 x 0.05 grams
per day.[22] Then Sioli moved on to malaria-therapy patients. These patients
he first infected with *vivax* malaria, injecting them with infected blood and
allowing their fevers to peak repeatedly. He then administered plasmochin
to quench the fever and kill the blood-stage parasites. The first patient was
treated with the maximum tolerated plasmochin dosage, 3 x 0.05 grams per
day for several days, and showed a remission of fever and no parasites in the

blood. Sioli then refined his dosage regimens downward, seeking a low dose (minimum effective dose) that would cure the injected malaria without risk of recurrence. This dosage seemed to be on the order of 0.0125 grams once or twice a day for up to eleven days. The next test for plasmochin would be against naturally occurring malaria.

Plasmochin moved quickly from the clinic out into the field. After Sioli, Peter Mühlens of the Hamburg Tropical Medicine Institute and other members of the Bayer team worked on the human testing of plasmochin. Hamburg was a busy seaport and saw a range of imported illnesses, allowing Mühlens to test plasmochin on malaria patients at the Institute.[23] Mühlens first received plasmochin from Bayer in August 1925. Roehl himself went to Spain in the summer of 1925 to test the drug against naturally acquired malaria in patients at local clinics.[24] Roehl was excited by the fact that plasmochin could eliminate the gametocytes from the blood of patients with falciparum malaria, something that quinine could not do. Werner Schulemann took the new drug to Tuscany in Italy for successful tests.[25] Almost immediately Bayer had outside interest in its new medicine. The U.S. multinational United Fruit Company, with operations around the New World tropics, wanted a large quantity of plasmochin to test in their plantation hospitals. In return they agreed to publish their findings in their annual report.[26] They also sought reprints of all the relevant literature for their medical superintendents. For each of their eight hospitals, they requested 45 tubes of 25 tablets each and 135 bottles of 30 pills (dragées) each, for a total of over 40,000 doses of plasmochin.[27] United Fruit had good reason for their interest in a new drug. In 1924, their hospitals had treated 10,998 cases of malaria.[28] With success in these early locales, the late 1920s saw plasmochin use spread, often in combination with quinine.[29]

With wider use, plasmochin's great promise was tempered by the emergence of side effects. The new synthetic killed gametocytes in the blood and seemed therefore to offer a route to block the transmission of the malaria from human to mosquito. Overall, however, plasmochin showed some critical toxicity issues. Physicians occasionally observed cyanosis (particularly blue lips later associated with methemoglobinemia, a biochemical disorder that decreases the blood's ability to carry oxygen), and more severe adverse reactions were observed in other patients (notably those with what is now known as G6PD-deficiency, a genetic mutation). Awareness of these problems only grew gradually during the 1930s. Though it was still used extensively by the U.S. military early in World War II, growing concerns with toxicity, especially in African Americans patients, caused it to fall out of standard use.[30] But this negative verdict was nearly two decades in the making.

In the meantime, wider adoption of plasmochin meant not just new opportunities for clinical observations but increased production. This scale-up and commercial development required skilled chemists. As noted in the previous chapter, British malaria worker S. P. James visited the Bayer facilities in 1931. James sent his Rockefeller handler, George K. Strode, the International Health Division representative in Europe, a report of his visit, which commented on not just the biological testing facilities but Bayer's chemical endeavors. While Werner Schulemann invited James, the Rockefeller Foundation paid his way to Elberfeld through their "Health Officials Travel Fund." The Rockefeller officers were clearly aware that certain portions of the report were "for the time being somewhat confidential."[31] James described the facilities at the Elberfeld site, noting the number of chemists employed in a range of departments. "There are separate buildings for the laboratories of the chemistry department, the department of pharmacology and toxicology, the therapeutic department, etc." He was informed "that no fewer than 40 highly qualified research chemists" were on staff.[32] Another note of interest was the importance of the scale-up and development. Bayer's abilities to convert laboratory-scale success into manufacturing success piqued James's interest:

> I was interested to see that quite apart from the chemical laboratories devoted to the discovery of new preparations there is a department devoted to research into the practical problems of preparing those new drugs on a commercial scale. I understood that the secret of plasmoquine (if there is a secret about it) lies in this department. It may be easy for a research chemist to prepare a small amount of any of the derivatives in the plasmoquine series but some of them, particularly plasmoquine, are very difficult to prepare in large amounts and much research to that end was necessary.[33]

Even before commercial production, chemists had to provide sufficient material for testing the new compounds in humans, whose larger bodies—relative to canaries—required substantial dosages. James also noted the integration of top academic scientists into the research and development chain within the company.[34] On this point, James was perhaps self-serving, as academic appointments of such industrial researchers were often honorary. If nothing else, the remarks show James's political acumen. Certainly, though, Bayer's top people—men such as Carl Duisberg and Heinrich Hörlein—were alive

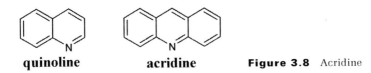

quinoline   acridine   **Figure 3.8** Acridine

to the importance of recruiting chemists and medical researchers from top university departments and institutes.

Second-Generation Synthetics

With plasmochin in hand, Bayer's scientists, Kikuth and Schulemann included, continued to mold the conception of drugs around chemical shapes and structures. Bayer's chemists developed structure-activity relationships for new series of potential drug candidates. As with plasmochin, they characterized these compounds with a therapeutic index—the ratio of the effective dose to the tolerable dose—using canaries and *P. relictum*. Here was an interface between chemical and biological models of disease, but, after the initial development of the canary model, most of the innovation centered on the chemical aspects of drug development while testing became routinized. Their most promising new starting structure, borrowed from a series of dyes, was the acridine nucleus. As the Bayer chemists explained in internal documents, the fundamental structural—chemical—difference between plasmochin and the new series was that plasmochin was built around the quinoline nucleus while their new compounds contained the acridine structure (fig. 3.8).[35] As in plasmochin development, a large series of compounds—more than 300 acridine-derived chemicals—were synthesized and tested. Two chemists, Hans Mauss and Fritz Mietzsch, supplied many of them.[36] Out of these, Bayer had a second synthetic success against malaria. In the early 1930s, Mauss and Mietzsch produced

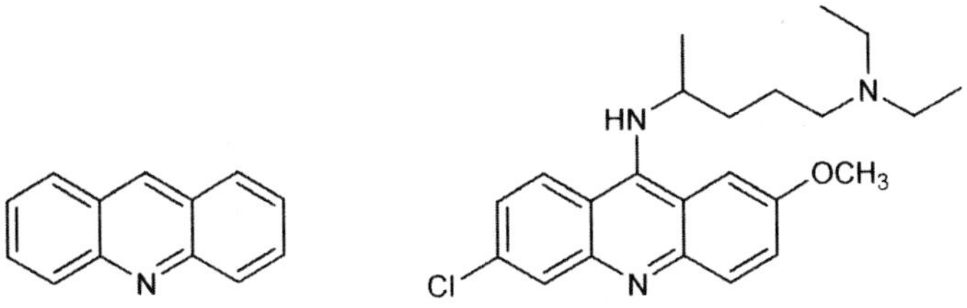

acridine   atabrine

Figure 3.9 Atabrine

atabrine.[37] The atabrine story paralleled that of plasmochin in key ways, although atabrine had unique problems and properties.

Kikuth identified atabrine using the Roehl canary test.[38] Far less toxic than plasmochin, atabrine was an acridine dye with a strong yellow color (fig. 3.9). The chemists' report on its preparation even included tassels of test fibers—cotton, wool, silk, viscose, and acetate—dyed bright yellow by the new "drug."[39] Bayer also screened the acridine compounds against streptococcal and staphylococcal bacteria, producing a number of antibacterial agents. Atabrine, like plasmochin before it, went first to Dr. Sioli for testing in paretics.[40] It was tested against naturally occurring malaria in the fall of 1930 in Romania.[41] For further trials against human malaria, atabrine traveled to the Hamburg Institute and on to Central and South America with Peter Mühlens and Otto Fischer, both of the Institute.[42] Following its travels and its successful tests against malaria, atabrine went on the market in 1932.

Bayer launched atabrine much like it had plasmochin a few years earlier. The drug firm collaborated with the United Fruit Company and sought to market the drug in the United States, working with a number of state and local health departments and soliciting business with the U.S. Public Health Service and in U.S. colonial possessions, such as the Philippines, Puerto Rico, and the Panama Canal Zone. As Winthrop Chemical moved slowly forward with plans to submit atabrine to the Council on Pharmacy and Chemistry of the American Medical Association, Bayer resisted their efforts for reasons of secrecy. The council, established in 1905, reviewed drugs and therapeutic claims and its approval was required for advertising in many medical journals.[43] Even by the 1930s, Bayer had not yet submitted plasmochin to the council because they wished to keep secret the salt with which they compounded the drug.[44] Atabrine's major negative departure from plasmochin was a reported, but not well established, neurological effect: some patients complained of hallucinations or induced psychosis. These reported side effects were echoed in recent years by another antimalarial drug, mefloquine.[45] Overall, though, atabrine showed far fewer toxicity problems than plasmochin. Whatever atabrine's potential drawbacks, Bayer marketed it in competition with the Netherlands-based monopoly Quinine Trust and kept an eye on potential clinical and commercial problems.

As with plasmochin, early adopters of atabrine were often left to develop their own treatment protocols, and, as with plasmochin, the League of Nations Malaria Commission—an interwar institution akin to the postwar World Health Organization—took an interest in atabrine, although these proprietary medicines were often too expensive for public health campaigns in the poorest areas of the world. The League of Nations Malaria Commission suggested a number of regimens for atabrine as a prophylactic and as a treatment for those already infected with one or another kind of malaria. For example, at the end of 1937, the commission suggested that a daily dose of 0.05 grams atabrine was not adequate for prophylaxis, recommending instead a twice-weekly dose of 0.20 grams.[46] The 0.05 gram daily dosing was elsewhere ascribed to "the inventors," meaning Bayer.[47] In August 1938, citing research conducted in Romania, Italy, and Malaya, the commission again endorsed a twice-weekly prophylactic regimen with a total dosage of 0.40 grams atabrine per week.[48] In 1939, Marshall Barber, working with the Rockefeller Foundation in Brazil, followed a different recommendation from the commission. There malaria workers employed a regimen with a substantially higher loading dose, 0.60 grams over three days followed by six days with no drug. Barber believed that atabrine "possibly saved me from malaria . . . it caused no discomfort and did not turn me yellow as atabrin is said to do sometimes. At the worst, better be yellow than sorry."[49] All these regimens varied in timing and loading as well as total weekly dose. Bayer's daily dosing gave the patient 0.35 grams per week, the commission's earlier recommendation gave 0.40 grams per week, and Barber's nine-day course averaged 0.47 grams per week. As Barber's comment, "better be yellow than sorry," suggested, atabrine's properties as a yellow dye were a potential problem for compliance with prophylactic regimens.

Like prophylaxis, treatment presented a specific set of problems. The Malaria Commission's treatment regimen for atabrine was 0.30 grams per day for five to seven days, divided into two or three doses a day. Their reports also addressed the pressing issue of how best to use atabrine to treat infants, a population highly susceptible to the disease: "This practical problem is of importance on account of the frequency and violence of the plasmodium infection in infants and the necessity of treating the swarming virus reservoir which they constitute." For those interested in preserving the health of populations, such as the League of Nations and the United Fruit Company, controlling transmission—and reservoirs of infection—was always in mind. For adults, the commission sounded a note of a caution with regard to atabrine use: "The effective dose of atebrin is close to the non-tolerable dose. Atebrin may cause epigastric pains and nervous or mental symptoms, which require further study. It has the additional disadvantage of turning the skin yellow . . . atebrin should be used only under medical supervision."[50] Without proceeding further into the intricacies of dosage and treatment, it is important to note that knowledge of atabrine's efficacy and toxicity was continually evolving.

Selling Synthetics

Since quinine, in spite of its side effects—such as blurred vision, nausea, and ringing of the ears—had centuries of tradition, legend, and use behind it, Bayer's agents had to convince doctors and patients that their new synthetic drugs were as good or better than the natural, traditional remedy. The new chemicals, plasmochin and atabrine, had to be safer and more effective, or better in some way—price, availability, and so on—or they could not compete with quinine. In the United States, a major market for Bayer served through their partner Winthrop Chemical, this meant the company and its detail men had to test and distribute the drugs in local, regional, and national markets; identify first movers in public health who could recommend the new drugs; and quash negative opinions expressed in any public forum. Bayer's detail men had a number of allies—and few adversaries—in their campaign for acceptance and sales. These allies, both expected and strange, included the Georgia State Board of Health, the United Fruit Company, and Henry Ford. Those in opposition were the occasional patient suffering from adverse effects and the monopoly Quinine Trust (Kina Bureau) and its associated agents, such as the Cinchona Products Institute in New York.

An example of Bayer's research and marketing networks is found in work of Daniel E. Seckinger. Seckinger, a Hopkins-trained MD and doctor of public health, worked for the Georgia State Board of Health as an epidemiologist. He conducted research on antimalarials, and his success with atabrine was reported back to Bayer's headquarters in Leverkusen. In 1933, agents of Winthrop Chemical met with Seckinger and supplied him with additional drugs for testing in Georgia.[51] As they reported, Seckinger "recently called at our offices to discuss with us the advisability of continuing his investigations during the next malaria season."[52] Seckinger also helped promote the use of the new synthetics. He met with medical directors from the Rockefeller Foundation and the United Fruit Company. The Rockefeller visit sought possible funding for atabrine in poor areas of the South. The United Fruit interview was "undoubtedly . . . of material benefit to Leverkusen."[53] Seckinger appears repeatedly in Winthrop's reports during the 1930s. Through Winthrop, Bayer kept itself apprised of who was who and what was what in U.S. public health and malaria control programs.

Winthrop's direct and primary agent was John W. Hart, who sent regular reports to Leverkusen via Winthrop Chemical. Hart was generally referred to as Mr. Hart and was variously described as associate research director of Winthrop's department of medicine or director of malaria research at Winthrop. A memorandum to the head office in Germany described him briefly: "our J. W. Hart, who is attached to our Department of Research Medicine, and a member of the National Malaria Committee."[54] Hart received his appointment to the National Malaria Committee—an organization "composed of national, state and county health officers for the study of treatment and control of malaria"[55]—at the recommendation of Louis L. Williams, the U.S. Public Health Service (PHS) officer who headed malaria investigations for the NIH at the time.

In 1933, Hart had traveled "through the South on behalf of Atabrine." He found that there was as much falciparum malaria in Florida and Alabama as there was in the southern parts of Georgia. Hart met repeatedly with Williams, who requested materials on plasmochin, Chinoplasmin (a combination drug compounded from quinine and plasmochin), and atabrine for the PHS display at the Chicago World's Fair. Most importantly for Bayer's material interests, Hart raised the issue of the need for drugs for malaria control, both directly with Williams and through Allen Johnson of the Federal Relief Commission. Thirty million dollars had been appropriated for malaria control, but unfortunately for Bayer "this sum was to be expended for ditching, draining, and screening." Hart raised the example of Daniel Seckinger's program in Calhoun County, Georgia, which had demonstrated that there were areas "in which the ordinary methods of mosquito control were impracticable and of no avail and that in such areas the only method of controlling malaria was through the administration of drugs."[56] Meeting with Williams and William H. W. Komp, who was conducting malaria studies in the Canal Zone for the PHS, Hart discussed the prospects of more federal money for the purchase of drugs: "These men agreed that certain sums should be diverted to drug control and promised to use their influence in having this measure adopted."[57] Some weeks following the meeting of the Southern Medical Association in Richmond, Virginia, Williams informed Hart that issue of atabrine and the Relief Finance Corporation had been reopened and that "they had agreed to allot sufficient funds for treatment of all persons working under the relief program in the Southern states who might become infected with malaria." Williams believed that some of this money might "also be diverted in selected areas" for buying atabrine to limit malaria "among others besides these workers." Williams urgently requested Bayer's continuing cooperation in "malaria control investigations in the state of Georgia, promising on his part to have Dr. Komp of the Canal Zone carry on his studies with Atabrine and Plasmochin for another year." With regard to Georgia, Hart replied to Williams that he and Seckinger would travel to New York City and discuss continued support of Seckinger's program directly "with the president of our organization." Seckinger also visited the Johns Hopkins School of Hygiene and Public Health in Baltimore to discuss collaboration with their personnel, the Rockefeller Foundation having already promised to continue salary support for him and his staff in the coming year.[58]

One earlier stop for Hart and Seckinger bears revisiting: the aforementioned annual meeting of the Southern Medical Association and a session of the National Malaria Committee held in Richmond, Virginia, in the third week of November 1933. Winthrop Chemical had a scientific exhibit at the meeting that "dealt solely with malaria and the drug therapy of this disease," which was separate from their commercial exhibit.[59] In the scientific exhibit, they presented large color charts of the life cycles of malaria parasites and showed where atabrine and plasmochin interrupted these cycles. Winthrop felt they were onto something new and important: "The interest shown by the many visitors who viewed this exhibit was really remarkable. The idea of a commercial house presenting a scientific exhibit of such accuracy of detail and instructive value was a new departure at medical conventions. Many comments were made regarding the data presented and the manner of execution of the charts and placards."[60] This may have been a self-promoting claim, but certainly it was more plausible in 1933 than today. One should recall that this was a time when the word "propaganda" did not carry negative connotations.

Hart and his colleagues were pleased with the response to their exhibit and the range of important visitors they received. Hart listed a number of "outstanding authorities on tropical medicine" as being among "the hundreds of physicians who visited this booth."[61] These included Colonel Charles F. Craig, professor of tropical medicine at Tulane University School of Medicine and retired from the U.S. Army Medical Corps; Colonel Edward Bright Vedder of the Army; Mark F. Boyd and Louis W. Hackett, assistant director of the International Health Division, both of the Rockefeller Foundation; L. L. Williams, Joseph A. Le Prince, William H. W. Komp, and Thomas H. D. Griffitts, director of the Division of Malaria Control Studies of the Florida State Board of Health, all four of the PHS; and Drs. T. F. Abercrombie and Henry Hanson of the Georgia and Florida State Health Departments. All were opinion and policy makers whom Hart and Winthrop must observe and convince. For example, Abercrombie had recommended atabrine to the Civilian Conserva-

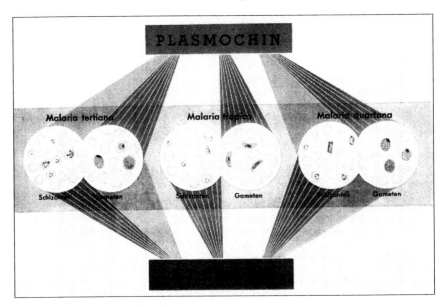

Figure 3.10   Illustration from Bayer marketing materials of the type displayed at the Southern Medical Association meeting. Courtesy of Bayer Business Services, Corporate History & Archives. (BAL Pharma Produkte A-Z, Plasmochin 1933–1937, 166/8).

tion Corps for their operations in the South. The CCC began successfully test-ing atabrine as a prophylactic among their enrollees as early as 1934.[62] Visits to the 1933 exhibit also resulted in many requests for copies of the charts, and the meeting report recommended that color duplicates be made (fig. 3.10). In all, more than one thousand members of the Southern Medical Association attended the meeting. The opinion leaders of the association were important to Bayer-Winthrop's promotion of the new synthetic drugs.

As the 1930s wore on, atabrine increased in acceptance and the Bayer-Winthrop marketing efforts proved a success, although not an unmitigated one. Nevertheless, they continued a strong political and scientific strategy of promotion, mobilizing allies, and identifying and neutralizing naysay-ers. Louis Williams of the PHS provides an example of the former, while George C. Shattuck of Harvard was reportedly one of the latter. With regard to Williams, in February 1935, Winthrop reported back to Leverkusen that it "would be of material advantage to our joint interests if Dr. L. L. Williams, who is . . . the American representative of the League of Nations' Malaria Commission, should attend the League of Nations' Malaria Congress in Madrid this year."[63] The problem facing Winthrop was that Williams was "not particularly anxious to make the trip," but he would if requested by the PHS surgeon general. The plan to bring him around? Bayer could ask Werner Schulemann "to exert some diplomatic pressure" and ask Lewis Hackett and another senior staff member of the Rockefeller Institute in Rome to write, "individually," to the surgeon general, Hugh Cumming, and suggest that Williams be designated to attend. Schulemann was able to get Hackett to write, and, in due course, Cumming's response was relayed from Washington, to Rome, to Leverkusen, and back to New York: "I shall be glad to bear your suggestion in mind."[64] The surviving Bayer records and Williams personal papers do not tell whether Williams did go to Madrid, but the incident gives an indication of how hard Bayer was prepared to work their networks to make the new synthetic drugs succeed.[65] We will see Williams in the following chapter as part of the PHS war mobilization.

Shattuck represents another type of intervention in which Winthrop's agents regularly engaged. As they reported in November 1935, "We regret to note that Dr. Shattuck made a somewhat slighting remark about Atabrine in a prominent Latin-American journal."[66] This was bad, but not as bad as it might have been. The report continued, "We do not believe that Dr. Shattuck is in any way related to the Quinine Trust, for he is a highly reputable physician whose ethical principles would not permit a commercial relationship." After some more background, the report concluded, "We are not very optimistic about our ability to make Dr. Shattuck a favorable partisan of Plasmochin and Atabrine. Nevertheless, we will continue to maintain contact with him through friendly connections at Harvard University." In spite of their negative projections with regard to Shattuck, they did bring him around. Just two months later they were able to report that a member of their Department of Research Medicine (perhaps their excellent Mr. Hart?) had "established friendly contact with Professor Shattuck, who readily admitted that he had very little information about Atabrine and Plasmochin."[67] In addition, Shattuck was known to have "suggested the use of both Atabrine and Plasmochin" when "asked by friends visiting the tropics for advice as to the treatment of malaria." Winthrop also took advantage of their new relationship to provide Shattuck with "a complete file" of Bayer's abstracts on their synthetic antimalarials. Winthrop's report concluded that "contrary to our expectations, we have evidently been able to make Professor Shattuck a favorable partisan of Atabrine and Plasmochin." In all circumstances, this was always the goal. But in spite of their efforts, they could not forestall the decline of atabrine: 1936 was to be the peak year for atabrine sales in the United States.

Winthrop continued to enroll allies in their fight to increase the market for atabrine in the United States and its territories. Their research department actively cooperated with many U.S. malaria control programs: "The State Board of Health in Georgia and the Civilian Conservation Corps in Arkansas are continuing in 1937 the programs instituted last year, covering both prophylaxis and drug control of malaria with Atabrine and Plasmochin. Thus far, 100% protection with Atabrine as a prophylaxis [sic] has been secured. In addition to these two programs a third will be instituted this year and continued through 1938 in Bryan County, Georgia, this being possible through the financial support of Mr. Henry Ford, who recently purchased the County."[68] Winthrop's officers felt that "Winthrop has done everything possible to promote Atabrine, distributing a great quantity of literature and concentrating the efforts of its Southern representatives on the product during the malarial season."[69] Nevertheless, it was "difficult to explain the lack of development, since Atabrine is an excellent drug. So far as the [U.S.] Government is concerned, the inclination is to fight malaria with sanitary means, such as screening, draining, etc., rather than by drug control." The emphasis on sanitary means—environmental interventions—kept Winthrop from fully engaging such allies as the U.S. government or even the Rockefeller Foundation.

In the United States, the makers of atabrine had also to fight against reports of side effects associated with their drug and the efforts of the Quinine Trust. Atabrine sales in the United States rose from $105,000 in 1933 to more $300,000 in 1936, though revenues softened in the following years.[70] In 1937, Winthrop Chemical reported back to the home office in Leverkusen that "although the sales of Atabrine reached $311,454.00 during 1936, representing an increase of 5%, the development of the product was not considered as satisfactory as has been anticipated."[71]

Among the problems to crop up in 1937 were personal injury claims. For example, they were sued for $10,000 in a South Carolina state court. The plaintiff claimed "to have been injured as a result of his use of Atabrine. Service of summons was made on our detail man, Mr. Demarest. The case has been removed to the Federal court in South Carolina and a motion will be made to vacate the service as improperly made." In another case, a claimant threatened to sue "alleging that he had suffered a psychosis" after taking atabrine. After a thorough investigation, Winthrop decided to settle the case for $400. Winthrop felt it would be "best to delay a test case" until they had updated their labels. The new labeling would exclude dosage information and add the statement "Winthrop products should be used only as prescribed by the physician."[72] The psychosis scare moved Winthrop toward a prescription-only position on atabrine. Bayer and Winthrop took the problem seriously, as its negative impact on business merited.

The reports of psychosis were one of several matters hurting atabrine. In general, however, the company did not believe the problem to be legitimate. "In some instances the psychosis was only a temporary condition and in others it was necessary to place the patients in an institution where they have had to remain. A careful investigation has been made by us of the cases reported, and it was found that in some there was a background of insanity."[73] They also pointed to a lack of medical supervision as a contributing factor. "In the majority of instances, it was learned that the individuals had bought the drug over the counter, believing they had malaria, although no diagnosis to that effect had been made. After the psychosis developed, a physician was called who attributed the condition to the drug without knowing what actually was wrong with the patient."[74] At worst, they thought the side effect to be real but

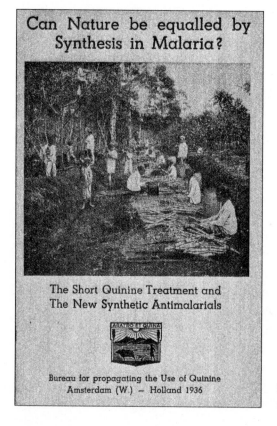

Figure 3.11 Booklet distributed by the Quinine Trust

transitory. Nevertheless, the drug's reputation was damaged. This side effect "more than anything else" kept back atabrine's "progress." Physicians were often aware of the psychosis problem, even though few reports appeared in the literature.[75] Winthrop and Bayer attributed the psychosis cases to exogenous issues particular to the patients in question—such as a history of mental illness, hereditary factors, or previous drug addiction—rather than to a general problem with their drug.[76]

Bayer and Winthrop remained convinced that they had a good drug and blamed the psychosis scare and the Quinine Trust for atabrine's failure to thrive in the United States, although the Trust's "activity" had also been felt elsewhere. The Trust published a pamphlet and distributed it "to every physician and druggist in the South." According to Winthrop, the pamphlet contained "very derogatory statements about synthetic antimalarial drugs as compared with quinine."[77] Indeed, the Quinine Trust was a recurrent problem. They mailed their "damaging pamphlets from Holland to avoid the official complaint which Winthrop lodged with the Federal Trade Commission." But Winthrop also believed that the Cinchona Institute in the Untied States had sent some of them (fig. 3.11). Faced with Winthrop's evidence, the Cinchona Institute agreed to stop the mailing. Winthrop hoped that the federal government would "soon issue an official 'desist order,' and that this will result in the publicity we desire."[78] Throughout these travails, Winthrop kept their filial promise: "Winthrop pledged their support to the I.G. [Farben, the German chemical conglomerate of which Bayer was a part] in the fight against the Quinine Trust."[79]

But Winthrop's efforts could not protect atabrine. By 1939, sales had not improved, though the Quinine Trust had retreated into the background slightly. The reports to Leverkusen that year concluded that "the main reason for the lack of progress in the last few years is the psychosis scare, which is far more important as a deterrent than the quinine competition or the variation in the incidence of malaria from year to year."[80] It is puzzling to note this near dismissal of the changing incidence of malaria. In contrast to the Quinine Trust or psychosis, Winthrop's reports rarely mentioned it, but this "variation" was actually a marked decline in the incidence of malaria in the United States during the late 1930s. The state of Georgia remained central to Winthrop's vision, as it "was the best Atabrine center in America." And here again in 1939, Winthrop faced neurological side effects. A number of reports of atabrine-related psychosis in Georgia yielded published reports in the state medical journal. Winthrop reported that "such publicity spreads like wild fire, and even though every effort has been and is being made to combat it through repeatedly circularizing physicians, giving lectures on the subject, etc., the damaging effects to the Atabrine business remain. Nothing can induce certain physicians to prescribe Atabrine or the laity in some sections to take the drug after it is prescribed. Naturally, Winthrop shall continue to do everything possible to build up this efficient product." The psychosis reports were not restricted to Georgia or even the United States, but their legitimacy abroad seemed even less compelling. For example, some cases had been reported in India, but "it was found that the condition was due to some complication of the disease. They all cleared up and the country (British India) which had reported them is buying the product in constantly increasing quantities." Apparently the antimalarial market in India was more elastic than in the United States.

Third-Generation Synthetics

While Winthrop worked on the U.S. atabrine market, Bayer's chemists and pharmacologists pursued new leads back in Leverkusen. Mauss and Mietzsch had supplied Roehl's successor, Walter Kikuth, and his group with the acridine compounds from which they selected atabrine. Two other chemical scientists, Fritz Schönhöfer and Hans Andersag, delivered a new series of aminoquinolines to Kikuth for screening.[81] In 1934, Andersag synthesized a colorless antimalarial, Resochin, later named chloroquine by the U.S. antimalarial program. The loss of the right-hand ring of yellow atabrine transformed this compound into the white (colorless) chloroquine (fig. 3.12). Resochin

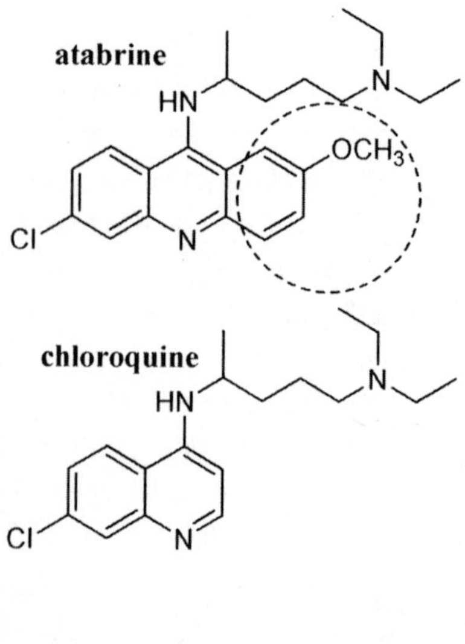

Figure 3.12 The loss of the right-hand ring (circled) of yellow atabrine transformed this compound into the white (colorless) chloroquine.

(chloroquine), unlike atabrine, never made it past Franz Sioli's neurosyphilit-ics. This compound's antimalarial activity may have been overlooked by the Germans because of their reliance on the Roehl test for preliminary toxicity data or because Sioli erroneously found toxicity in his paretic patients. After the war, Schönhöfer and Kikuth suggested that the latter explanation was correct, saying that the "toxicity of this substance [was], however, so great in comparison to its effect, that it was treated no further."[82]

But this series of 4-aminoquinolines was promising, and another com-pound, sontochin, closely related to chloroquine, moved forward in Bayer's program. Sontochin was a methylated chloroquine (fig. 3.13). After Kikuth had tested sontochin in animals, Sioli tested it in paretic patients in 1937. Believing sontochin to be less toxic and just as effective as Resochin, the Bayer workers dropped Resochin (chloroquine), producing less than a kilo-gram of this compound. By the end of 1938 and beginning of 1939, Peter Mühlens and his collaborators at the Hamburg Institute for Tropical Medi-cine successfully tested the new methylated drug against naturally occur-ring malaria.[83] Neither of these chlorinated aminoquinolines—sontochin or chloroquine—would be marketed in the United States before the outbreak of war in Europe. The antimalarial program at Bayer continued through the war, producing little of the novelty that it had before the war.[84] Of course, the Bayer network was increasingly isolated and deprived. Even the Hamburg Institute was bombed. With regard to the new series of compounds, it would be left to the U.S. wartime antimalarial project to identify chloroquine as the postwar drug of choice.[85] World War II saw the United States and Britain pursuing their own programs,[86] while the Axis developed sontochin for wartime use.[87] In spite of their apparent overlooking of chloroquine, the interwar German effort remained the first large, systematic attempt to identify a synthetic sub-stitute for quinine and was a model from which future efforts would draw.

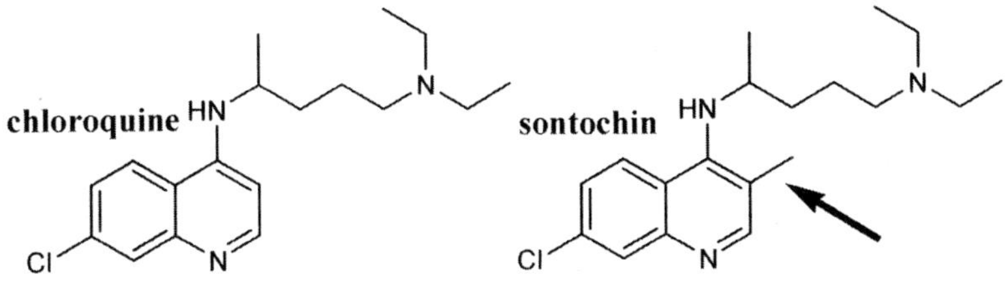

Figure 3.13 Sontochin was chloroquine with a methyl group added at the arrow.

From Peace to War

In the first half of the twentieth century, Rockefeller money and research moved biomedicine into new and critical areas. For malaria research, Rockefeller-funded people and institutions bridged the disjunction between the interwar period and the sudden changes brought on by World War II. Before moving on, we should examine their antimalarial efforts through the lens of Winthrop, Bayer, and their new drug atabrine.

Along with the League of Nations, the Rockefeller philanthropies were variously engaged with malaria control and research during the interwar years. Most important were the Rockefeller Foundation's International Health Division (IHD) and the Rockefeller Institutes in New York and Princeton. Winthrop's agents listed the Rockefeller Foundation among the important institutions with whom they must deal to successfully promote synthetic antimalarials.[88] They were careful to distinguish the "Rockefeller Institute for Medical Research" as "absolutely distinct from the Foundation," with its "own endowment, also from Rockefeller." Winthrop and Bayer personnel were much less interested in the institute, presumably because it was "devoted exclusively to research." With public health and the sale of drugs as their business, they focused on the International Health Division as the Rockefeller philanthropy that merited attention. The IHD "lends assistance, through financial grants and the loan of expert personnel, to programs for the eradication of communicable diseases, the principal campaigns so far having been directed against hookworm disease, yellow fever and malaria in Italy, Albania, Bulgaria, Greece, Spain, Portugal, Columbia, Central America, Virgin Islands, Jamaica, Porto Rico, Philippine Islands. The Foundation believes that it can make its most lasting contributions in the public health field through new knowledge on ways of controlling disease and through new methods of prevention 'within the means of the communities concerned.'" Unfortunately for Bayer's sales, the "officials of the Foundation are generally not interested in Plasmochin and Atabrine, because these drugs are considered too expensive for mass control of malaria in all regions of the world." As Paul F. Russell of the IHD put it in 1936: "Quinine is a rich man's remedy in the Tropics, where ordinary country people cannot afford it. Plasmochin and atabrine are even more expensive and have to be handled more carefully."[89] Of course, the period from 1939 to 1941 would bring further strains and estrangement for Bayer and even its most enthusiastic U.S. partners.

While economic efficiency was a central tenet of Rockefeller public health initiatives—like those of the League of Nations—the closing years of the 1930s brought new geopolitical realities. In particular, Japanese military advances in China and perceived threats to all of East Asia and the Netherlands East Indies (today's Indonesia) focused more attention on quinine and the Quinine Trust, who controlled the world supply from their plantations on Java. The Rockefeller Foundation—and indeed the Rockefeller Institutes in New York and Princeton—turned their antimalarial efforts more and more toward drug development and its required infrastructure of animal and clinical testing. Much of the testing of new drugs in the United States at the end of the 1930s and beginning of 1940s was coordinated or facilitated by the staff of the Rockefeller Foundation and Institutes. And the Rockefeller philanthropies were not alone in renewing and broadening their interest in malaria. They and other U.S. institutions interested in public health and national security took a fresh look at antimalarial drugs with threat of war looming. Critical among these newer players in malaria was the National Research Council (NRC). Meeting in Washington, DC, in April 1939, NRC's Division of Chemistry and Chemical Technology reached the timely conclusion "that research work should be stimulated in the field of quinine substitutes and synthetic antimalarials."[90] NRC would focus efforts of the U.S. medical and public health researchers on quinine substitutes. In 1940, their new Committee on Chemotherapy published a brief manifesto on the subject in both the *Journal of the American Medical Association* and *Science*. The first author on the manifesto was a young MD, a malaria researcher at the Rockefeller Institute in New York City named Lowell T. Coggeshall.

Chapter 4

Preparing for War

When the war in Europe began in September 1939, researchers and health officials in the United States were already trying to address the shortcomings and potential shortfalls of quinine, cinchona, and the existing synthetic antimalarials. This period prior to U.S. entry into the war showed some of the weaknesses and strengths of the National Research Council's approach to scientific research. The NRC had begun to take an interest in malaria chemotherapy some months before the invasion of Poland. Meeting in Washington, DC, in April, NRC's Division of Chemistry and Chemical Technology (Chemistry Division) asserted the need for, and committed itself to, stimulating research "in the field of quinine substitutes and synthetic antimalarials."[1] Originally formed by the National Academy of Sciences in 1916, the NRC was composed of leading scientists. Its mission was to employ science and technology in the promotion of both national welfare and national security—two pressing concerns in the run-up to U.S. entry into World War I.[2] With a second great war looming, the NRC established a temporary committee to look into the status of malaria and antimalarial drugs. Like Albert Einstein's 1939 letter to President Roosevelt urging him to conduct research on the atomic bomb, this NRC committee meeting was part of the United States' first slow mobilization for war.[3]

National Research Council

The story of how a small, underfunded subcommittee of the NRC grew into a major research program has implications for much postwar biomedical research.[4] The institutional transformation was confused rather than systematic, characterized after the war by William Mansfield Clark (1884–1964), a professor of physiological chemistry at the Johns Hopkins School of Medicine and wartime chairman of NRC's Chemistry Division, as "kaleidoscopic":

> The changes in organization were sufficiently kaleidoscopic to give the impression of an unstable pattern. Indeed, a person concerned only with the superficial aspects of organization might be tempted to use the record in support of the contention that a similar emergency in the future had best be handled by a predetermined body in accordance with a pre-formed plan. But this would be to misread the record. It is a record of research in which organizational matters were continually adjusted to meet the demands of scientific advances.[5]

Much as Roosevelt's modest Advisory Committee on Uranium first moved federal nuclear research onto the wartime path, so did NRC's chemotherapy initiative launch the antimalarial program. Prewar federal resources and expertise in science, technology, and medicine were relatively minimal.

During the first years of the NRC's involvement with malaria chemotherapy, 1939 to 1941, the Chemistry Division operated largely as an independent, professional organization in concert with other such bodies, such as the American Association for the Advancement of Science (AAAS), the American Medical Association, and the American Chemical Society. In 1941, the Chemistry Division and the NRC's Division of Medical Sciences (DMS) were co-opted by federal government programs for emergency management, specifically the Office of Scientific Research and Development (OSRD), which was a component of the Office of Emergency Management (OEM). Much of the work prior to large-scale federal intervention relied on the networks of the Rockefeller Foundation, which cooperated with commercial firms such as the United Fruit Company, the Squibb Institute for Medical Research, and Parke Davis and Company, to identify drug candidates and test them for efficacy against malaria. Lowell T. Coggeshall (1901–1987)—a physician/researcher of the Rockefeller Institute, the University of Michigan, and later the University of Chicago—was a pivotal figure. He was one of a handful of malariologists who successfully bridged the prewar and wartime regimes and made critical contributions to the development of a U.S. antimalarial program.

NRC was motivated by the conflict already raging in Asia and imminent in Europe. They knew three things: that quinine was inadequate as a remedy; that synthetics might provide a way around U.S. dependence on threatened quinine supplies; and that malaria was out there—waiting—in a world at war.

Promoting their research agenda required them to remind American medical and scientific audiences that malaria was a persistent danger. They publicly asserted, "Contrary to popular belief, malaria is still one of humanity's major scourges. India, with a population of some 320,000,000, has a yearly average of from 70 to 80 million sufferers."[6] In making their case for the expanding and imminent threat of malaria, NRC cited the prominent president of the Rockefeller Foundation, Raymond B. Fosdick. Emphasis on scale was important for illustrating the actual and potential impact of malaria: In some parts of the world, malarial incidence was 100 percent. And malaria directly killed around one million people every year.

The Chemistry Division unanimously agreed that "research work should be stimulated in the field of quinine substitutes and synthetic antimalarials" and that, while "quinine, plasmoquine, atabrine, and a few other drugs have been useful, there is in the judgment of the medical profession, great need for something better."[7] None of these compounds—quinine, a natural product, and the others synthetic drugs—were entirely adequate either for the prophylaxis or treatment of malaria. They could not entirely destroy the parasite in vivo, leaving patients at risk for relapse, and none gave 100 percent prophylactic protection at safe dosages. Other concerns also weighed against the earlier treatments: plasmoquine was toxic to some patients even at low doses and continued prophylactic use of quinine often resulted in blurred vision, nausea, and ringing of the ears. Atabrine had mild toxic effects—such as vomiting, nausea, and diarrhea—and tended to dye the patients' skin yellow, both of which hindered compliance with prophylactic regimens.

In other words, the drugs available to treat or suppress malaria were, for one reason or another, inadequate. The NRC had established a temporary survey committee on antimalarials and malaria to decide whether the field merited a standing committee to examine—along with the DMS—"the whole problem of the chemistry and synthesis of antimalarials."[8] This modest beginning was one indication that creating large-scale, state-sponsored biomedical research was neither as easy nor inevitable as it might seem from our contemporary perspective.

As a follow-up to the formation of the NRC's Committee on Chemotherapy, Surgeon General Thomas Parran Jr. of the PHS convened a national symposium on malaria in Atlanta in May 1940. Among others, Coggeshall and the NIH's Lyndon F. Small were in attendance. No doubt the German blitzkrieg into Belgium and the Netherlands earlier in the month—marking the end of the so-called phony war on the western front—focused attention on change in the larger world. The conferees identified a number of problems hindering antimalarial research. In particular, chemists could not get their compounds tested, while biologists lacked compounds for their assays. This pointed to "an urgent need for coordination to bring such groups in contact and arouse their interest."[9] Coordination was also necessary to prevent the duplication of efforts. In the area of chemotherapy, the conference called for a pursuit of structure-activity relationships (SAR), bypassing quinine and atabrine, which failed to act against sporozoites or to act on the non-blood stages of the parasite, and pursuing leads such as plasmochin, which showed promise of reducing relapse by attacking the parasite in its exo-erythrocyte stage (outside the red blood cells). As commercial firms—predominantly Bayer—had conducted much of the early SAR work, the conferees called for some mechanism to promote communication between those in the industrial research laboratories and those outside. Finally, the conference produced "an incomplete outline of essential research in the field of malaria," as its purpose had not been "to formulate a program of research but rather to discover opportunities for coordinated effort in a program toward broader horizons of thought and research service."[10] The conference's rather diffuse suggestions emphasized cooperation between the natural and medical sciences and the acquisition of basic knowledge of the parasite and its control. Surgeon General Parran's gathering did not concentrate efforts but widened the conversation.

For Parran and his military counterparts, malaria was more than a global enemy. Malaria was a threat to war mobilization at home. Louis Williams, an ally of Bayer in the efforts to market atabrine in the United States, was seconded to the U.S. Army by the U.S. Public Health Service. He assisted the Fourth Corps Area (later the Fourth Service Command) in Atlanta, Georgia, in their efforts to control malaria in and around military camps. In this position, he also coordinated state and local efforts with those of the army, not only with regard to malaria control measures but also with regard to venereal disease—a historically recurring PHS combination of concerns. Once the United States had formally entered the war, Williams was relieved of these coordination duties and ordered to organize a new public health agency, Malaria Control in War Areas (MCWA). Within two months, Williams had the office up and running, still based out of Atlanta. Protecting workers and servicemen in twenty states, Puerto Rico, and the District of Columbia, MCWA was a major success on the home front, evolving in 1946 into the Communicable Disease

Center, the first instantiation of today's CDC.[11] Williams, like Parran, believed in the government's ability to impact public health on a grand scale. Domestically malaria could be controlled, even eradicated. But in India-Burma, North Africa, and the Pacific—especially in a shooting war—the military faced a far less tractable public health situation. They needed better tools.

On the R&D front, the combined enthusiasm of the NRC and the Public Health Service yielded much discussion and at least some attempt at retooling existing research agendas to international concerns. For example, in June 1940, William Taliaferro of the University of Chicago wrote to Parran to suggest an interdisplinary research team. Taliaferro had missed the meeting in Atlanta the previous month, but had spoken with his Rockefeller colleagues, Coggeshall and Mark F. Boyd of Rockefeller's Tallahassee, Florida, research station. He understood from them that most of the proposed work would be directed towards the development of new drugs, first in animals models and then in human subjects. Taliaferro thought that his colleagues could rise to these challenges. He suggested a number of his coworkers in the University of Chicago's Division of Biological Sciences, including Clay Huff, as potential participants in a multidisciplinary project: "one compact group working on the question of the mode of action of plasmodicidal drugs in the body," involving "detailed studies" on drug metabolism. This would further the service of chemistry in medicine because, "if any real leads were discovered they might greatly facilitate the work of the synthetic chemists."[12] The Chicago group was not alone, but these early calls for the coordination and expansion of malaria research moved only a few workers.

In August 1940, the Committee on Chemotherapy published its malaria manifesto in *Science* and in the *Journal of the American Medical Association*. The new committee would "concern itself not solely with antimalarials," but they would be "its first assignment." The committee outlined six objectives. First among them was "Chemistry in the service of medicine, with special emphasis on the discovery of new and useful synthetic drugs."[13] The remaining five objectives—for the promotion of chemotherapy in general and antimalarial chemotherapy in particular—showed the scope and limitations of the NRC's capabilities and vision.

The second goal of their initiative was to increase cooperation between the chemists who made new compounds and the pharmacologists who could test them. They observed a common problem of coordination: "It often happens that an organic chemist synthesizes a new compound of therapeutic possibilities but does not know to whom to turn to have it tested. Similarly, a pharmacologist discovers that a certain chemical exhibits hitherto unsuspected physiologic effects but has no information as to which organic chemists could help him in the preparation of the compound and its more promising derivatives."[14] To coordinate such work, they called upon the committee to act "as a general clearing house for the collection and classification of information as to the chemists, manufacturers, pharmacologists and others in the United States who are now at work in this field, the special lines of investigation they are following, and any other pertinent data." Again, coordination would also help the problem of duplication.

The final three objectives were largely logistical in nature. They should not be "too ambitious" at the early stages and should, at least initially, limit themselves to only malaria chemotherapy. They should "prepare a compact semipopular presentation of the malaria situation throughout the world, particularly in our own land, including a summary of what is going on here and how it is retarded and handicapped by lack of funds, for the purpose of enlisting public appreciation and support." This last bit was crucial; they needed money. The manifesto called for them to "secure funds from interested individuals, institutions, foundations, firms and others for the support of the work of the committee, the establishment of research fellowships and such other activities as will advance and expedite the achievement of the results sought."[15] The federal government was not explicitly mentioned as a possible source of funding. Coordination—to encourage cooperation, to identify those who could move the research forward, and to avoid duplication—was first and foremost what the NRC set out to do. They also kept firmly in mind the necessity of not expanding the project too quickly and, of course, the need for support: scientific, moral, and financial.

Rockefeller's Role

Lowell T. Coggeshall was a crucial node between the NRC's and the Rockefeller Foundation's malaria networks. Though he was listed first alphabetically on NRC's August 1940 manifesto on malaria chemotherapy, he was not a member of the original NRC temporary committee on malaria and malaria chemotherapy. This temporary committee was first convened by, and staffed from, the NRC's Chemistry Division and so consisted of three organic chemists: Leonard Cretcher, assistant director of the Mellon Institute of Industrial Research; Lyndon F. Small, PHS and head chemist of the National Institute of Health; and Marston T. Bogert, a professor emeritus from Columbia University who chaired the committee.[16] Subsequently the Medical Division of the NRC nominated two members—both MDs—to the temporary committee: Torald H. Sollmann, dean of the Western Reserve University School of Medicine; and Coggeshall, whose institutional affiliation was given as International Health Division, Rockefeller Foundation, New York. At the Chemistry Division meeting in November 1939, the temporary committee reported on the urgency of the problem, and the NRC duly discharged the temporary committee and established a regular, standing committee, the Committee on Chemotherapy. U.S. Surgeon General Parran approved the continued service of Lyndon Small on the standing committee, which proceeded with the same personnel as its predecessor.[17]

Coggeshall had wide-ranging malariology experience. He was born in 1901 and educated at Indiana University, earning his MD there in 1928. He had spent summers during his university years studying limnology in the streams and lakes of Indiana and later conducting mosquito surveys in Georgia with Samuel Taylor Darling, the eminent American malariologist.[18] In 1939, Coggeshall was working at the Rockefeller Institute in New York City. His work was typical of the International Health Division's growing direct involvement in laboratory science for public health purposes.[19] He was one of several Rockefeller-supported scientists conducting biological and clinical research on malaria, including precipitin tests for diagnosing malaria.[20] The precipitin test was an immunologic tool to supplement or supplant the microscopic examination of blood and mosquitoes. Also working on malaria immunology were William and Lucy Graves Taliaferro—husband and wife—at the University of Chicago. They were funded by Rockefeller Foundation grants, and William would be an active member on NRC committees throughout the war.[21] Coggeshall knew the Taliaferros from his Rockefeller-arranged internship at the University of Chicago, where he served prior to his appointment to the Rockefeller Institute.

Coggeshall soon became involved—along with John Maier, his Institute colleague, and John Ferrell, associate director of the IHD—in a growing program of facilitation, coordination, and actual testing of novel antimalarial drugs. Where they had previously eschewed synthetic antimalarials as economically unsuitable to domestic and international public health, the Rockefeller officers—like the NRC—took a fresh and approving look in the light of changing geopolitical circumstances. In the NRC's words, "so far as quinine itself it concerned, the world is practically dependent for its supply on Java and the Kina Bureau [the Quinine Trust]." This was nothing new, but there was an emerging risk that "the world . . . might be cut off from this supply or perhaps compelled to pay exorbitant prices, if Java should be seized by some other nation."[22] War could shift the economic equation away from quinine and toward synthetic antimalarials.

The Committee on Chemotherapy, its individual members, and the NRC launched a road show and publicity campaign to enlist the support of professional organizations and promote awareness of their initiative. Coggeshall was the committee's malariologist. The first stop was the joint meeting of the National Malaria Committee, the Academy of Tropical Medicine, and the American Society of Tropical Medicine at the end of November 1939 in Memphis, Tennessee. Other cooperating institutions and organizations included the AAAS, the American Chemical Society, the Tennessee Valley Authority, the Public Health Service, the War Department, and industry groups such as the American Drug Manufacturers Association and the Manufacturing Chemists Association. As these allegiances were largely rhetorical, Coggeshall and his Rockefeller colleagues remained central to antimalarial efforts.

Coggeshall's plans for testing drugs at the Rockefeller Institutes moved forward during the summer of 1940. Issues of how to coordinate and collaborate between the nonprofit, for-profit, and government actors arose. Successfully resolving these issues would continue to be critical to the research and war efforts. Abbott Laboratories of Illinois had contacted Coggeshall in July with regard to getting their compounds tested against malaria parasites. Abbott's program was a year old and had generated nearly fifty compounds. Abbott was "distinctly interested" in having the Rockefeller group test their putative antimalarials. They also had a number of questions about Rockefeller's testing plans: How many compounds could they test? Must the submitted compounds have some proven, or at least theoretical activity?[23] Coggeshall responded that the Rockefeller researchers were interested in testing any new compounds that "might logically have an effect on the malaria parasite." He added that most of the compounds that they had tested to date were ones that showed some activity against bacteria and were "not too toxic."[24]

In consonance with NRC's forthcoming manifesto, Coggeshall and Rockefeller had "developed a routine for testing all sorts of drugs," justifying these investments on the basis of the wartime threat to existing antimalarial drug supplies and the fundamental weaknesses of these drugs. These facilities allowed Rockefeller "to test a large number of different preparations, and our program is set up so as to run indefinitely." All that would be required for the submission of compounds would be some preliminary information on toxicity and solubility.[25] Abbott sent Coggeshall two compounds that had shown some activity—and some toxicity—when administered by injection to canaries. They also supplied Coggeshall with structural formulas of the two chemicals, which they asked him "to keep confidential."[26] One was a quinoline compound, the other an acridine compound. The Rockefeller group also tested compounds for Squibb,[27] where their collaborator was Harry Benjamin van Dyke, head of the pharmacology division of the Squibb Institute for Medical Research. Van Dyke had good Rockefeller credentials, having been a professor at the University of Chicago and more recently a department head at the Rockefeller-sponsored Peiping Union Medical College in China. The testing program continued throughout 1940, even as Coggeshall made expanded plans for wartime work.

By October 1940, Coggeshall was again reassessing the Rockefeller malaria programs. The war was now an explicit context for ongoing research. It seemed to Coggeshall "that in view of the present conditions our organization might now give some thought to a plan of action relating to malaria and war." Rockefeller was uniquely placed to do this. "There is no single organization in this country, including the federal services, that has spent as much time or money on malaria as The Rockefeller Foundation. Therefore, we can be expected to be called upon for advice and aid in the event of any minor or major emergency." Just two weeks earlier, Imperial Japanese forces had begun their occupation of Indochina. War and malaria had historically co-occurred, with troops and refugees exposed to new climates, conditions, and diseases. "The trend of events seems to be such that considerable activity might be expected to occur in regions where malaria exists. In the past the concentration of nonimmune individuals in areas of endemic malaria has had serious consequences. For example, in Macedonia in 1916 . . . there were times when 40 percent of the men were incapacitated for duty because of malaria." Nonimmune people were those who had not been repeatedly exposed to malaria, a process that could provide partial natural immunity to the worst symptoms disease. In the United States and the Americas more broadly, Coggeshall saw mobilization for war as immediately putting military units in jeopardy: "It is almost certain that the rapid localization of troops in Southern United States, Caribbean area, or South America will be attended by epidemics." In his opinion, public health measures and research should precede the outbreak of disease. Previous studies of "war malaria" had been too slow and took place only after the epidemic's peak. Coggeshall wanted Rockefeller mobilized for war.[28]

Given all this, and that "the medical departments of the government services will have the responsibility of caring for troops," what should Rockefeller and the International Health Division do? Coggeshall proposed a plan. "Our part could be the study of malaria epidemiology and control with troops in the field. The concentration of these nonimmune individuals would provide unlimited investigative possibilities that can never be had with a civilian population. It would be possible to conduct controlled investigations in chemotherapy, new serologic diagnostic methods [precipitin tests, for example], prophylaxis, and many other related studies." Coggeshall counted twenty-six staff members in the IHD who had "a considerable amount of experience with malaria, many having limited their activities to this disease alone." He advocated the formation of a well-rounded "study unit" that "should include individuals with clinical, immunological, and epidemiological experience . . . supplemented in the field by men with entomological experience." Coggeshall believed that "an exceptionally strong unit" could be assembled "from the staff of the IHD and can justifiably be expected to uncover new information in a field that has been considerably muddled." He was ready to begin immediately: "If we do intend to do anything, the necessity for planning ahead is the most important item."[29] This was a critical inflection point between the prewar world of biomedical research and public health, and its postwar successor. Would Rockefeller's IHD be able to step up to the new scale of research and intervention?

Wilbur Sawyer, the director of the IHD to whom Coggeshall had addressed his proposal, could already see problems with Coggeshall's vision of IHD's role in the coming conflict. He read Coggeshall's memo with "great interest" and wanted Coggeshall to "develop the idea further."[30] However, his "first reaction" was somewhat defensive with regard to IHD's staffing. This reaction was "one of surprise that you feel that our Division is rich in malaria staff, as one of our outstanding personnel problems now is to create a few more field malariologists." A shortage of qualified staff and their training were critical issues in Sawyer's view. As to Coggeshall's field-research agenda, Sawyer felt it premature given the current state of knowledge. He noted Coggeshall's "suggestion that valuable observations can be made on troops in the field, particularly as to the value of prophylaxis and chemotherapy," but felt that these would require "improved methods" of testing, methods that they had yet to develop.

Sawyer made two suggestions of his own as to what IHD's response to war should be: "1) the finding and recommending of improved methods, and 2) their application in the field."[31] Even with regard to his own plan, Sawyer saw manpower as a major hurdle. Rockefeller simply did not have the staff to operate in this field on this scale. Sawyer did not want IHD to pursue its "present lines" of research and public health outreach in the context of war mobilization. He felt that they already had "infinite opportunities for testing any procedure," not just among the U.S. military "but also in regions like southwest China, India, Africa, etc." Having written this, Sawyer could not in good conscience turn away entirely from the terrible impact that war would have on public health. Sawyer wanted to put innovation in methods ahead of field work. In Sawyer's view, the scale of wartime needs would easily outstrip the capabilities of the Rockefeller Foundation. Events were already proving Sawyer's vision true. The United States was moving to a war footing. Two days before Sawyer's memo, the federal government had placed an embargo on the export of scrap steel and iron, a move intended to counter Japanese advances in Southeast Asia and the ongoing occupation of China.

Sawyer's caution notwithstanding, chemotherapy remained on the agenda at the Rockefeller Foundation. On 27 November 1940, officers from IHD conferred with their colleagues in the foundation's Natural Sciences Division, including Warren Weaver, director of the division, and Frank Blair Hanson, its associate director. Moving through the general field of chemotherapy, its methods, and content, they discussed anti-syphilis-drug research at Johns Hopkins. This program had begun from two leads, arsenic and sulfanilimide. Malaria chemotherapy was central to the discussions.

Chemists and compounds were crucial to any area of chemotherapy. Warren Weaver said "that it would be easier to suggest an organic chemist for malaria work if those interested could decide on the substance with which to begin their study."[32] John A. Ferrell, associate director of the IHD, cited the German work on atabrine and plasmochin and use of quinine as a lead compound in their development. It was Coggeshall's opinion that it would be better to start from a compound other than quinine, but he "had no particular one in mind."[33] The discussion then moved to possible organic chemists with whom to collaborate. Suggestions included Louis F. Fieser at Harvard and Roger Adams at Illinois, both eminent organic chemists at arguably the two top departments in the country. Weaver pointed out that James Conant, as "chairman of the National Defense Research Commission's committee on chemistry," had "undoubtedly made an extensive study of talent in all the fields of chemistry." Conant was a well-known organic chemist before becoming president of Harvard University and before his years of national service. Weaver felt Conant would be well equipped to offer suggestions, a convergence of Rockefeller's needs with those of government.

In December 1940 and January 1941, Ferrell and Coggeshall continued to discuss how Rockefeller might expand its antimalarial program. They consulted closely with Eli Kennerly Marshall Jr., a chemist and pharmacologist at the Johns Hopkins School of Medicine. A rising star at a favored institution, Marshall was member of Rockefeller's networks. Marshall was educated at the College of Charleston, South Carolina, and Johns Hopkins University, where he received his PhD in chemistry in 1911 and his MD in 1917.[34] Marshall and the Rockefeller staff settled fairly quickly on additional points of collaboration. Coggeshall believed that Taliaferro and his group at Chicago were "not particularly interested in the chemotherapy of malaria, *per se*."[35] And they selected Harvard's Louis Fieser as a primary chemical collaborator. Fieser had earned his doctorate at Harvard, working with James Conant whose crucial role in wartime science and technology Warren Weaver had alluded to. Fieser, too, was not new to Rockefeller. On 9 December 1940, the scientific directors agreed to allocate up to $23,400 "for studies of chemotherapy in relation to malaria."[36] These funds would allow the IHD to supplement their skills and facilities in the area of malaria chemotherapy, as they were "not equipped to determine the pharmacological properties of such drugs in laboratory animals" or "to synthesize new drugs to the end that an antimalarial substance of superior merit may be created." They would fund Marshall at Hopkins to determine "the toxicity, absorption, excretion, and tissue distribution of selected compounds in birds."[37] With Marshall, they brought a new face and a new approach to antimalarial research. They would also free the IHD from its "almost complete dependence on commercial companies for new compounds" by supporting Fieser's work at Harvard in "the synthesis of new compounds, and the further regrouping of the active principle in drugs which have already shown some therapeutic properties."[38] This was much like the process that the Bayer chemists had used, developing multiple series of drugs based on different leads and different nuclei, for example, the quinoline compounds and the acridine compounds. In January, Coggeshall had an opportunity to meet with Fieser while on a trip to Boston. He found Fieser to be very interested in malaria chemotherapy and ready to send materials to Rockefeller for testing. Coggeshall and Ferrell were both prepared to move ahead, working with Fieser and testing his compounds.[39]

Rational Drug Development versus Random Screening

Discussions with Marshall made clear another reason, apart from mere independence, that they wanted their own synthetic chemists. Marshall thought that unless they could work "on a large scale by the hit and miss method," it was "essential to have a thorough basis . . . for suggesting what new compounds . . . should be synthesized." According to Marshall, this was how they would set themselves apart from, and outperform, commercial programs. Marshall continued, "A planned study . . . on a small scale cannot hope to compete with the type of studies conducted mainly by commercial companies where hundreds of drugs are synthesized and crudely tested for activity. However, this hit and miss method of the manufacturer [owes] future results largely to chance." Rockefeller and the university workers would not and could not compete with the commercial chemists in manufacturing, but their research resources remained deep in comparison with the prewar U.S. pharmaceutical companies. Marshall believed that, although one could not compete against the companies with regard to scale, "it is quite likely by careful planning and adopting a rational approach to the problem one can outthink those who are dependent upon mass production."[40]

The same day that Marshall wrote these words to Rockefeller's Ferrell promoting the rational approach to drug discovery, Coggeshall sent Ferrell his own impressions from a meeting with Marshall. He found Marshall "deeply interested" in chemotherapy. Marshall was "highly trained in physiology and pharmacology, as well as in organic chemistry" and had "extensive experiences in bacteriological chemotherapy (which involves the same general principles regardless of the pathogenic agent involved)." Coggeshall's report refined what Marshall meant by a rational approach. Marshall believed "that the correct approach to the malarial problem is to select the potential effective drugs on the basis of their physiological and pharmacological action; for example, those readily absorbable from the gut with low toxicity and with the capacity to penetrate red blood cells."[41] Coggeshall described this approach in opposition to a more random—what Marshall had called "hit and miss"— approach. Coggeshall here was most likely reporting on Marshall's opinion, not offering his own. The "indiscriminate trial and error method" of testing whatever materials were at hand was distinct from a more considered and rational approach. Antimalarial work gave Marshall, an innovator in pharmacology, a large new audience for his rational approach to drug testing and drug metabolism.

Coggeshall also passed on a theory regarding Marshall's approach to drug screening, one advanced by Marshall to both Coggeshall and Ferrell. Extending his experience with bacterial chemotherapy, Marshall suggested that an initial screen should be against the most susceptible strain of malaria that they could identify, perhaps the monkey malaria *Plasmodium knowlesi*. Marshall suggested in vitro testing against this parasite—testing in blood outside a living body—rather than in vivo against the parasite in a living primate. Whether Marshall realized it or not, this was not technically as simple as in vitro screening against bacteria. Marshall's argument for using the most susceptible strains—those organisms most easily killed by available drugs—was based in simple logic: compounds not active against the most virulent bacteria might be active against some other strains, and the use of easily killed strains in a screen would reveal potential leads most readily.[42]

Whether or not this observation in bacteria could be extended to malarial parasites, Coggeshall recommended Marshall to Ferrell, "Regardless of the correctness of this theory, a man of his ability and experience should be of great aid to us. The plan he suggested of the synthesis and subsequent testing of the pharmacologic action and toxicity for the correct dosage of test drugs takes away a high degree of the guess work associated with the routine test method." With Marshall in charge of synthesis, basic pharmacology, and toxicology, the Rockefeller staff would then test the drugs against various stages of malaria parasites, as Marshall had "neither facilities [n]or the experience" for such work.[43] Rockefeller was interested in drugs for both treatment and prophylaxis. Coggeshall's final sentence of his memorandum suggested that he was not entirely ready to abandon the routine—hit and miss—testing methods of the commercial enterprises: "As far as Dr. Maier and I are concerned, it is an ideal plan as we will proceed in the same fashion as heretofore, obtaining drugs from individuals within the commercial house, but in addition we will have available this valuable assistance from an expert in the phases of the work least familiar to us."[44] This strategy of testing whatever compounds were available would persist even as others propounded and practiced a rational approach to drug development.

Marshall and Coggeshall pointed to a major divide in drug discovery: the choice between the rational and the random approaches. Marshall clearly desired to move away from "hit and miss," routine testing—by trial and error—to a rational approach for the construction of chemical structures for chemotherapy. One contemporaneous view on rational methods can be found in a May 1940 *Lancet* article, "A Rational Approach to Chemotherapy," which dealt with the antibacterial action of sulfa drugs.[45] Its author suggested that an "antibacterial substance" may "have a chemical similarity" to an "essential metabolite." Therefore, "research might then reasonably be directed to modification of the structure of known essential metabolites to form products which can block the enzyme without exhibiting the specific action of the metabolite."[46] Indeed, the sulfas worked by blocking the uptake of a chemically similar nutrient (p-aminobenzoic acid) that was essential to bacterial growth. This activity earned these drugs the descriptor *antimetabolites*. Marshall himself had worked extensively on the sulfa drugs from 1936 onward, but antimalarial chemotherapy had not reached such a state of sophistication, for the simple reason that much about the basic biology and metabolism of the malaria parasites remained a mystery.[47]

Even without such detailed knowledge, Marshall's interest in the biological activity of antimalarials, such as their ability to enter red blood cells or their breakdown in vertebrate hosts, showed a strong move toward the rational, biochemical approach to drug development—a move supported by the Rockefeller Foundation. For example, the Rockefeller Foundation's 1945 *Annual Report* noted that IHD had supported Fieser's work "on chemotherapy in relation to malaria" since 1940.[48] IHD and the Natural Sciences Division both saw something novel and valuable in Fieser's approach. Fieser was "trying to break away from the conventional and purely empirical scheme of chemotherapeutic research and to develop a rational method for the discovery of new chemotherapeutic agents through research that will provide some understanding of the phenomena of drug action and metabolism."[49] Fieser's rational method was consonant with Marshall's call for a rational approach that could outthink random, routine screening. In scale, they could not compete with industry, but in intellectually flexibility and innovation, Marshall believed they had a real comparative advantage. In the end, when government resources increased their capacity, Coggeshall and others adopted both Marshall's "rational approach" and the "hit and miss method" that Marshall wanted left to the commercial houses.[50]

Restructuring the Research Network

Coggeshall knew that Marshall had strong feelings about collaborations with commercial firms, and Coggeshall took these concerns seriously. Marshall believed that cooperation between academics and companies was "extremely important," but those from academe must be "absolutely free to conduct and publish their investigations as they please."[51] Marshall worried that commercial firms would seek to take advantage of naïve or inexperienced researchers. One had to adopt "a firm stand." Marshall advised Coggeshall to insist that companies provide structural data and names for all the materials that they supplied. In certain cases, the companies wanted to protect their proprietary interests by withholding the chemical details of their compounds. This could be to shield these compounds from direct competition as antimalarials or to hide from competitors compounds developed for entirely other purposes. Coggeshall found this advice "very useful" and felt that, as he and his colleagues gained more experience with the companies, they would follow Marshall's advice and steer clear of "disagreeable messes." Thus, Coggeshall "formulated the policy of telling them that all results will be turned over to them when we are ready and not before."[52] For Coggeshall and Marshall, avoiding disagreeable messes in the area of medical research meant keeping the upper hand with regard to information and publication.

In January 1941, Coggeshall and John Ferrell of the IHD sought to design a research program to incorporate other collaborators and expertise with their own programs in clinical, pharmacological, and immunological research. Primary among these collaborators were Fieser at Harvard and Marshall at Hopkins, as well as commercial firms with distinct needs and resources. They had to establish basic tests for activity and toxicity before new compounds could be usefully solicited or synthesized. Marshall was also interested in a more sophisticated approach to pharmacology, probing the physiological and biochemical behavior of the drugs in mammals and birds. For the U.S. program, Marshall's innovations were a small change from the interwar work at Bayer. But Rockefeller's plans were by no means a radical departure from what had gone before. The institution shifted from a public health perspective bounded by economic limitations to a research agenda that in many ways embraced Bayer's industrial research network.

Looking forward, Coggeshall and Ferrell produced a research outline that was more than superficially similar to one provided to Rockefeller by S. P. James some ten years previously as part of his report on Bayer's Elberfeld facility. This report had been sent by the English malariologist James to George Strode, who coordinated Rockefeller's European operations from Paris. (Strode had returned from the Paris office to become associate director of the IHD in 1938.) Both the 1931 and the 1941 outlines emphasized the role of chemists in developing assays, the synthesis of new compounds, the use of animal models, the testing of promising drugs on paretic patients, field testing in malarial areas, and, implicitly for Bayer, the need for commercial participation in the manufacture and sale of drugs. There were certain differences as to levels of association between individuals and firms and to the centralization of control, but both plans seemed to suggest a scale of only dozens of workers in a handful of laboratories. For Rockefeller, the commercial partners appeared explicitly under two of the six headings, and other nonacademic collaborators can easily be read into headings on human (clinical) testing: Initial human trials typically took place on paretics in private or state hospitals, and Rockefeller worked with Gorgas Memorial Institute in Panama, the United Fruit Company, and the U.S. military for field tests against natural malaria.[53] Bayer's efforts in the 1920s and 1930s were crucial to the first developments in synthetic antimalarials, so the IHD's interest them was natural. (See table 4.1.)

Within a few days of receiving Ferrell's letter, Coggeshall had fleshed out the outline of Rockefeller's "Chemotherapeutic Program." Though Coggeshall felt the program to be "very self-sufficient," he suggested that the outline might be shared with Surgeon General Parran or Lyndon Small of the PHS, and he listed a number of outside collaborators.[54]

Coggeshall began with the synthesis of new compounds and named three academic and five industrial collaborators for this phase of the work: Marshall, Fieser, and Robert C. Elderfield of Columbia University; and, on the industrial side, Squibb, Parke Davis, Calco Chemical, Eli Lilly, and Winthrop Chemical. Coggeshall and Maier would conduct animal testing at the IHD laboratories at the Rockefeller Institute, while Marshall continued studying metabolism, toxicology, and pharmacology. For testing against induced malaria (paretics with neurosyphilis), he proposed Mark Boyd's Rockefeller-funded clinical research center in Florida and a New York collaboration between the IHD laboratories, Bellevue Hospital, and possibly the Manhattan State Hospital at Ward's Island. For field trials, Coggeshall nominated five IHD doctors working in the New World tropics, including Fred L. Soper in Brazil. Coggeshall suggested that the hospitals of the United Fruit Company and Standard Oil of New Jersey might be used "by courtesy"; both companies ran hospitals in malarious regions.[55] As we saw in the previous chapter, United Fruit worked with Bayer to test atabrine and plasmochin. Standard Oil had conducted its own investigations into the new synthetic drugs.[56]

With regard to preliminary drug screening, Coggeshall included a final table: "Malaria Infections of Lower Animals Currently Used and Available in This Country for Therapeutic Studies."[57] He listed three monkey malarias and three bird malarias. The simian varieties were *Plasmodium knowlesi*, *P. inui*, and *P. cynomolgi*. The last two were both originally isolated at the IHD laboratories from "naturally infected monkeys from local animal dealers." Also claimed for the IHD was the avian malaria *P. lophurae*, isolated from a "naturally infected pheasant at the Bronx Zoo Park." Missing from

Table 4.1 **Organizational Outlines**

Bayer 1931	Rockefeller 1941
The organization concerned with antimalarial drugs at Elberfeld is as follows	Chemotherapeutic Research for Prevention and Control of Malaria; Lines of Study; Plans for Individual and for Group Work
1. Chemists devise and make the preparations and do "chemical assays."	1. Production and selection of synthetic compounds to be tested. Aid obtainable from (1) Organic chemists (2) Pharmacologists (3) Commercial Companies

2. The therapeutic department (Dr. Kikuth) evaluates curative and prophylactic efficacy in bird malaria . . . according to Roehl's method. About 300 canaries per week are used.	2. Laboratory and animal tests: Coggeshall, Maier
	(1) Warburg apparatus
	(2) Laboratory animals
	    Canaries
	    Ducks
	    Monkeys

3. Pharmacologists and toxicologists (Dr. Weese and others) investigate the pharmacological action of the drugs when administered intravenously and orally to research animals and whether the action of the drug is cumulative or not.	3. Pharmacological test: Marshall at Johns Hopkins Medical School (1) Toxicity (2) Absorption (3) Distrubution
4. Drugs are tested in inoculated human malaria (paretics) in arrangement with Dr. Sioli (in charge of a mental hospital at Düsseldorf).	4. Human tests: induced malaria, paretics (1) Prophylaxis (2) Cure (3) Dosage, etc.
5. A whole-time traveling medical officer (Dr. Peter) tests the therapeutic action of the drugs on natural cases of human malaria at the malaria clinic at Gurbanesti in Roumania.	5. Human tests: natural malaria, field conditions (1) Prophylaxis (2) Cure (3) Dosage
6. Further trials on natural malaria in arrangement with Prof. Mühlens and Dr. Otto Fischer at the Tropical Diseases Institute, Hamburg. Commercial production, sale, and distribution of compounds undertaken by Bayer.	6. Commercial production, sale, and distribution of compounds of proven value

Sources: Left column: S. P. James's report to the Rockefeller Foundation, James to Strode, 12 November 1931, p. 3, folder 675, box 51, series 401, Record Group 1.1, Rockefeller Foundation Archives, RAC. Right column: letter, John Ferrell to Lowell Coggeshall, Inter-Office Correspondence, 27 January 1941, folder 491, box 50, series 100, Record Group 1, Rockefeller Foundation Archives, RAC. Outlines slightly rearranged for clarity.

the list of significant avian malarias was *P. gallinaceum*, as its use was not—yet—allowed in the United States. Along with vector and host information and the laboratories that used these various parasites, Coggeshall included another piece of data on each: whether it was "affected by sulfanilamide," Coggeshall's current favorite lead compound.

During 1940 and 1941, it was the Rockefeller Foundation itself, particularly John Maier and Coggeshall, who coordinated much of the testing of compounds for industrial partners. They and their Rockefeller-funded collaborators conducted animal studies at the Rockefeller Institute and Johns Hopkins (E. K. Marshall's laboratory), and they coordinated clinical work with United Fruit Company hospitals and Gorgas Memorial Hospital in the Canal Zone.

Coggeshall himself worked closely with the industrial collaborators, especially the Parke Davis Company on their sulfa drug Promin (chemically a sulfone). Parke Davis had shown Promin to be well tolerated in humans when they studied it against streptococcus. Coggeshall had found that it was active against both avian and simian malarias and against induced malaria in paretics in New York. In March 1941, Coggeshall was prepared to assert two points: that Promin was more active against *Plasmodium* parasites than any drugs except quinine and atabrine and that it was able to terminate an induced *vivax* infection.[58] These claims were positive but not definitive. Coggeshall still considered Promin "only as a lead in the field of malaria chemotherapy," and he felt it was time for "clinical evaluation in natural infections."[59] After negotiations with the United Fruit Company and the Gorgas Memorial Hospital, Coggeshall set out for Panama and Colombia to test it in the field. His results, published later that year, were suggestive but not outstanding. Coggeshall and his coauthors concluded that Promin and another favored sulfa were especially promising as representing a whole new class of antimalarial, yet there were "no reasons for giving the drugs in preference to quinine or atabrine for the treatment of malaria."[60]

Even as Coggeshall took these crucial clinical steps with Promin, the ground was shifting. Between Coggeshall's arrival in Panama in April[61] and the appearance of his Promin paper in the *Journal of the American Medical Association* in September 1941, much changed in Coggeshall's world and in malaria research. The expanding war would alter the scale of resources available and crucially alter the federal research infrastructure for biomedicine.

Rapid change was all around. At the end of August, Coggeshall resigned from the IHD and departed for the University of Michigan. President Franklin D.

Roosevelt's administration was generating new agencies in response to the war. And many began to heed NRC's plea for research coordination and funding. Although Roosevelt had established the National Defense Research Committee (NDRC) as a part of Office of Emergency Management back in June 1940, the NDRC did not originally cover medical research. Roosevelt extended it to medicine with a new executive order in June 1941, when he created the Office of Scientific Research and Development (OSRD) under the OEM. OSRD in turn spawned the Committee on Medical Research (CMR) chaired by Alfred Newton Richards. By this time, too, the Chemistry Division had a new chairman, William Mansfield Clark, professor of physiological chemistry at the Johns Hopkins School of Medicine. Clark was born in 1884 and educated at Williams College and Johns Hopkins University, where he received his PhD in 1910. Returning to Hopkins in 1927, he served there as a professor of physiological chemistry for twenty-five years, including his NRC service and his war work for CMR.[62] As CMR chairman, Richards wrought the first change upon the NRC's original Committee on Chemotherapy, when he decided to co-opt the NRC's existing advisory committees to support the work of his newly formed CMR in the summer of 1941.[63]

The Limits of NRC

That summer, as the likelihood of U.S. involvement in World War II increased—and with it the potential threat to U.S. troops of malaria—specific plans with regard to malaria research, prophylaxis, and treatment remained diffuse. In response to the continued concerns of the medical officers of the U.S. armed services and the Public Health Service, on 8 July 1941, the Division of Medical Sciences of the NRC held a conference on malaria chemotherapy. Many of the attendees at this first conference would repeatedly reconvene either as the "Malaria Conference" or the "Conference on Malaria Research." Among the seventeen present at the first meeting in July were Mark F. Boyd (Rockefeller Foundation), William Mansfield Clark (Johns Hopkins), G. Robert Coatney (PHS, NIH), L. T. Coggeshall (Rockefeller Foundation), H. W. Florey (Medical Research Council of Great Britain), E. K. Marshall (Johns Hopkins), L. F. Small (PHS, NIH), W. H. Taliaferro (University of Chicago), Lewis H. Weed (chairman of DMS), and three U.S. Army colonels, including James S. Simmons. According to Clark, chairman of the Division of Chemistry and Chemical Technology of the NRC, it was the post-conference report of E. K. Marshall that "foreshadowed what was to become the principal line of work."[64] Marshall's report, "Tentative Methods for Preliminary Testing of Antimalarial

Drugs," emphasized the use of avian malarias in canaries, chicks, and ducks for testing antimalarial activity and the use of ducks, chicks, or mice for the testing of toxicity.[65] At the time of this first meeting, the principle funding source for antimalarial chemotherapy remained the Rockefeller Foundation and federal support of intramural research at the NIH, represented by Coatney and Small.

In spite of discussions at the Malaria Conference, other organizational issues persisted, and NRC's weakness as an underfunded talking shop was apparent. Contributors raised concerns about the distribution of findings and about the level of control that the committees and panels would exercise over research. Some, like Taliaferro at Chicago, felt that progress would be best if specialists pursued their own lines of research unfettered by overarching agendas. Taliaferro's malaria work had been funded with Rockefeller money since 1925.[66] At the first Malaria Conference meeting, he asserted his belief "that studies along fundamental lines were of equal importance to the actual testing of new compounds."[67] Urging more fundamental research, Taliaferro reacted negatively to Coggeshall's suggestion that a way of disseminating information be found, "so that our attack on chemotherapy of malaria would be more efficient." Taliaferro wanted there to be "no attempt at regimenting research along this line, but that individuals and organizations with special ability and equipment should attack phases of the problem for which they were best suited."[68] In terms of research values, this debate—pitting research regimentation against the individual pursuit of fundamental lines of research—paralleled Marshall's divide between routine, large-scale testing and rational drug development. Both arguments involved issues of scale and independence. These debates, soon muted by U.S. entry into the war, continued after the Axis surrenders. But the interplay between personal idiosyncrasies, technical problems, and institutional constraints would continue to shape the growing program.

From a practical standpoint, further refinement of the animal models of malaria was immediately the rate-limiting step in the effort to find a substitute for quinine. Lewis Weed, chairman of the Division of Medical Sciences, had told Clark in August 1941 that the preliminary testing of new compounds was their pressing concern and "until these methods of rapidly sifting are devised it seems that there is already ample activity in the field of synthetic chemistry on the problem of malaria."[69] From the fall of 1941 through the spring of 1942, the development of adequate avian malaria screens retarded their progress.

The conference and the NRC were particularly interested in importing *Plasmodium gallinaceum* from Mexico and safely distributing it to the screening labs. With assistance from the U.S. Department of Agriculture, they eventually managed this. As a disease of domestic chickens, *P. gallinaceum* was a potential threat to U.S. farmers and the food supply. Taliaferro believed that its presence in the United States should be kept secret, not so much to limit enemy knowledge of research methods, but for fear that it might be acquired by enemy agents within the United States and used for sabotage.[70] By the end of 1941, the infection was established in five laboratories around the country: the National Institute of Health (Coatney and Small), the Department of Pharmacology of the Johns Hopkins Medical School (Marshall), the Rockefeller Institute (Maier), the University of Michigan (Coggeshall), and the University of Chicago (Taliaferro).[71]

In the laboratories, the establishment of antimalarial drug screening was an early priority. Safety and sabotage aside, the pressing issue in avian malarias was the quality of research animals and some sort of standardization for the model systems within and across laboratories. Earlier problems with the supply and quality of canaries had dogged the Rockefeller testing efforts. John Maier had to change the method of testing used in the IHD laboratory because it was "increasingly difficult to get canaries from the animal dealers, and those canaries which are obtainable are far from a uniform stock. We felt that the fact that our test animals could not be considered biologically uniform was probably making our tests difficult to interpret." Faced with supply difficulties, Maier turned from canaries to ducks: "It has recently been found that *P. lophurae* is very virulent for young ducks, and therefore we have been trying to standardize this infection as a basis for our further testing, using known antimalarial drugs."[72] Even earlier, Coggeshall had also commented on problems with canaries: "At the present time the difficulty in receiving canaries is slowing up our work."[73] By the middle of 1941, Marshall, too, was looking critically at canaries, but for other reasons than their quantity and quality. Looking back to Roehl's work, Marshall found Bayer's use of the therapeutic index—the ratio of the effective dose to the tolerable dose—in canaries to be flawed, as the toxicological data for birds did not translate well to mammals, including humans.[74] Again, as he would with the use of mosquitoes, the outsider, Marshall, challenged a basic assumption of previous antimalarial researchers.

With discussion of canaries and mosquitoes, malaria chemotherapy research had not yet gone too far from its foundations. But change was rapidly accelerating. The organizational shift during the late 1930s and early 1940s from Rockefeller, to NRC, to the emerging U.S. government Committee on Medical Research reshaped malaria research. The lack of coordination of research efforts between chemists and biologists, raised by the NRC and the IHD, remained a hindrance to progress. Addressing the coordination and money issues would transform research funding and management in the United States for decades to come.

From NRC to OSRD

Before the Malaria Conference could address the coordination of research efforts—the how and who of the project—it would have to solidify its goals and content, and resolve the issue of funding that had been in suspension for more than two years. In September 1941, the second Malaria Conference convened. Coggeshall, chairing the meeting, announced that OSRD funds were now available. With federal money in the offing, the program's goals needed clarification. Coggeshall called for a plan of investigation and said that NRC "was anxious" for the Malaria Conference "to draw up a general program of work to be done and to approve specific projects."[75] Anxiety over the lack of focus was justified.

The Malaria Conference could not reach an overall consensus. Marshall, again, pressed for the development of standardized chemotherapy research. This would require the determination of two preliminary findings: First, "someone should settle one way or another the question as to whether sporozoites and trophozoites react differently to drugs," which readers will recall was S. P. James's assertion in 1931. James believed that potential prophylactic drugs should be tested against the sporozoites injected by the infectious mosquito. Others thought that activity against the blood stages of the parasite was sufficient. It is interesting to note that Marshall, an outsider to malaria whose previous expertise was in antibacterial (antibiotic) research, questioned the necessity of mosquitoes in the biological models of malaria. "Secondly," Marshall said, "since these drugs were ultimately to be used in human malaria, we should know definitely how the experimental [animal] disease compares with the disease in man." Taliaferro, who at the previous meeting had expressed his concern with overregimentation, made a number of suggestions for further research. Following these remarks, the minutes dryly noted, "There was a general discussion of whether we should draw up a general program but no one had definite enough ideas to carry this further."[76]

Marshall's position on toxicity was taken up by the wartime program, which employed activity against avian malaria as its primary screen. As Clark later wrote, "The use of avian malarias for tests of antiplasmodial action leaves open the question of a drug's toxicity. Since the ultimate object of preliminary toxicity studies is to provide the basis for judging whether a trial of the drug in man is permissible and advisable, it would seem wise to pay less attention to the toxicity of the drug in the bird and more attention to the toxicity of the drug in mammals, which in some respects may subject a drug to processes more closely analogous to those in man."[77] This distinction marked Marshall's departure from the toxicity assumptions inherent in Roehl's model and required the expansion of non-avian model systems for toxicological screens. Amid the rigors of wartime research aimed at drug development for human use, avian malarias were found to be essential but limited in their utility.

With the Rockefeller researchers and most of the NRC committee members still discussing the establishment of a screening process and the development of new drugs, the U.S. military was clearly looking for a compound that could be put into the field as soon as possible. The military and the OSRD bureaucracy were competing with NRC as the prime movers in antimalarial research. At the September conference meeting, asked about the Army's main concern with malaria, Colonel James S. Simmons "said he thought that the development of a field prophylactic was most important and pointed out that up to the present time malaria had not been attacked from this point of view."[78] The U.S. Army's need for a field prophylactic against malaria would lead Richards's Committee on Medical Research to reexamine atabrine in detail even while it continued the search for new drugs. Thus CMR would foster the routine, the random, and the rational, pursuing the routine development of a known drug, atabrine, the random screening of available compounds, and the rational innovation of novel compounds.

In the fall of 1941, the NRC's Committee on Chemotherapy, extant since 1939 and a driving force behind the increased awareness of the importance of malaria chemotherapy in a changing world, was honorably discharged by NRC.[79] After its dissolution, the committee's members remained available for further efforts, such as the other NRC committees that advised CMR. With its CMR in ascendance, OSRD first made money available for malaria research in September 1941. By year's end, the Japanese had bombed Pearl Harbor and the British base at Singapore, and the Japanese offensive in Southeast Asia had disrupted quinine supplies. With the United States at war, the federal taps opened. Over the winter of 1941 and into the spring of 1942, the CMR approved and the OSRD funded various investigations in malaria research: chemical syntheses, life cycles of parasites, immunology and histopathology of malaria, cytological effects of drugs, parasite biochemistry, and drug metabolism. "The chief interest of the period, however, lay in the development of testing procedures with which to screen new compounds for antimalarial activity in avian infections."[80] This emphasis brought the conference more fully in line with Marshall's proposals and with the Rockefeller Foundation's internal recommendations with regard to the best way forward. Rockefeller's efforts in 1941 and 1942, an extension of their prewar programs, were similar in type to the rising CMR program but much smaller in scale, involving only a handful of collaborators and compounds. Meanwhile, with Coggeshall and Marshall as a crucial pivot for an overall yet-to-be-finalized strategy, the U.S. antimalarial program proceeded only slowly in a kaleidoscopic and ad hoc manner.

Chapter 5

Cooperation and Coordination

The National Research Council's fear—that the world might be cut off from its quinine supply if Java were seized by a hostile nation—became reality early in 1942. As the worst came to pass, the federal government would ramp up its involvement in malaria research in an aggressive but scattered fashion. The crisis was too soon upon the United States for any preformed plan of action.

Squeezed by U.S. trade sanctions, the Japanese advanced into Southeast Asia, toward Dutch colonial possessions in the East Indies. On their way, they attacked the centers of Western naval power in the Pacific: the British base at Singapore, which they captured and occupied, and the U.S. base at Pearl Harbor in Hawaii, which they hit hard in a surprise attack on 7 December 1941. The Japanese had planned this attack on the U.S. Pacific Fleet, parallel with their southern advance in Asia, to preempt U.S. interference in the conquest and exploitation of the Netherlands East Indies (Indonesia). The commodity of interest to the Japanese was not quinine or rubber but the major oil fields on the island of Java. The western powers had other supplies of oil. Prior to the Japanese advance, however, more than 90 percent of the world's supply of quinine and cinchona bark had come from Java. After Pearl Harbor, quinine and cinchona bark would become still more precious. In 1940, the rising threat to Java from the Japanese expansion in Asia had prompted the United States to increase its imports of crude cinchona bark from less than 750 tons per year to more than 2,700 tons. By 1941, the exigencies of war had pushed world demand for quinine itself to over 1,000 tons, up from around 700 tons per year during the 1930s.[1] Suddenly in the winter of 1941–1942 (summer in the Southern Hemisphere), the world's supply of quinine was plunged into the midst of war.

With Pearl Harbor bombed and Singapore in enemy hands, the Allies tried desperately to retain Java by intercepting the Japanese invasion fleet, but the Japanese navy defeated the Allied task force under Dutch rear admiral Doorman at the Battle of the Java Sea, 27–28 February 1942. The United Nations commander, Vice Admiral Helfrich, had ordered the Allied naval units to attack at all costs (at this time, the term *United Nations* was often used in reference to Allied joint operations). The costs were high indeed. The Allied military reported mixed losses, but a Japanese communiqué, reported in the *New York Times,* far more accurately depicted the situation: "Imperial Headquarters claimed today that five United Nations cruisers, including one United States warship, and six destroyers had been sunk in two great week-end sea battles off Java." The report added that the United Nations fleet was "virtually annihilated" and the Japanese fleet "is now engaged in mopping up remnants."[2] Java surrendered on 9 March, with the Japanese taking 60,000 prisoners. The Allies were cut off from Dutch quinine and rubber supplies, both strategic commodities. But the American program to replace quinine as the antimalarial of choice was still just getting started.

The United States Goes to War

In 1942 and 1943, the antimalarial program would find itself with three main scientific (and clinical) priorities: synthesizing new compounds, understanding atabrine, and developing chloroquine. As the animal screens, particularly the avian malarias, came up to speed in a range of laboratories, the supply of new or interesting compounds would soon fall behind testing capacity. In addition, the military urgently needed atabrine stabilized and regimented for use in the treatment and prevention—or at least suppression—of malaria. Winthrop Chemical, shorn of its German attachments by U.S. entry into World War II, assisted the American war efforts. On the heels of atabrine's development as the drug of choice, superseding quinine, would come chloroquine, a drug with newfound promise. As the war progressed, chloroquine research would expand, but it would not emerge from clinical testing until after the end of hostilities. Much organizational evolution was required for all these pursuits.

Throughout the war, shifting priorities and organizational structures produced a program constantly in flux. William Mansfield Clark described the antimalarial project as kaleidoscopic, giving the "the impression of an unstable pattern" while "organizational matters were continually adjusted to meet the demands of scientific advances."[3] Clark's kaleidoscope allowed flexible responses to emerging needs and knowledge. This was a bottom-up approach to research organization, one not necessarily well suited to a government program. To feed federal dollars to the growing research and development projects, CMR and NRC created a large number of committees, subcommittees, and panels to address a widening range of topics. Heading the initial efforts were Alfred Newton Richards, chairman of the CMR, and Clark, chairman of NRC's Division of Chemistry and Chemical Technology (Chemistry Division). The research they sponsored with OSRD money created innovations in military medicine and drug discovery. Volunteers and paid contractors, guided by the proliferation of panels and committees, produced new compounds, testing methods, dosage regimens, and clinical findings. These, in turn, were underwritten by organizational innovations, chiefly in three areas: communication, scale, and administration.

Following the pattern from 1939 to 1941, the U.S. antimalarial program took shape in an ad hoc way. With more than eighty research and development contracts and still more corporate and academic volunteers, thousands of people were eventually involved in one aspect of the program or another. One needs to examine only a relatively small number of committees and panels and a selective view of research programs to get an essential understanding of the whole enterprise. Permutations were common throughout the program's history. The panels formed under the various coordinating committees were flexible in their roles—advisory or administrative—and in their subject matter, following new leads into new areas of specialization. A complete catalog is not necessary to grasp the nature and overall structure of the wartime program. From early 1942—the months immediately following Pearl Harbor—the national emergency and the federal government pushed the scale from the prewar Rockefeller and NRC realm to a size and scope of biomedical research not seen before.

The spring of 1942 saw Rockefeller's networks pushing up against organizational limits. John Maier of the Rockefeller Institute assessed the situation in the expanding area of malaria chemotherapy. He identified six laboratories that screened antimalarials: Maier's own IHD laboratory; Marshall's laboratory at Johns Hopkins in Baltimore; Small and Coatney's NIH facility in Bethesda, Maryland; Coggeshall's at the University of Michigan, Ann Arbor; Arthur P. Richardson's at the University of Tennessee, Memphis; and Taliaferro's at the University of Chicago. In addition, he identified two sites with industrial connections, research institutes funded by Merck and Squibb.[4] These laboratories had plenty of spare capacity—the "bottleneck" was in the supply of chemicals to be tested. Most of the compounds feeding into these screening labs came from chemical and pharmaceutical companies, with the result that the labs were competing with one another for compounds and in many cases were duplicating each others' efforts.[5] To expand the number of new compounds available, Maier advocated increased cooperation with "an independent organization," one not associated with industry.

Traditionally Rockefeller turned to its academic collaborators for program expansions. Maier discussed his plans with Professor Louis Fieser, an organic chemist from Harvard University with whom the foundation had had a long relationship. Again, IHD already supported antimalarial synthesis in Fieser's lab. Now Fieser was interested in converting all his research activities to war-related work. His suggestion to Maier was to increase the current IHD commitment fourfold. Initially, Fieser pursued this support in preference to a grant from the newly formed Committee on Medical Research of the OSRD. Maier concurred, finding their relationship "very satisfactory." An academic chemist funded by Rockefeller dollars was more biddable and more committed than potential corporate partners with agendas of their own. Maier favored "expanding the program at Harvard, both as a means of increased independence from commercial companies, and, more important, as a means of increasing the number of chemicals for testing."[6] Yet by the middle of 1942, Rockefeller's efforts were being eclipsed by the CMR and its rapidly proliferating NRC advisory committees.

Personal preferences aside, Fieser was soon involved with the CMR program; his OSRD synthesis contract began in October 1942.[7] Fieser had provided Abbott Laboratories samples of various compounds from his stocks. (Abbott had been collecting materials from many sources for the NRC malaria program.) Early in 1943, Arthur Richardson in Memphis screened Fieser's compounds against the avian malaria *P. lophurae* in ducks. Three compounds showed activity, all quinones "bequeathed" to Fieser by the late chemist Samuel C. Hooker.[8] The compounds attracted attention not just for their—rather limited—antimalarial activity but for their simple chemical structures and their lack of either sulfur or nitrogen atoms. This lack set them apart from most other classes of active compounds, and these new leads appealed to NRC. Fieser submitted additional related chemicals from his collections for testing and went on to synthesize hundreds of compounds in the naphthoquinone series.

Fieser's program expanded with government patronage. He and his coworkers published more than a dozen papers after the war on the synthesis and biochemistry of the naphthoquinones.[9] During the war, Fieser's compounds were successful enough to be among the eighty compounds tested in humans by the CMR, but as a class they did not yield a drug for many years to come. Fieser's involvement showed the determination of the NRC to scour the country's chemistry laboratories for compounds to screen. And while Fieser's work points to continuity between Rockefeller's efforts and those of the CMR, Harvard would be just one of more than thirty colleges and universities to receive CMR antimalarial synthesis contracts during the war.[10]

Fieser's experience with CMR and NRC was not unique. Overall, this multiplication of efforts within existing networks—and expansion to new collaborators—was typical of the program. Bureaucratic growth tracked intellectual expansion. CMR and NRC took on the solicitation, synthesis, and testing of compounds and expanded into other areas. The period from May to December 1942 saw a burst of ad hoc Chemistry Division committees on "special and pressing problems," such as the Survey of Antimalarial Drugs in July, the Committee on the Synthesis of Antimalarial Drugs in December (later known as the Panel on Synthesis), and the Conference on the Synthesis of Quinine during that fall. To coordinate all this activity, CMR created the Subcommittee on the Coordination of Malaria Studies in December 1942,[11] which was replaced in November 1943 with the Board for the Coordination of Malaria Studies and the emergence of the Panel of Review. Of all these new entities, three merit more detail here: the Survey of Antimalarial Drugs; the Committee on the Synthesis of Antimalarial Drugs (Panel on Synthesis); and the Subcommittee on, and its successor Board for, the Coordination of Malaria Studies. As the list suggests, 1942 and 1943 would see a whole new creature grow from the seeds that the NRC and Rockefeller had planted.

By June 1942, progress on avian malarias was well advanced, and the Malaria Conference shifted its emphasis from biological systems back to chemical questions. As Maier had pointed out a month earlier, the push for chemical compounds came as animal systems for testing expanded in many places. The NRC collaborators had established a number of model systems, "animal infections": *P. lophurae* in ducks, *P. gallinaceum* in chickens, *P. cathemerium* in canaries, and, on a more limited scale, *P. knowlesi* and *P. cynomolgi* in monkeys. Lyndon Small and G. Robert Coatney had *P. gallinaceum* in chickens at NIH's Beltsville, Maryland, facility; Marshall had *P. lophurae* in ducks at Hopkins; and Richardson and Redginal I. Hewitt at the University of Tennessee Medical School employed *P. lophurae* in ducks and *P. cynomolgi* in monkeys.[12] In time, the use of *P. cathemerium* in ducks was extended to Marshall at Hopkins, Richardson at Tennessee, and Harry Benjamin van Dyke at the Squibb Institute for Medical Research.[13] As William Taliaferro, now chairman of the Malaria Conference, reported on 20 June: "Testing facilities for animal infections have now outrun available drugs. Emphasis should, therefore, be placed on the synthesis of new compounds, on the isolation of naturally occurring substances, and especially on obtaining possible active chemicals from the stocks of commercial houses."[14]

June was also a turning point in the Pacific war. With the Japanese Navy losing four fleet carriers at Midway, U.S. war plans would soon deploy marines and soldiers on many malarious islands and atolls of the Pacific. The antimalarial program would turn more to chemical and organizational matters as the war progressed.

The Survey of Antimalarial Drugs

By late in the spring of 1942, the Conference on Malaria realized that they needed a mechanism for handling information. Clark proposed the establishment of a central office for all information, with the handling of "in confidence" data to be carried out to the satisfaction of the commercial partners. "In confidence" information was data about compounds contributed by commercial firms who reserved their proprietary interests in the compounds tested. This designation restricted the circulation of certain data on chemical structure or biological activity. Clark felt that CMR supported this policy, though later, as we will see in chapter 6, it would come to poison his relationship with CMR and its chairman A. N. Richards. Clark later recalled that Richards "emphasized" the importance of "the proper protection of commercial interests."[15] This was an early instance of the tension between good communication and proprietary interests. As William Taliaferro, chairman of the conference, reported at the time: "*There should be a freer exchange of information* between investigators on OSRD contracts and especially between those testing drugs. An ideal solution for the latter group would be the compilation and maintenance of a catalog of the various drugs tested, but this presents a considerable number of difficulties, among which is the need of maintaining secrecy among the competitive commercial firms supplying drugs" (emphasis in the original).[16] On 1 July 1942, Clark brought to the Malaria Conference a draft letter for circulation to the chemical firms, "outlining the scope of the project." That morning, the conference discussed the letter at length, leaving its "specific details" to Clark.[17] Clark's letter would pave the way for a new office to control and ease the flow of information.

In July 1942, the NRC and CMR established the Survey of Antimalarial Drugs by recommending and approving contract OEMcmr-186 with the Johns Hopkins University chemistry department ("OEMcmr" was the abbreviation for Office of Emergency Management, Committee on Medical Research). William Mansfield Clark was the "responsible investigator"—what we might today call the principle investigator—for the first year of the survey.[18] Clark also became the official "intermediary between the Survey office and the representatives of commercial and academic institutions." To implement his policies and organize the survey, Clark put in place people he knew and trusted. First was Frederick Y. Wiselogle, a colleague from the Hopkins chemistry department. Clark put Wiselogle "in immediate charge of the cataloguing of information, of the preparation and distribution of the Survey tables, special reports and bulletins," and Wiselogle "handled the correspondence in matters of detail." [19]

By the end of August, the Malaria Conference had agreed to two categories for compounds, a general class for "those requiring no particular secrecy" and another for "those which were confidential." [20] That month, over the signatures of Richards, Clark, and Lewis Weed, chairman of NRC's Division of Medical Sciences (DMS), the CMR sent a letter to all participants in the program outlining the procedures of the newly formed survey. "If you wish to co-operate, we request that you send to Dr. Wiselogle the information specified below, provided that you are willing in each instance to have this information circulated among those who are engaged in research on antimalarial drugs. While the free exchange of all information might lead to the more rapid progress, the limitation stated above is made in recognition of the fact that legitimate reasons for restricting disclosure exist in specific instances. Judgment thereof is left to the informant." [21] This letter served as the basis for interactions with the survey.

The August letter did not fully address the status of "in confidence" information on commercial compounds. Clark took this issue to the research directors of several firms and worked out an agreement over the handling of their proprietary interests. The CMR signed on to Clark's plan on 14 November 1942, and the survey and the companies moved into a trial period under this understanding.[22] The survey controlled the flow of material and various classes of information between workers and the committees coordinating the work. "Restricted," "confidential," and "secret" were categories the government used at various times for defining the status of information that was not "open," a normal process for protecting sensitive information from the enemy during wartime. Following Clark's suggestion, the survey designated another category, "in confidence," for information that a commercial firm did not wish openly distributed in survey tables.

Essential to maintaining trust and communication, the survey had two contradictory responsibilities: the distribution of findings and the maintenance of appropriate confidentiality and secrecy. Many of the compounds tested as antimalarials came from chemical and pharmaceutical firms who had commercial interest in any successful antimalarial compounds.[23] Furthermore, many compounds came out of unrelated research programs, both civilian and military, such as chemical warfare. For these reasons, chemical structures often had to be held "in confidence" by the survey, while critical data were distributed to only those whose work required such knowledge. This careful handling created trust in the survey and in the program among all parties. Beyond national security and proprietary interests, other factors offered motivation and built trust among the participants. As Clark said, "The pharmacologists had selfish reasons as well as reasons of honor for observing these confidences strictly; for in certain instances the firms synthesized on request, and at great cost, many compounds needed to follow 'hunches.'" He added, "There was good will on both sides, and its maintenance was essential."[24] In due course and as a complement to the survey, the Panel of Review would emerge as an essential clearinghouse for funding decisions.

It is interesting to note the contrast here between the malaria program and the war's other large pharmaceutical program on penicillin. Clark worked hard to protect proprietary information and interests, while the penicillin program was ostensibly open, sharing all information among all participants, commercial or otherwise. We will return to penicillin later when Clark's efforts come under critical scrutiny. But for now, let us note that Clark's diligent confidentiality on behalf of commercial participants was a unique situation emerging from values shared between industrial and academic chemists. Clark was a strong proponent of a scientific ethos common to researchers that the intellectual integrity and property of all involved should be protected. The survey embodied this spirit.

On 11 February 1943, the CMR discussed the "centralization of information in the Survey, relations with commercial firms, synthesis program and volunteers."[25] CMR sought to upgrade the survey and boost its staffing. At the time, CMR saw no reasons to change the relationships between its antimalarial group and the commercial firms or between the group and individual investigators. According the minutes, CMR attached "great importance" to the antimalarial program and would "give sympathetic consideration" to any proposal for speeding its progress. At this meeting, Richards presented and the CMR approved a letter in response to a letter from Clark to Lewis Weed asking CMR for input on funding and the appropriate scale of the project. The NRC advisors, including Clark, "should not hesitate to contemplate projects in the chemical field." CMR and OSRD would fund the hiring of laboratory assistants and happily expand or revise existing contracts. More specifically, Clark was authorized to request additional monies for the expansion of the survey staff.[26]

Clark wasted little time in securing assistance. In February 1943, Clark added Kenneth C. Blanchard, a professor of biochemistry from New York University. Housed with the survey in Hopkins's Welch Medical Library, Blanchard served as the liaison between the survey office and the Biochemistry, Chemistry, and Pharmacology Panels. Blanchard's contributions included scientific input. Combing through the data assembled at Welch Library, he made a number of recommendations to the Chemistry Panel about future synthetic work, to the Biochemistry Panel regarding studies of the mechanism of action of antimalarials, and "to the Pharmacology Panel regarding the sorts of data needed for appraisal of drugs."[27] The survey staff also included two chemistry graduate students, Emmett L. Buhle and Elinor Hartnell, who catalogued chemical and biological data. Several clerical staff handled the correspondence, recorded pharmacology data on "Survey cards," and prepared tables. Their names were recorded in the survey reports: Mrs. Allan Erskine, Mrs. Leonard Jones, and Miss Catherine Fowler.[28] With words, personnel, and money, the CMR supported Clark's modus operandi.

The CMR continued to endorse Clark's priorities. When their discussions with CMR were once again brought to a satisfactory conclusion, Clark and Wiselogle codified their mutual understanding in Survey Bulletin #3, issued 4 May 1943.[29] Thus, the survey divided all information into "restricted" and "in confidence": The former represented the general classified nature of this wartime research, and the latter indicated the release of information only to those designated by the firm involved. Following discussions with Clark, Richards wrote on behalf of the CMR, "It is proposed that in the future, confidential classification will continue to be applied to the commercial products mentioned above. In addition, chemists who supply drugs will be directed to label as confidential, when submitted to the office of the survey, any substance described by pharmacologists as having sufficient activity against bird malaria to warrant the assumption that it may prove useful in the prevention and treatment of human malaria. Such substances will be included in the 'confidential' list. Data regarding the less potent materials will be circulated in a 'restricted' category."[30] Richards was mixing the official meanings of "confidential." Clark understood the distinctions: "The term 'in confidence' was used for classification by the supplier." This was distinct from the sometime official government term "confidential." "In confidence" had replaced the earlier "confidential" when the survey had adopted the government term "restricted."[31] It should be noted that, because of these arrangements, the survey tables—which were all classified by the government as "restricted"—did not constitute publications from a legal standpoint, and, at war's end, the survey separately sought permission to publish the data as a monograph.

For Clark, the survey was at the center of a professional community with shared values. As Clark later wrote, "It was assumed that all who co-operated with the Survey would do so in order to contribute of their own free will scientific information of potential value to a problem of military importance." Clark used the adjective "scientific" alongside the positive values of cooperation and free will to emphasize the community of trust in which he operated. "The level of operations being set at the scientific, there was no questioning of other considerations which determined the choice made by the supplier himself as to which . . . classifications he would place on information he supplied to the Survey."[32] At least in the early days, Clark himself functioned as the liaison between those who needed more information and those companies who gave their compounds "in confidence." Clark was never disappointed by his commercial colleagues.

Survey Bulletin #3 remained Clark's baseline document for his understanding of the survey, yet by the end of the year, Clark began to have doubts about Richards's support for him and his role as mediator with the commercial chemists. As we will see in the next chapter, the first four months of 1944 would be a time of crisis for Clark and his professional ethos. Defending the "in confidence" treatment of proprietary information, Clark wrote to E. Cowles Andrus, assistant to the chairman of CMR and visiting physician at the Johns Hopkins Hospital, and copied the letter to the entire Subcommittee on Coordination of Malarial Studies: "The present system of handling *confidential* information is simple and safe. . . . In practice the confidential information is treated almost as if it were *secret*." In this letter to Andrus, Clark made clear the values of individual scientists—"the chemist" and "the pharmacologist"—arguing that the scientists themselves were best qualified to know what information should be shared. "In any event the chemist, who knows the potential supply of the raw material, the problems of synthesis and the possible variants of a compound and the pharmacologist who knows the pharmacological value of the compound are jointly the best censors." [33] Clark wanted to avoid a "clumsy" solution—"another form of censorship"—such as the formation of a new panel or board to regulate this information. The ethical exchange of necessary information among professional scientists was, for Clark, both sufficient and elegant. While Clark defended the professional values of his fellow scientists and fought against clumsy bureaucratic solutions to the "in confidence" problem, the survey continued to function.

Kenneth C. Blanchard and E. K. Marshall, both at Hopkins, worked to create a meaningful scheme for numbering compounds and reporting activity in a range of screens and tests. [34] Blanchard had joined the survey in February 1943, while Marshall headed up pharmacology efforts in the Johns Hopkins School of Medicine and the School of Hygiene and Public Health. One of the first orders of business was a review of both the data collected by the survey and that available in the published scientific literature. Soon it emerged that the designations—such as positive, negative, the same as control, or inducing anemia—used for rating activity were not consistent enough between different tests and labs to produce usable structure-activity relationships. To normalize results between diverse screening procedures, the survey introduced quinine as an internal standard into all tests. All activity was measured against "quinine equivalents." As Marshall wrote after the war, "The quinine equivalent of an antimalarial drug is the ratio by weight of the dose of quinine to the dose of the drug under assay when both drugs, administered under identical conditions, produce the same response in parasitized birds." [35] So a compound three times as active as quinine in a particular screen would be given a score of "3" for that test. Work in bird malaria and other tests showed that such measures relative to quinine were generally good to within a factor of two. [36] By this method, the survey standardized the data relating to all compounds and distributed this data to project participants, taking care to seek the permission of those who had submitted their compounds "in confidence." Periodically, the survey issued reports, solicited input on promising compounds from testing groups, and, later in the war, saw to it that the Panel of Review got all the pertinent data in specially prepared, systematic tables.

As the program grew and spread, the need for a centripetal force to bind it all together became increasingly apparent. The survey office was the workhorse of the antimalarial program: It catalogued and indexed chemical compounds, kept records of testing data, and distributed reports, all with an eye to avoiding the duplication of efforts among participants. It also prevented duplication by reviewing proposals. Clark wrote, "As the need for centralization in the interests of efficiency increased, the Survey had an ever-increasing load in the collection and transmission of compounds to testing laboratories, the collection and transmission of reports on the tests, the checking of data, inquiries regarding possible mistakes, and the following up of neglected promises."[37] Blanchard and other survey staff "served as emissaries on many special missions," helping Clark maintain the essential good will and spirit of cooperation that kept the program functioning. The survey distributed confidential reports supplied by industry, such as Lederle Laboratory's *Chemotherapy of Malaria* and Parke, Davis, Inc.'s *Antimalarials: Natural and Synthetic*.[38] Its final product was the two-part, three-volume, 2,500-page summary of "factual data," published as *A Survey of Antimalarial Drugs, 1941–1945* and edited by Frederick Wiselogle. One should note that the program received compounds from more than one hundred institutions, and in some cases from more than one person or group at each institution. These bodies included more than twenty government and nonprofit laboratories, more than fifty companies, more than fifty universities and colleges, and a number of foreign governments; tracking all these materials and the data associated with them was a major enterprise. The growth in biological and clinical information handling was a major innovation for the antimalarial program and a requirement—even before the use of computers—for large-scale research. The survey's creation and its facilitation of communication were essential to conducting R&D on this new scale and with a diverse and widely distributed network of collaborators.

In general, Clark's personal involvement with the survey led to smooth operations, with lead researchers granted access to all data on the compounds with which they worked. For example, he took emergency responsibility for Australian Neil Hamilton Fairley's chloroquine work (about which we will say more in chapter 7) and ruled that Fairley be given access to reports and meetings about chloroquine. In most instances, those doing the testing were in direct contact with the suppliers of compounds, were they corporations or academics. On a small scale, at the level of the committees and panels, chairs could facilitate communication. But as the program grew and the data streamed in, Clark found it harder to channel information to those who supplied the program with compounds for clinical testing.[39] The volume of reports aside, the CMR had other growing pains about which to worry.

Coordination and Military Needs

While the survey could publish data and help make useful connections between various laboratories and investigators, a higher level of coordination and decision making was needed to keep all the committees and panels functioning together. This was the role initially attempted by NRC's Malaria Conference. Coordination of different scientific disciplines remained a challenging priority. Soon, the growing number of compounds successful against avian malarias and ongoing work on the human pharmacology of atabrine necessitated a new body, "a central committee" to facilitate "the processing of new compounds from synthesis, through screening, on to special pharmacological studies, and thence to the clinical testing."[40] Therefore, the CMR created the Subcommittee for the Coordination of Malaria Studies (December 1942 to November 1943)—later the Board for the Coordination of Malaria Studies superseded the subcommittee—that reported to NRC's Committee on Medicine.

Issues before the subcommittee were largely biological, clinical, or immunological, but the major preoccupation was the need to shepherd new compounds through the system efficiently. And military requirements remained paramount. The need to extend limited pharmacological studies to larger clinical studies became clear relatively early with atabrine and new potential drugs. The subcommittee formally recommended that the armed services conduct field studies of atabrine regimens.[41] With regard to military collaboration—particularly in the conduct of clinical research—Clark believed the malaria program to be distinct from other wartime research. Military liaison officers were contributing members of all NRC committees. For the malaria program, NRC and the military not only exchanged information, they extended clinical research from "civilian clinics" to "the enlarged facilities of the services."[42] The active participation in the program by the Army and Navy would become one of the pressures leading to the evolution of the subcommittee into the Board for the Coordination of Malarial Studies. To advise in specific areas, the subcommittee established a number of new bodies: the Committee on Methods for the Quantitative Determination of Atabrine in Body Fluids, the Biochemical Panel, and the Panels on Pharmacology, Clinical Testing, and Synthesis—this last was chaired by Clark himself.

While they waited for new therapeutics to emerge from the synthesis program, the military still needed to replace quinine. The survey's Bulletin #3 opened with a quote from Brigadier General James S. Simmons: "The greatest contribution that can be made to American Medicine at this time is the development of an effective method for the prevention of malaria among troops in the field."[43] This need drove the subcommittee to pursue atabrine. Reporting as chairman of the clinical panel to the Board for the Coordination of Malaria Studies in March 1944, James A. Shannon characterized the program's first years: "The direction of the early work (1942–1943) was conditioned largely by the early loss to the United Nations of their normal sources of supply of quinine, by the lack of adequate stock-pile of quinine, and by the lack of information which would permit the intelligent use of quinacrine [atabrine]. Those who were intimately concerned with the malarial problem during the first year of the war may recall the gravity of the situation."[44] Shannon added that concern about the adequacy of atabrine compounded the worries about quinine. Shannon was an MD-PhD at New York University working at New York's Goldwater Memorial Hospital.

Early reports from the field had suggested that atabrine could not acutely terminate a clinical attack of falciparum malaria (control the symptoms) nor cure either falciparum or vivax malaria (kill all the parasites in the patient). As atabrine was the synthetic drug available, the antimalarial program conducted clinical and toxicological investigations of atabrine with the goal of optimizing its prophylactic use by the U.S. military. As usual, committees and conferences followed the work, yielding another "branching of organization": the Committee on the Toxicity of Commercial Atabrine, serving from May to October 1942 under the Chemistry Division, and the Conference on Atabrine, serving from October 1942 to November 1943 under the DMS. These were followed by the Committee on Methods for the Quantitative Determination of Atabrine in Body Fluids (Chemistry Division) in November 1943.[45] The synthesis of new compounds and the screening of old and new ones continued as work on atabrine proceeded.

The Committee on the Toxicity of Commercial Atabrine arose, as one might imagine, from fears about the quality and safety of the atabrine available in 1942. As Clark pointed out in his postwar history of the program, this concern was voiced during a meeting of the NRC Subcommittee on Tropical Diseases on 9 May 1942. Unnerving reports of "toxic effects" of U.S. atabrine— "characterized chiefly by nausea, vomiting and diarrhea"—had come to the NRC. And it remained unclear, even with Winthrop Chemical's cooperation, "as to whether the method of manufacture was precisely the same as that followed in Germany."[46] The concerns expressed by the Navy and the Army led CMR and NRC to look into the matter further. NRC duly constituted the Committee on the Toxicity of Commercial Atabrine. On 3 October 1942, the committee reported to CMR the findings of their investigation. As standards for analysis, three groups of chemists prepared pure samples of atabrine by three different methods. E. K. Marshall then tested various commercial samples of atabrine from a number of countries against these standards in pharmacological studies. With no significant differences in toxicity found in animal tests, the baton passed to James Shannon who oversaw clinical studies at Ohio State University, the New Jersey State Reformatory in Rahway, and New York's Sing Sing Prison. These human tests also found no significant differences in toxicity among the various samples and the standards. Winthrop Chemical and British Imperial Chemical Industries, Ltd., assisted in this investigation. Winthrop Chemical, through prewar patent arrangements with I. G. Farben, held the U.S. rights to the drug and its manufacture.[47]

Although commercial atabrine seemed as safe as could be, Clark noted that "a strange result" emerged from the three large clinical studies. The Ohio State researchers had observed an incidence of toxic symptoms in one-third of the subjects, while both the Sing Sing and Rahway studies reported that only single-digit percentages of patients showed toxicity. These ratios varied not with the source of the atabrine but with the location of the study. The U.S. military saw this toxicity difference across locations as well. This was indeed a strange result, and Clark acknowledged that it produced much consternation. NRC and CMR were torn between a desire to study this phenomenon—to determine scientifically why different large-scale study populations responded so differently to the same drug—and a fear that too much emphasis on the toxicity of atabrine could exacerbate existing problems with prophylactic compliance by military units. In the end, they left the strange findings unstudied and sought to reassure the troops that atabrine was safe when used as directed.

Nevertheless, military personnel often resisted atabrine prophylaxis. The military referred to the patient compliance issue as "quinacrine discipline," quinacrine being atabrine's generic name. As Clark explained, "The maintenance of routine administration of quinacrine proved to be extremely difficult and that not until several cases of neglect led to disasters did some field commanders impose that rigidly controlled administration of quinacrine which was to reduce greatly the incidence of malaria among troops."[48] Overall, the military and the civilian committees and researchers agreed that atabrine's usefulness outweighed its side effects, and the successful, controlled use of atabrine in the field moved forward. The Committee on the Toxicity of Commercial Atabrine asked to be disbanded and recommended the creation of a new body to pursue the remaining issues of atabrine. So emerged the Atabrine Conference.

Concerns over atabrine popped up again from time to time. The Atabrine Conference and the Panel on Pharmacology—chaired by E. K. Marshall—worked together on studies of the acute and chronic toxicity of atabrine. Worry about acute toxicity diminished with a growing number of positive reports coming in from military units in the field. Acute toxicity was formally dropped as research topic in May 1943, as "representatives of the Army and Navy had declared the matter to be of minor importance."[49] As for chronic toxicity, atabrine's widespread use kept this topic one of interest. The refinement of atabrine required new analytic tools. The Atabrine Conference initiated wider studies on the metabolism of atabrine in the body, looking into how atabrine was broken down and how they might measure levels of the drug and its metabolites in various bodily fluids. In November 1943, the NRC established the Committee on Methods for the Quantitative Determination of Atabrine in Body Fluids (Chemistry Division). The proximal cause of its creation was another request from the military. Shannon's group at Goldwater Memorial Hospital addressed this problem.

One reason for this continued interest was a desire to extend dosage standards from quinine to atabrine. James Shannon and his group had established guidelines for the use of quinine, correlating clinical responses to measured levels of the drug in patient plasma. To created new guidelines around atabrine, Shannon and his group needed a parallel quantitative analytical technique. Bernard "Steve" Brodie and Sidney Udenfriend, working with Shannon at Goldwater Memorial Hospital, developed a method that could be routinely used in the study of atabrine in patients and research subjects.[50] This was a quantitative method for studying how experimental dosage regimens translated into drug levels in the body. Looking back at these "rationalized regimens" after the war, Clark characterized this work as "the most important practical accomplishment made in the program."[51] Brodie and Udenfriend's work was an innovation that allowed rationalization. From standardized measurement came rational clinical interventions. With atabrine's growing reputation of reliability, it began to appear more and more as a baseline or standard in clinical tests, displacing quinine in many instances. And in the field and clinic, atabrine was it.[52] Atabrine production for 1943 was slated to reach 2.5 billion tablets.[53]

Brodie and Udenfriend's techniques allowed for other important work on the chronic toxicity of atabrine and on the metabolism and degradation of atabrine in the body.[54] They also provided valuable tools for any future understanding—and optimal use—of new antimalarials. Using a Coleman fluorometer, Brodie and Udenfriend helped pioneer the use of physical instruments in pharmacology and biochemistry. Simply stated, the assay methods involved extracting water-based biological samples—plasma, feces, urine— with organic solvents and then shining light of specific wavelengths through the samples. Key to the technique were identifying good solvents and finding a specific wavelength that would precisely reveal the chemical compound that one wished to measure. With the assay, as Brodie explained to an NRC Division of Chemistry conference, it was "possible to determine both atabrine and quinine together in the same final solutions."[55] Light of one wavelength (420–430 millimicrons[56]) caused atabrine to fluoresce—to glow in a measurable and quantifiable way—while quinine fluoresced at a different wavelength (365 millimicrons). Measuring both wavelengths with the fluorometer allowed the determination of both drugs in a single sample.

Brodie and Udenfriend developed fluorometric assays for atabrine, quinine, and chloroquine, among other compounds, and were able to detect biologically active compounds in blood, urine, and other biological materials. These methods, tuned and standardized by the NRC committees, were essential to the numerous clinical and field studies of antimalarials during the war. To make this technology more widely available—to allow clinical research and to determine patient compliance anywhere in the world where patients, especially soldiers and marines, might be taking antimalarials—the Navy worked on a tougher, more portable version of the fluorometric instruments.[57] As chairman of the Clinical Panel, Shannon coordinated much of the work on plasmochin, atabrine, chloroquine, and dozens of other compounds. In subsequent years, after their major contributions to the malaria program, Brodie and Udenfriend pursued this instrumental work further while once again working for Shannon, this time at the NIH's National Heart Institute.[58]

As chairman of the Clinical Panel, Shannon coordinated much of the program's research in this area. Typically, Shannon's own clinical investigations involved the use of both paretics (neurosyphilis patients) and prisoners. In March 1942, Shannon had started his malaria chemotherapy work under OSRD contract OEMcmr-112. Although Shannon had made arrangements with the New York City Board of Health to have all candidates for malaria therapy channeled to him, the amount of "clinical material" available to Shannon was limited, and most of it, at least in the early months, was used for research on the determination of atabrine and quinine in blood.[59] Beyond atabrine and quinine, Shannon's group worked on the clinical development of dozens of other compounds during the war, including plasmochin, sontochin, chloroquine, and pentaquine. These were tested in more than 1,100 psychiatric patients at three New York hospitals and in more than 500 prisoner volunteers.[60] The NIH's Robert Coatney ran a prison-based clinical program at the Atlanta Federal Penitentiary in addition to his avian malaria program in Maryland.[61] Alf Alving of the University of Chicago headed the third major prisoner program, based at Illinois's Stateville Penitentiary.[62] The Chicago program's most famous participant was Nathan Leopold, who, along with Richard Loeb, had murdered Bobby Franks in 1924, creating a nationwide scandal.[63] As people whose care had been given over to the state, the psychiatric patients had little say in their participation. The prisoners participated voluntarily, at least by the standards of the time. Their motivation is difficult to recover, although Leopold plausibly suggests a mixture of patriotism, curiosity, and a desire for favorable treatment. These and other hospital and prison programs—alongside the military testing of drugs—allowed the wartime program to vastly scale up its clinical work in a very short time.

Growth, Bureaucracy, and the Board for the Coordination of Malaria Studies

In the closing months of 1943, the Subcommittee for the Coordination of Malaria Studies found itself overburdened by growth. The demand for increased facilities for clinical testing and the drain on civilian medical personnel by the draft meant reassessing the division of labor between civilian and military organizations. It should be noted that while NRC and CMR participants were mostly civilians, the program had an enormous contribution from the armed forces. Dozens of reports flowed in from India-Burma, the South Pacific, and military hospitals all around the country.[64] Collaborative work with the Australian military—particularly through the offices of N. Hamilton Fairley in New Guinea—determined the optimal dosage regimen for atabrine as a field prophylactic.[65] Clinical feedback on atabrine and other drugs from the armed forces was a major contributor to progress.

In response to an increasing role for the military, Lewis H. Weed, MD, chairman of NRC's Division of Medical Sciences, sought to bring together the armed forces, the Public Health Service, and the civilian agencies. Aside from his NRC duties, Weed was a professor of anatomy and director of the School of Medicine at Johns Hopkins. In October 1943, Weed wrote to Major General Norman T. Kirk, surgeon general of the U.S. Army, moving to replace the subcommittee with a board that would include representatives of the OSRD and the surgeons general of the Army, Navy, and PHS. One aspect he emphasized for the military was that they must carry out "the final field tests" of any drugs developed.

> To consolidate the rapidly evolving knowledge and to make the maximum use of existing facilities, it is essential that closest cooperation and coordination between the federal agencies and the civilian enterprises be achieved. It appears that the principle requirement is the formulation of a comprehensive plan by which the extensive civilian and service investigative program are integrated. To secure this with the rapidity that the urgency of the situation demands and without confusion of present administrative relations, it is essential that civilian and military personnel and facilities be regarded as constituting a single mechanism within which specific tasks could be apportioned.[66]

The Board for the Coordination of Malaria Studies, including the chairmen of the NRC's committees, replaced the Subcommittee, with certain distinctions. As Weed asserted at its first meeting, the board would operate independently—unlike the NRC committees. The board's members would directly convey its recommendations to their parent organizations. The NRC's Committee on Medicine would still approve any changes to established therapies prior to their recommendation to the surgeons general, and the OSRD would continue to fund the board's operations.[67]

The board—as "final arbiter of recommendation originating in the panels and forwarded to CMR regarding contracts"[68]—would oversee all the panels, committees, and structures that had been developed over the preceding four years of haphazard, decentralized, and kaleidoscopic growth and evolution. With the growth of chemical synthesis and screening of drugs, even the reconstituted board might not be able to keep up with the pace of research coordination. In fact, lag in the board's decision making created problems. Because clinical and toxicology data arrived slowly in comparison with the number of promising leads found against avian malarias, the chemists were often in front of the preclinical data. As Clark put it, the synthesis program had to continue "on the basis of extreme empiricism."[69] There simply was not enough information on the performance of compounds against human disease and on their toxicity to steer the synthesis program rationally. Extreme empiricism was a negative counterpart to a more rational approach. It meant that the program often had to resort to the random—blind—screening of compounds without any feedback of test data to guide compound selection. Even as the subcommittee became the board, progress slowed because of the absence of feedback on the performance of tested drug candidates. This failure created the need for another panel, a Panel of Review, "advisory to the Board," which could review all the data on a series of compounds and give the synthesis program "systematic direction." The Panel of Review consisted of the chair and secretary of the board and the chairs from the Panels on Biochemistry, Clinical Testing, Pharmacology, and Synthesis. The survey's senior staff participated on the Panel of Review and facilitated the "disclosure of 'in confidence' information to members of panels . . . as needed." [70] The rise of the board sent change rippling through the panels and committees.

With such growth and focus—and the creation of the Panel of Review—Clark eventually withdrew as chairman of the Panel on Synthesis. The old Subcommittee for the Coordination of Malaria Studies had established this panel as the Committee on Synthesis in December 1942. The Panel on Synthesis dealt with synthetic organic chemistry and guided work on what new compounds should be made. Clark had chaired the new group as he was already "privy to the 'in confidence' information in the Survey" and could therefore prevent duplication of effort, particularly from commercial partners. Clark's panel had only advised CMR and coordinated research efforts. There was still no "central management" and "administration was decentralized." [71] He had selected three regional directors from academic institutions: Robert Elderfield (Columbia University), Eastern Area; Joseph B. Koepfli (California Institute of Technology), Pacific Coast Area; and Ralph L. Shriner (Indiana University), Middle West Area. These regional coordinators assisted Clark and those in Washington, DC, with recruiting and organizing chemical efforts. With many chemists volunteering their materials and services and expressing a need for chemical intermediates, the OSRD had contracted for chemical syntheses, but money alone was not sufficient to the needs of the program. As 1943 wore on, coordinating between those synthesizing new chemicals and those testing them would prove taxing.

Clark had seen trouble with his leadership in synthesis since the winter of 1943–1944. Originally Clark wanted to offer the chemists a free hand. He wrote to his friend, Robert F. Loeb, the professor at Columbia's Medical College of Physicians and Surgeons who had replaced the first board chairman, Frederic Hanes of Duke University, "Fundamentally there has been no theoretical guiding principle in the synthetic work. Therefore I had hoped that a certain degree of freedom on the part of the chemists plus repeated prodding from me would result in the design of new leads."[72] Yet with "nothing much having come of that policy" by that winter, he searched with no success for other chemists: "A good many of the top 'organizers' are theoretical men with no penchant for the type of thought we need," and practical chemists were already "up to their necks in contract work." And the malaria program already had "a goodly number of the men noted as makers of compounds," many of whom had been working with Clark on a voluntary basis even before the OSRD contracts, from the time when the only government-funded and -organized synthesis program was Lyndon Small's at NIH.[73] Loeb agreed with Clark's assessment of the synthetic picture: by May 1944, he was certain that the chemists were now running behind. Loeb argued that it was time to bring the chemists to the fore. "I feel now that they can be told that this is a problem of first importance, and it may be possible to give a little better orientation to synthesis than it was two years ago." In sum, however, he felt that the synthetic program, along with the other demands on Clark's time, was more responsibility "than one man should be asked to carry at one time."[74]

In July 1944, under pressure from Loeb and Richards, Clark stepped down and the Panel on Synthesis got a new chairman, Carl Shipp Marvel of the University of Illinois.[75] "Speed" Marvel also added the Columbia University chemist Arthur Cope to his staff. Both Marvel and Cope were organic chemists of wide reputation, and, unlike Clark, specialists in synthesis. For Clark, though, Marvel's appointment came down to him as a "virtual order" from CMR chairman A. N. Richards through board chairman Loeb.[76] It should be noted that Clark and Loeb were good friends, so the routing of this "order" was most likely deliberate (Clark's relationship with Richards was, as we will see, much more fraught). Clark obeyed: "In accordance with your wish . . . I called up Speed Marvel and without allowing him to talk too much I got him to promise to come on Wednesday. . . . I do hope that you can be present at the conference for I anticipate that we are going to have a hard job persuading Marvel."[77] Marvel did indeed come on board, replacing Clark as chair of the Panel on Synthesis.

Loeb sought to shake up other panels as well. His earlier communications with Clark suggested that the expanding program would need to augment its first movers in more fields than just chemistry. Loeb wrote that the "Biochemical Panel, as you say, had not received the support which you and I agree it should receive from Marshall and Shannon. I feel, however, that this is no deterrent to its expansion, and I am sure that they will not 'buck' it, and that they would be very glad to sit in on meetings of that group."[78]

Clark proposed to Loeb that the expanding biochemical work be organized by dividing it in two categories: "(1) Theoretical work in which plans are left largely to the judgment of the individual investigator in accordance with the underlying policies of peace-time research. (2) 'Service work,' principally upon methods of analyses, study of degradation of drugs, etc. Problems in this category should be fairly well lined up under central direction and since the results of such investigations are directly connected with the demands of the clinicians I would advocate that the direction of such research be under the Clinical Panel."[79] Here Clark made a distinction between what might later be called grant work and contract work, and perhaps between creative, innovative work of the kind espoused by William Taliaferro and the directed, routine work also essential to clinical investigation.

This was not a distinction that Clark was willing to let go of lightly, hitting it again in the postscript to the same letter. "Starting with no illusions of grandeur, but with the idea that a beginning must be made, I got four contracts for work that, in my judgment, had best be carried out with a good deal of freedom of action. However, there have now entered two biochemical problems needing coordination with the work of the pharmacologists and clinicians: (1) general service work on analytical methods; (2) studies of degradation, etc., which require talents of a kind different from those possessed by most of the present contractors in the biochemical field. If the biochemical work is to be on a broader basis, as I think it should, there must be a better coordination and sympathy on the part of the Pharmacological and Clinical Panels."[80] The "general service work on analytical methods," exemplified by the work of Brodie and Udenfriend, was essential to the clinical understanding of atabrine and other antimalarials. The interplay of the rational and the empirical, the fundamental and the routine were subtle and shifting, but work directed toward specific program goals was taking precedent over "theoretical" work pursued at the discretion of the individual scientists.

From Coordination to Administration

Structures for coordination and communication could not substitute for actual management. For example, the expanding survey was an essential innovation for the coordination of this large-scale program. But the survey, even with more staff, was only in the business of communication and coordination; it could not provide administration. Neither, in the end, could the networks and committees of NRC. Clark's NRC connections, through the Chemistry Division and its committees, were not the only links between the government program and NRC. As suggested above with Lewis Weed's NRC service, the Division of Medical Sciences continued to have input with regard to clinical work. The DMS's Committee on Medicine was not "intimately connected with the program," but the committee did review the work of the Malaria Conference, the Subcommittee on Coordination of Malarial Studies, and the Subcommittee on Tropical Diseases, "and such recommendations of the Board for the Coordination of Malarial Studies as concerned therapy."[81] Yet for all the interconnections and coordination, and the creation of the board and the Panel of Review, the NRC proved inadequate to the CMR's needs. The NRC could advise CMR and coordinate data, but it could not manage research. The board's lag was one symptom of this lack. The government's CMR program needed to address this gap.

With the creation of the board and an impending reorganization of the CMR along the lines of the National Defense Research Committee (NDRC), the antimalarial research program moved on with established routines and a steadiness reinforced by Allied victories and a growing vista of the postwar world. This world would be a very different one, not least because of the growth of government administration and bureaucracy during the war and the end of the state of emergency that had eased cooperation among competing interests. The emerging postwar vista and the need for administration drove changes in the culture of R&D, changes that would sorely test the professional ethos represented by William Mansfield Clark.

Chapter 6

Trust and Transition

The war began to turn dramatically in favor of the Allies during 1943. The surrender of the German army at Stalingrad in February and the Allied invasion of Sicily in July were two indicators of this shift. With the postwar world clearly in their sights and the growing complexity of wartime research demanding more administration, government functionaries looked to new bureaucratic structures for the management and control of projects like the antimalarial program. They worked changes not just in scale, organization, and methods of drug development but in the values of science and the scope of government involvement in biomedicine. What did it mean for prewar values that the government became deeply involved in the management of biomedical research? Growing government bureaucracy impinged on the promises of confidentiality that NRC had made to commercial firms. It also created a drive for centralization. Personalities, egos, and values had to accommodate themselves to changing organizational parameters and new power structures.

The transition from the professional ethos of NRC to the bureaucratic realm of wartime government work was not an easy one for the antimalarial program or its main NRC protagonist, William Mansfield Clark. Some of this difficulty was even visible in the official, triumphalist history of OSRD published after the war. Stewart Irvin, deputy director of OSRD, wrote,

> There were disadvantages to this relationship between CMR and NRC, stemming from the dual functions which the NRC committee members were required to exercise. They had been appointed by the NRC to NRC committees. Insofar as they sat around a table and formulated

advice for the Surgeons General they were functioning in their capacity as members of the NRC committees. When, sitting around the same table, they recommended proposals for research to CMR, they were functioning as advisors or consultants of CMR. When they advised the Surgeons General on the basis of CMR research it would be difficult to define their capacity. This situation led to some confusion; several members of NRC committees went through the war only vaguely familiar with CMR, unaware that it paid the expenses of their meetings and incompletely aware that the ultimate responsibility and entire expense of the research program was its province. It is fair to say that this confusion was an annoyance rather than a hindrance to the success of the program and that it was minimized by general confidence in the integrity of the principals.[1]

Words such as "disadvantages" and "confusion" suggest that the melding of the NRC advisory committees with the CMR bureaucracy created a disjuncture between the academics and professionals (employed primarily in academic and industrial settings) on the one hand and the bureaucrats and soldiers (employed by the government) on the other. The NRC was originally founded to address the demands of the nation during a period of national crisis, emerging as it did from technological boom years of World War I.[2] Yet, as Irvin suggested, NRC's members were not accustomed to the government structures they encountered during World War II. Things only held together because of the "integrity of the principals."

Emblematic of the culture clash was a conflict between William Mansfield Clark and A. N. Richards, chairman of CMR. Although they were both academics engaged in extracurricular service, Clark's and Richards's contrasting roles in the antimalarial program brought Clark to a crisis of conscience over the sharing of proprietary information. This "Feud," as Clark termed it, directly illustrates a major shift in research culture in the United States. The professional, individual—even gentlemanly—ethos of Clark and NRC offered a stark contrast to the regimented, legalistic networks of Richards and OSRD. The ascendancy of government bureaucracy was a major example of the shifting culture of R&D at large scale. Both sides of the feud bear detailed attention: though the bureaucracy largely prevailed, essential elements of Clark's ethos survived the war. The tension remained even as the balance of power shifted. Understanding the postwar organization and funding of biomedicine requires an appreciation of this balance and how it is maintained. At stake, in a time of national emergency, were issues of centralization, growing government bureaucracy, and potential conflicts of interest between private entities and the government.[3]

For the antimalarial program, Clark stood firmly on the side of professional ethos over government bureaucracy. With his personal commitments to industrial chemists, he felt the changes around him most acutely. Clark stood for both scientific freedom and intellectual property rights. He was born in Tivoli, NY, in the Hudson River Valley south of Albany. His father and maternal grandfather were both Episcopal clergymen. Clark attended Williams College, where he received BA and MA degrees in 1907 and 1908. He went on to earn his PhD in chemistry from the Johns Hopkins University in 1910. Clark worked in government laboratories for a number of years, first with USDA and then as chief of the Division of Chemistry of the Hygienic Laboratory of the PHS from 1920 to 1927. The Hygienic Laboratory was a precursor of the National Institutes of Health. In 1927, Clark returned to Johns Hopkins as the DeLamar Professor of Physiological Chemistry in the School of Medicine. Clark remained a Hopkins professor for twenty-five years, until his retirement in 1952.[4] It was from this position that he served the National Research Council as chairman of the Division of Chemistry and Chemical Technology from 1941 to 1946. As Chemistry Division chairman, Clark fought for the proprietary interests of chemists and corporations and against efforts to make him a government official. These issues defined him as a champion of NRC's prerogatives as a professional organization and drove him into conflict with CMR chairman Richards.

Centralization and Communication

A motion toward centralized control accompanied efforts at coordination and later administration. For a time, Clark's survey office exerted this centripetal force. The survey was the clearinghouse for data and compounds, but Clark did not want it to provide direction to the research. "All the Survey office pretends to do is to serve those who cooperate by circulating that information which the individuals concerned allow to circulate and to file notice when we detect duplication of effort. The notice is not by way of *direction*."[5] Clark expected that properly notified participants would "make adjustments" without the "further participation" of the survey. Clark believed that the survey had neither the time nor the desire to vet proposals for future work. They sought only to avoid duplication of work already underway. They would not block the pursuit of "hunches" or reserve whole classes of compounds to certain firms or laboratories. "We could not become party to a system of staking out claims if it should interfere in any way with efforts to get an improved antimalarial to our armed forces. That is the prime objective." For Clark's purposes, centralization was coordination that met military needs and optimized output by minimizing duplication.

Yet research administration quickly became a concern, and a new centralizing force was needed to provide direction. For this purpose, Lewis Weed, chairman of the NRC's Division of Medical Sciences, proposed to assemble a board of representatives from the NRC committees, the OSRD, and the surgeons general of the Army, Navy, and Public Health Service. In the fall of 1943, as we saw in chapter 5, these representatives organized the Board for the Coordination of Malarial Studies chaired by Frederic Hanes of Duke University. All these men, including the chairs of the NRC committees, were voting members of the board, which was financed by OSRD. As Weed wrote that October, "Considerable coordination of the joint efforts has been achieved but the work could be accelerated by more rapid centralization of reports from the field, by the assignment of adequate highly-trained personnel, and by better integration of the field studies, one to the other, and to the body of knowledge already collected in this country."[6] To speed this along, "coordination must be made at once." Weed wanted a group that could "effectuate an overall program of study." Tellingly for an organization driven by the centralizing impulse, Hanes soon had to step down as he "felt that he was too far from Washington to maintain adequate contact."[7] Robert F. Loeb, professor at Columbia's Medical College of Physicians and Surgeons, replaced Hanes as chairman of the board.

The creation of the board and the course of its subsequent development were not predetermined. The structure of the entire program was contingent and spontaneous, a product of the national emergency. Even the most basic relationship, that of NRC with CMR, seemed driven by necessity. According to OSRD deputy director Stewart Irvin, CMR seized an expedient solution: "Given the situation as it existed in July 1941, the collaboration was an obvious and desirable arrangement. The advantages outweighed the disadvantages by far. Initiation of research was expedited by months at a moment when time was of the essence. CMR gained the advice of several hundred men, who were specialists in their fields, already organized, and somewhat familiar with the needs of the military."[8] Irvin put this slapdash approach to R&D organization down to expediency; Clark, however, felt it was a virtue. Future emergencies need not "be handled by a predetermined body in accordance with a pre-formed plan."[9] The malaria program's organic and ad hoc development was a good thing. Clark believed that the program had emerged to meet specific and evolving medical and scientific needs: that it had emerged from his Chemistry Division and NRC's scientific community.

Trust was the value that held Bill Clark's community together.[10] The maintenance of trust was important to Clark, and it was central to his own perception of his role in the program. As the program grew and the role of the military increased, Clark would find this more and more of a challenge. Trust meant that Clark had to keep his promises to the commercial chemists. Clark saw a clear distinction between the early days of program—before the synthesis contracts had gotten fully underway—and a later period when OSRD paid for the making of new compounds. In the first period, it was chemical and pharmaceutical companies that provided the vast majority of compounds to be screened as potential drugs. As we have seen, Clark allowed companies to submit compounds "in confidence," meaning that data on the compounds would be kept on a strictly need-to-know basis, with the company retaining final say over who might be allowed to see such data.[11] Clark and the survey oversaw the maintenance of these verbal gentlemen's agreements.

Personal and professional interactions maintained trust and facilitated exchange within the project community. As Clark observed, "Dr. Wiselogle, in charge of the Survey, took every precaution to preserve inviolate the obligations, and all prayed that no accident would happen. Obviously, risks were taken on both sides. They were frankly discussed and were willingly assumed both as a necessity in the emergency and as a matter of statesmanship on both sides superseding fear of obvious legal complications that might result from accident."[12] While Clark found some colleagues wanting in their grasp of his conception of individual responsibility and trust, Loeb, E. K. Marshall, and James Shannon seemed kindred spirits even during Clark's conflict with the CMR. This example is from a later letter to Shannon, but it illustrates Clark's conception of his community's values. Clark took upon himself "the responsibility of authorizing you to reveal 'in confidence' information to those whom you have named, providing that you will impress upon them their responsibility and providing that you will take it upon yourself not spread before them *all* the 'in confidence' information available to you . . . simply use good discretion." Clark promoted this as "a common sense attitude," suitable for dealing with whatever objections would arise. Clark also embraced his colleagues, expressing his "appreciation of the fact that you and Marshall have impressed responsibility on all your workers. Thereby we have kept the faith so well that we may attribute the leaks that have occurred to industry itself rather than to our group."[13] In the later days of the program, bureaucracy and legal definitions overtook such personal representations. Eventually, the Panel of Review required access to all "in confidence" information. Even so, with a single, temporary exception, all suppliers granted the panel this access as a general operating principle.

As Clark pointed out, risks were taken by many participants, risks required by the urgency of the matter and the times. Far-flung collaborations with numerous institutions and individuals required flexibility and the action of a good-faith broker of information. From the outset, Clark put himself in this role. It was a role he treasured, as his intervention on behalf of Brigadier Neil Hamilton Fairley in 1944 suggests. Fairley was the Australian medical officer who had overseen the testing of atabrine in Australia and New Guinea and whose organization would also test chloroquine late in the war. Informed that the visiting Fairley would not be included in upcoming Panel of Review meetings for fear of revealing "in confidence" information, Clark discussed the matter with Marshall, who in turn took it up with Shannon. The three urged George A. Carden Jr., secretary of the board for the Coordination of Malarial Studies, to invite Fairley to the meetings "on the basis that he is actually working with a series of compounds and contributing brilliantly to our knowledge thereof."[14] Clark further refined the subtle terms of inclusion. Fairley could be included "on the basis that he is an actual worker, whereas some of his associates cannot be invited because they are not on the same basis." Fairley, as an active collaborator, was "entitled to knowledge pertinent to his researches, provided he be made familiar with our systems of treating information 'in confidence' and respect it as we all know he will." Shannon and Marshall would "eliminate from the Panel discussions references to compounds with which the Brigadier will not be concerned and Marshall, who knows the Brigadier well, will see him before the Panel meetings and explain the situation." Personal knowledge and professional interactions guided the handling of "in confidence" data. To Clark, this was just "a common sense policy to follow." To get the job done, Clark emphasized social accommodations and common sense over the rote observance of rules.

The Feud

In spite of his diplomatic efforts, Clark's assurances of confidentiality and his efforts on behalf of participants to preserve their proprietary interests were undercut from many directions. He often found himself defending these arrangements. For example, the Panel on Synthesis requested that Clark pursue the possibility of "broader disclosure." Clark demurred. He had already raised this issue in one-on-one discussions with various research directors. He felt it unwise to raise such delicate matters in writing "as there are numerous angles which cannot well be taken up by correspondence."[15] For Clark, these were, by definition, personal interactions. Disclosure was something to be mooted between colleagues. And his conversations revealed "a great variety of opinions ranging from those who are willing to enter into complete disclosure to those who think of something comparable to arrangement regarding pooling of information on rubber, to those who doubt seriously whether any arrangement will be satisfactory." The synthetic rubber program, like the penicillin program, was one where participants agreed to fully share all pertinent information.[16] This diversity of opinion was further complicated by instances in which industrial collaborators were happy for program workers to share all information about their compounds, but still displayed "extreme reluctance to afford any information whatsoever to rivals."[17] Clark was ever sensitive to the legalistic turn and the personal touch, such as his judgment to confine himself to "conversations" and avoid "correspondence."

Clark detailed the pressure he was under to alter his arrangements with the firms. In this, he viewed CMR chairman A. N. Richards as his main antagonist. According to Clark, "The matter was brought to a head by Dr. Richards, who suggested that exchange of information might be arranged through some form of contract with the Government." In this pursuit, Richards enrolled Clark's friend Robert Loeb, chairman of the Board for the Coordination of Malarial Studies. Clark attributed Loeb's willingness to undertake this urging to his initial ignorance of "the history or the operations of the Survey." Clark felt "a great deal of pressure from all sides toward broader disclosure." Clark again had to explain his position in order to "clarify the atmosphere and to inform Dr. Richards regarding both the operations of the Survey and the nature of the problem we have to face." Yet the CMR wielded far more power than Clark, and it was already flexing new bureaucratic muscles: "The new Board for the Coordination of Malarial Studies, recently organized, includes in addition to the chairmen of the Panels, official representatives of the Army, Navy, Public Health Service, and the OSRD, each empowered to act on behalf of his organization. Signs of its new power are already developing."[18] This new power would centralize decisions—scientific, clinical, and financial—in a single body.

On the matter of confidentiality, Clark was almost pugnacious. Clark demanded of Richards, "As soon as higher statesmanship permits, I should like a decision on the future policy regarding disclosure and exchange of information on antimalarial drugs."[19] And Clark felt obliged to reiterate that his confidentiality policy made cooperation work: "If the Survey is to continue under existing policy, Wiselogle and I can proceed promptly to solicit the necessary cooperation of commercial firms on the basis that they understand. I judge it to be unwise to give the necessary assurance that these plans are within the framework of established policy if a radical reform of basic policy is to be proposed to suppliers and is to require reorganization of the Survey." Clark did not favor the contractual basis on which the rubber and penicillin programs were run. "Should a new policy in substantial degree take the form of contractual relations between Government and commercial firms, such as have been elaborated in the penicillin case, it might be advisable to have both the scientific and the legal affairs under one administrative head. Even spatial separation of the scientific and legal branches might be dangerous because constant guidance on the legal implications of decisions might be required in this field, which is one of great detail." Should a more legalistic framework of cooperation be instituted, legal and scientific decisions would blur together. Clark wanted to keep the lawyers at a distance from himself and NRC. He believed that NRC's "province" was "exclusively that of science, but whether this be true or not, I am unfitted by training and disposition to exercise leadership in any matter that is conditioned by the minutiae of legalistic arrangements." For Clark, lawyers and science were not a good mix. Richards would have to decide whether to take a legalistic path and lose Clark or to do things the NRC way and put science and trust first.

As leverage, Clark brought to Richards's attention the schedule of NRC's nominating committee, which would be taking action on new division chairmen in early April. In essence, this was a threat to resign if the position of chairman of the NRC division no longer appealed to him. Richards must decide for or against the legalistic policy—but finalize the decision—or remove the malaria project from the NRC.[20] The nominating committee would want Richards's decision so that they could select an appropriate chairman. Clark was frustrated that Richards would not, or could not, render a decision. Indecision had delayed the clinical program—the expansion of Shannon's work—because those in power could not authorize additional personnel. Clark's feelings of betrayal over the confidentiality issue did not go away, nor apparently did his anger towards Richards. Clark was emphatic that Richards, in the early going, had been as enthusiastic as Clark himself for "proper protection of commercial interests." Now, having threatened these arrangements, Richards was silent.

Clark was anxious that this problem not be allowed to spread. "I fear the consequences of having indecision extend to the matter of disclosure especially at the very time when the Panel of Review is working out its plans for an acceleration in all branches."[21] Certainty of procedure was essential for increasingly rapid growth. Clark sharpened this point still further, emphasizing to Richards that making a decision—any decision—was as important as which policy CMR might choose. Whatever Richards decided with regard to further disclosure, it must decide quickly to avoid further delays to the project. Richards met Clark's demand for a decision with a month of silence.

The OSRD legal attack on the "in confidence" agreements was compounded by the proposed reorganization of CMR. Early in the spring of 1944, OSRD began circulating plans for a new CMR. Two outcomes were sought: first to bring the CMR more into line with the formal bureaucratic organization of the older National Defense Research Committee (NDRC), and second to relieve the stress on Richards as chairman of CMR.[22] As part of this reorganization, Vannevar Bush, director of OSRD, wanted to install a layer of administrators directly under Richards.[23] Each of these chiefs would head a new division of CMR. If Clark were to become a CMR division chief, he would become a de facto government official. This was an additional title and position beyond Clark's chairmanship of NRC's Chemistry Division. If Clark did not accept a CMR division, he felt he would be squeezed out of the process and his previous agreements and relationships undermined by the new order. The reorganization would make Clark's position between CMR and NRC— and between the OSRD lawyers and the commercial chemists—unbearable.

In Clark's view, his feud with Richards and Bush's reorganization of CMR were not his only problems. The argument with Richards often made work impossible. With regard to expanding the synthetic chemistry program and the problems of coordinating it with testing and pharmacology, Clark made implicit reference to his differences with Richards: "It must be remembered that we started on a volunteer basis before CMR granted financial support. And at that time the only comprehensive program of synthesis was [Lyndon] Small's. The Feud made it impossible to obtain complete cooperation. I had hoped that the show-down would result in more definite directives from the Board but what the Board resolved was virtually a green light for the continuance of a large part of the Small program and with no well developed plan to take its place."[24] Another problem for Clark was the growing pressure from the legal division of OSRD to protect public investment in research. This pressure focused on increasing the distribution of data within the antimalarial program and ensuring that private firms would not unduly benefit from government-funded clinical research. By March 1944, these converging trends had created a crisis of conscience for Clark.

On 4 March 1944, the OSRD's memorandum "Recommendation Regarding Exchange of Information between OSRD Contractors and Commercial Firms" was read into the minutes of the Board for the Coordination of Malarial Studies. The recommendation had originated in the OSRD patent office under Captain Robert A. Lavender, USN (ret.). Lavender believed "that serious confusion will result and that the Government's interest will not be protected (1) unless all parties are advised that reported information may be disclosed to others and (2) unless all parties are under contract providing for patent rights." Lavender wanted to toss out the "in confidence" agreements and move all relationships onto a contractual basis. Furthermore, he wanted the volunteers out of the loop. Those not under contract would no longer receive survey reports. For Lavender, "full and complete cooperation including exchange of information between laboratories working in the all important antimalarial field" was not practical without contracts.[25]

Clark's "in confidence" restrictions were in the line of fire, but at least some on the Panel of Review stood up for the rights of the those not under contract. The panel's recommendations to Richards with regard to the OSRD memo were, in turn, read into the minutes and approved: The panel asserted that the existing information exchange was "essential to the progress of research on new antimalarial drugs." They found Lavender's changes to be "incompatible with the advancement of the program of malaria research."[26] Clark was not entirely alone in his battle.

At the beginning of March 1944, Clark tendered his resignation as chairman of the Division of Chemistry to the NRC. The resignation was effective at the end of his term of office, 30 June 1944. He sent a copy of this letter on to Richards, with an explanation for his action. Clark's words show his intensity and deeply felt beliefs. "As anticipated when I gave you my urgent memorandum of January 31st, there came up on March 1st the organization of an intensive drive to develop two series of potential antimalarial drugs. . . . All effective action appeared to be blocked by the directives of your legal advisors. I joined in the protest which was subsequently transmitted to you as the deliberate action of the Board." Robert Loeb, too, tendered his resignation as chairman of the Board for the Coordination of Malarial Studies. His action "inevitably brought into the open conflicts of administrative authority far more deep-seated than those which were apparent in the immediate fracas."[27] Loeb—his protest registered—quickly relented. Loeb felt that agreeing to serve as a government official was a professional sacrifice that he must make in order to get on with the urgent work at hand. In the coming weeks, Loeb and Clark would debate such matters in detail. Clark's feud with Richards simmered on.

In search of a connection with Richards, Clark pursued the personal touch. He wrote to the CMR chairman that he trusted in "the strength of our friendship."[28] Clark felt cut off from his network of colleagues by Richards's failure to include them in the reappraisal of the survey. "What I foresee will inevitably obstruct it [cooperation] is your inability to let friends, who, by reason of office, may rightfully share your responsibility, assume their fair share of responsibility. Thus I have learned . . . that Weed, [A. Baird] Hastings, and [Alphonse R.] Dochez, the latter representing O.S.R.D. on the Board, have been left in such ignorance of your thought regarding the Survey that I am unable to use their advice. Not having been privy to your thought for a period of over six weeks on matters that I consider to be of critical importance, I regretfully have come to the conclusion that I cannot pretend to have the responsibility not actually entrusted to me." One senses more than just matters of proprietary interest behind Clark's hurt tone. Whatever his final motivation, Clark—feeling betrayed by a friend—resigned when his authority was undermined by indecision and a lack of a shared policy.

The restructuring of the CMR continued, as well. On 18 March, new plans were issued for the reorganization. Vannevar Bush wrote to Frank B. Jewett, president of the National Academy of Sciences (NAS), on the reorganization of "the medical affairs of OSRD in order to relieve Dr. Richards of many administrative affairs." (NAS was NRC's parent organization.) This "serious burden" had accumulated with the tremendous growth in CMR's activities.[29] In Clark's copy of this letter, the following passage was marked with a question mark, and the phrases "advisory capacity" and "is in no way altered" were circled: "Under the present contract the various committees of the National Research Council act in an *advisory capacity* to the Committee on Medical Research and its Chairman. Under the new arrangement this *is in no way altered*, but it is expected that they will also advise the [CMR] Division Chiefs concerning the conduct of research in their respective fields." Attached to this letter was the Memorandum Reorganizing the Administration of the OSRD Medical Research Program, dated 20 March 1944, calling for the establishment of four Division Chiefs, who would presumably shoulder much of the administrative load for Chairman Richards. Clark's copy of the

Memorandum has one sentence underlined: "Similarly, a Division Chief may hold an appointment as a member or as Chairman of an advisory committee of the National Research Council." These markings all indicate Clark's misgivings about becoming a government official.

Clark, the chemist, also believed that there might be intrinsic barriers to legal definitions. Having seen the thousands of the structures tested, Clark felt their interconnectedness might set a natural limit on possible legal claims. The chemical structures, the modeling of active compounds, and their division into classes suggested that proprietary interests might be difficult to disentangle in the chemical landscape. "It is my personal opinion that contractual relations for the exchange of information, made with a view to protecting equities on the one hand and Governmental interests on the other would be immeasurably complicated because of the fact that so many common features run through so many of the 7,500 compounds listed in the last report of the Survey." Clark believed it was impossible to sort out proprietary interest and priority of discovery. Beyond this chemical argument, Clark articulated a professional argument against legalistic solutions and in favor of personal interactions embedded in the shared ethos of the chemist and NRC. As a professional and a representative of NRC, Clark had worked out the "in confidence" procedures with CMR's blessing. This was not a role appropriate to "a Government official armed with the potential or suspected weapons of a Government agent." If CMR wanted to interfere with Clark's personal relationships, he would have to leave, and the survey would require "new general management." Any new system, Clark emphasized, would have to incorporate the values of decisiveness, trust, and honesty. "It is impossible to handle delicate matters except with frankness and impossible to be frank while radical changes are in contemplation." With Loeb and others protesting, the ensuing atmosphere of uncertainty left Clark feeling that "affairs of pressing importance are going to the dogs rapidly."[30]

Clark wrote to Frank Jewett on 27 March 1944 following a call from Roger Adams the previous Friday with regard to Clark's nomination for another three-year term as chairman of NRC's Division of Chemistry. Adams was an academic chemist of wide repute who worked for the NDRC. Jewett was president of the National Academy of Sciences. To Jewett, Clark emphasized his consistent message to Richards: Clark could not and would not deal with the commercial firms on a contractual basis. As evidence of Richard's understanding, he cited his reaction when Richards had attempted to name him to the CMR's penicillin committee the previous year. Clark had demurred, as this would have necessitated his dealing "with commercial people on a basis quite different from the way in which I had dealt with them in the malaria program."[31] With regard to the penicillin committee, Richards wrote Clark "a very nice letter showing his appreciation of my stand." From this Clark concluded that "Richards knew of my disinclination to deal with commercial people on any basis other the purely scientific." Clark was surprised that Richards should fail to once more appreciate his position. Would Clark be allowed to continue as before? Or would he be forced to proceed in malaria in accordance with the penicillin program policies? Clark would stay on as chairman only if the Division of Chemistry were no longer in charge of the survey or if his policy of confidentiality were maintained.

Penicillin—like synthetic rubber—was a wartime program often compared to antimalarials. In both projects, information was freely shared between participants.[32] Against this model and in support of the maintenance of "in confidence" information, Clark solicited the input of fellow chemists involved in war work. To keep things clear, Clark wrote to Roger Adams about some remarks that he (Clark) had made to Richards about the use of contracts and disclosure. With regard to the penicillin contracts, Clark had heard "hints that the commercial people were not entirely happy."[33]

Adams's response was marked "Personal & Confidential." Adams did not find Clark's negative characterization apt. He himself had not found the firms "too unhappy about the present set-up," with regard to penicillin. Though he would not go so far as to say "that the penicillin contracts have worked beautifully." Adams found them to have "worked unusually well in view of the fact that some eight or nine concerns have been called together under government control in a cooperative project." With regard to penicillin work, the contractual system and the pooling of all findings was a functional compromise. Adams could not give Clark the support he needed. As to Clark's query "concerning the question of wider disclosure in the malaria field," Adams was far more sympathetic. Malaria was a different field from penicillin. Malaria had a "central committee" distributing research problems and had little duplication of effort. In Adam's view, further "mimeographing of reports and distribution would merely add a tremendous burden to your office without furnishing any pertinent aid to the contractors." Adams thought that the two projects were sufficiently different that there would be "no advantage" in wider disclosure in Clark's project "due to the fact that for the most part the various laboratories are working on the synthesis of different types of compounds." For Adams, it did not "seem appropriate to compare the malarial field with penicillin since all of the laboratories in the latter are attempting to prepare molecules of one or two very definite structures. By interchange of information much effort and time will be saved in elimination of duplication."[34] Chemically, penicillin was a distributed research project on a single, narrow subject rather than the simultaneous pursuit of thousands of new compounds. For antimalarials, the scientific problems and putative solutions under investigation were broader and less well defined than for the penicillin project. In terms of R&D, malaria had a much larger research component while penicillin focused on development.

Crisis and Reconciliation

By early April, Vannevar Bush was actively engaged in damage control with regard the OSRD-NRC rift. In a letter to Frank Jewett, NAS president, and copied to Clark, Bush repeated that the CMR restructuring was an internal OSRD matter only. OSRD was an emergency wartime organization not intended to interfere with the internal operations of the NRC or its parent, the NAS. As an emergency organization, OSRD was set up "with the full authority residing in the Director." Bush could "operate intelligently only by appropriate advice and delegation." OSRD had two distinct functions that had to remain separate: "(1) of initiation of programs, their periodic review, and the establishment of proper policy to govern them, and (2) the definite and detailed administration of contracts." This first function was a matter of consensus and was "performed at all points by committees, and the meeting of minds, first by committees of specialists and second by committees chosen to be representative of the various interests involved. The second must of necessity, both by reason of law and for the establishment of clear responsibility in the expenditure of government funds, be delegated either directly or through channels, to individuals within the organization." Bush wanted "the business and the scientific phases of administration" separated, with the business end of things kept to OSRD. Bush portrayed the threatening reorganization of CMR as an effort "to relieve Dr. Richards by the appointment of new officers, and the delegation to them of . . . the supervision of contracts from the professional and scientific point of view." This would not impact the business "of initiation, review, and policy." Bush wanted forceful administrators: "We need strong men, who will take and exercise responsibility, and see that results are attained."[35] In spite of these efforts, Clark's mental and emotional condition were deeply impacted by the threat of becoming an ethically compromised bureaucrat, shorn of his scientific independence and integrity.

On 18 April 1944, Robert Loeb met with Clark in Baltimore; in Loeb's words, it "was a hard day with Bill Clark. He's about the dearest, finest and most lovable soul that ever lived but his soul is being tortured by a problem which I do not believe is ours. I, too, *hate* to become an official of the Government . . . because I hate not to have independence as a free and untrammeled individual and because I too have distrust of certain governmental motives. But, if it's the law that it be so to do the work at hand and if I do not have to compromise my personal integrity, I can accept it. I tried hard to tell this to Bill, but he won't or can't see."[36] Loeb felt his intervention was not helping Clark: "I can do no more about Bill but feel that his position must be handled by Dr. Bush and Dr. Jewett—particularly as Bill says he will under no circumstances go on in any capacity other than his present one and because he feels so strongly that one of the motives involved is that of 'doing in' of the N.R.C. by the governmental agency, i.e., the O.S.R.D." This was a critical point for Clark, the professional organization losing power to the governmental. Loeb would report back to Richards and Bush on his meeting with Clark: "I just hope he (Bill) knows that I am devoted to him and that I am sympathetic with his point of view, but feel we *must* get on with what the lawyers say is the mechanism for action. The great mistake was made when N.R.C. and C.M.R. were set up as *different* groups . . . that's, however, water over the dam." On 18 April, Bush requested some direct clarification from Clark. He felt he had only heard Clark's concerns "indirectly." He hoped "that when you find it possible to do so you will plan to drop in to see me some day soon."[37] Clark replied to Bush almost immediately, copying the letter to Adams, Jewett, Richards, Weed, and Ross Harrison, chairman of NRC.

The 18th and 19th of April were difficult and thoughtful days for Clark. On the 19th, he wrote to Bush that he had received his "kind invitation" of the previous day—the same day that Loeb and Clark had met in Baltimore. Loeb had told Clark that the reorganization would redefine his service to the program. Clark also complained to Bush of the new legal encroachments on his earlier policies. "Dr. Richards had previously informed me that a memorandum by Mr. Connor on the Survey of Antimalarial Drugs expresses the present attitude of OSRD"; Connor and Richards laid down "the conditions under which [Clark] would have to operate in this particular field."[38] John T. Connor was a lawyer. He had joined the legal division of OSRD in April 1942, had become head legal advisor that October, and was the first general counsel of the OSRD until June 1944, when he joined the U.S. Marines.[39]

In a letter to Jewett the same day, Clark described his motivations as "not being determined by anything other than the desire to put science to the service of the war effort." He feared that the lawyers were "heading us for strict regimentation." Clark worried that Connor, too, was pushing him to become a government official. Connor might be "a sane and capable fellow," but he was "hardly in a position to judge a situation *first* from the point of view of a statesman." Clark did acknowledge that with CMR organized into divisions along the lines of NDRC, he could expect new power to run the program. Yet he still found the government-official issue particularly troubling. Clark told Jewett that Loeb and the Panel of Review wanted him to step down as chairman of NRC's Panel on the Synthesis and to focus on the survey—"a job of which they and I are proud, while administrative officers ask me to do so in a capacity entirely different from that which, in my judgment, has determined the success of the venture."[40] Clark continued to argue that becoming a government official would undermine his effectiveness at the survey.

With the pressure on, Clark only had "room only for a 'yes' or 'no.' . . . The writing on the wall is plain." Unable to convince his colleagues and superiors of his position, Clark now begged "a final consideration." Clark was coming to his wit's end, and, wishing to "be spared the agony of any further discussion," he asked to be relieved of his "duties on behalf of the CMR." He also wrote to Jewett, begging "to be spared any further discussion with Dr. Richards or Dr. Bush," as he had "been unable to convince anyone that I am reasonable in this matter and having found that discussion only muddies the water at a time when the water is clearing." Something had to be done to save the malaria program: "Indecision has brought the malaria program to an all-time 'low.' Prompt action is essential to getting on with this vitally important program."[41]

With Clark's complaints and protests registered, Bush revised the plan for reorganizing the CMR. Clark reviewed Bush's revisions. They impressed him "as a great improvement over the first." Nevertheless, Clark distrusted the legal regimentation. The putative reconstitution of the malaria program as a division of the NDRC might undercut or distort the advisory role of the NRC committees. Clark knew the work needed to get done, but he was disturbed "that anxiety for legalities allows plain courtesy to be overridden. There is danger that there will be lost the good will which is worth a regiment of workers." Courtesy and honesty, the values of the statesman and the scientist, were cast down in favor of legal necessity. Clark pleaded with Jewett: "I am convinced that everyone in high authority except yourself has gotten hold of the central problem at the wrong end but only with the best of intentions."[42] Clark asked Jewett, too, that he be relieved of his CMR duties.

Vannevar Bush, in receipt of Clark's 19 April letter, remained perplexed. On 21 April, he wrote to Clark to express his confusion. Bush again reemphasized that he wanted only to reorganize CMR in a way that would remove as much of the administrative burden as possible from Richards. He pointedly stated that the matter of how this was to be done had not been settled or finalized, and he asked again—though he had read Clark's memos—for Clark to speak with him in person on the matter. Bush wanted Clark's "direct thoughts." These might well be glimpsed in some undated drafts of a letter that Clark wrote and saved but never sent (more on these below). Bush asserted that Connor's memorandum on the Survey expressed only his views and was only one of the "documents that are involved in the present consideration." With matters not yet finalized, Clark's letter did not—in Bush's mind— "meet the actual existing situation."[43] Bush felt Clark was overreacting to the proposed reorganization.

Meanwhile, on Saturday, 22 April 1944, Clark wrote a "strictly private and confidential" letter back to Loeb. Clark seemed more than ever filled with doubt and perhaps even self-pity or loathing: "I shall ever prize your letter. You may be quite sure that I know everyone has acted with the best intentions and motives, if not too wisely. I am happy to have worked with men who can scrap among themselves without rupturing friendship. Your letter helps a great deal because, when one stands alone on conviction, there is always the creepy feeling that one's ego has allowed special matters too much emphasis." Clark still lamented that the CMR involvement undermined the gentlemanly cooperation of the NRC initiative. Clearly he felt betrayed, at least by Richards. Clark remained a champion of NRC's prerogatives. For Clark, freedom and responsibility were core values and essential for moving war work ahead. As chairman of the Panel on Synthesis, he had sought to accommodate rather than administrate. "It is on the basis of wishes more than on the basis of formal organization that I like to work and on which I have offered the facilities of the Division of Chem." He advocated the exercise of "garden variety of common sense" and urged all "to make the best of what was available without assuming all will be ideal."[44] Clark made the case that he and the NRC had done the best under the circumstances and that NRC was, by its nature, special.

At heart, Clark saw NRC as a professional body. Clark's NRC had initiated the chemotherapy project, and CMR had given it additional responsibilities. Clark's Division of Chemistry was egalitarian with regard to all chemists regardless of their employers. "Whether or not, as someone remarked, the commercial people realize it, the fact remains that the Division represents all the leading chemical societies of America and particularly the American Chemical Society which is noteworthy for drawing no line of distinction between academic and commercial chemists. Were there occasion to do so I could place my policy before the Division, representing the chemists of America, and I think I know their temper with regard to certain expressions of opinion within the Panel of Review and Board."[45] Here Clark explicitly cites the professional nature of his understanding with the commercial chemists and, by extension, the commercial firms. "Whatever may be the final official directives, the pressure from the high administration and the attitude within the Panel of Review combine to render impotent in practice a spirit in which I feel I would have the overwhelming support of the chemists of America were I to bring matters into the open." The bureaucratic impulse of the high administration did not sit well beside the professional spirit that animated the Division of Chemistry.

Nevertheless, Clark was sensitive to the medical as a well as the chemical nature of the program. Questions about private gain versus the public good surrounded the medical output of the antimalarial program. Academic inventors often licensed inventions of medical importance in a nonexclusive way.[46] Clark wrote to Loeb, "Now it is a fact that you and I and all others who live a medical environment hate to see any thing covered up especially when it concerns the healing art. Therefore it is natural to demand an opening up even when we feel we must keep an agreement, which is to the contrary."[47] These concerns reiterated those Clark had written to Alphonse R. Dochez, a civilian member of CMR and a friend of Clark's, four weeks earlier: "Like everyone with an academic training and medical environment, I would have preferred some arrangement whereby all information on antimalarials could have been pooled. I had to be realistic."[48] Clark's expediency and NRC's egalitarianism underwrote a policy whereby commercial chemists could contribute to the program but not have the intellectual property rights compromised.

Clark saw himself as not just practical in the face of the emergency but a fair dealer in a fine American tradition. "It is also natural to be suspicious when profits are involved. On the other hand there is an agreement and there is the American principle that none should be judged guilty unless and until convicted on sufficient evidence. . . . Since, as of this date, there has been no holding out of which I have good evidence and since every case of suspicion that I have investigated has turned out contrary to the allegations, I have been very much disturbed by the repeated evidence of suspicion on the part of all members of the Panel of Review other than myself. . . . Thus it has become increasingly difficult for me to operate in accordance with Division policy and spirit and Panel attitude."[49] Clark's NRC division had a policy of fair-dealing and a presumption of innocence, while Clark felt the Panel of Review, a creature of the CMR, was pervaded with an attitude of suspicion. But Clark had had enough of being second guessed. He warned Loeb that, even in his absence, the board should honor the confidentiality agreements and that they should cease all talk of failures to cooperate until they had firm evidence of such. Clark pleaded, "Please be realistic."

With regard to the voluntary cooperation of commercial firms, Clark was also on the spot with the firms themselves, as the example of the Squibb Institute for Medical Research suggests. Clark had a "long conversation" with the institute's director, George Harrop: "George's worry is that during 4 years his institute has devoted 7/10 or 9/10 (I forget the figure) of its resources to malaria in addition to the services of his best man [Oskar Paul] Wintersteiner in the cortical hormone synthesis program with nothing of practical value to the war effort to show for it. In money the malaria work has been to the tune of between $200,000 and a quarter of a million. What he wanted first was some assurance that this effort was not seriously out of line with [what] other institutions had done so that he could make a plea to his directors to carry on with malaria work. What he wanted second was some perspective of the program as a whole so that he could direct intelligently."[50] Clark had reassured Harrop that Squibb's contributions were "not out of line," adding that if resources were too tight, quality could substitute for quantity; fewer novel compounds would be less labor than many similar ones. "Brain power" could substitute for "man power." Elsewhere in the commercial world, things were similar. Ken Blanchard characterized the survey relationship with Winthrop Chemical: "Full spirit of cooperation under difficulties." Blanchard weathered the storm at the survey, assuaging concerns, offering advice, and passing on information, but Fred Wiselogle and others were as harried as Clark or more so.

Clark complained to Loeb about the damages he and the survey staff had suffered. Wiselogle had resigned for reasons of health. "The boy is exhausted and has had on his hands a revolution in his staff due to the pestering the Survey has had in a period during which every body was going in circles. I advised him to take a vacation and when Marshall heard the reasons he, like Blanchard, said 'good' on the announcement that Fred was off for a rest."[51]

Clark was doing damage control with regard to his own NRC duties as well. He told NRC chairman Harrison "that I would accept the Chairmanship of the Division for another term merely to avoid embarrassing questions but provided that I take care of the routine work by only infrequent visits to the office. I hate to think of three more years of this just to avoid a scandal. I have burned my bridges behind me in the malaria field." Even while lamenting the apparent outcome and his own failure, Clark still expressed his regard for Loeb. "With the kindest personal regards and the very best of good wishes that your bravery and sense of duty and knowledge and judgment and skill in dealing with people will make you a triumphant leader in a most important job I remain . . . lovingly yours."

As much as March and April 1944 were months of stalemate and crisis for the antimalarial program, May was a month of reconciliation. As April turned to May, Clark and Bush finally met. As Bush wrote to Richards, "I have now had a very pleasant discussion with Dr. Clark."[52] The only major change to the CMR reorganization was the addition of a medical administrative officer under Richards and above the new division chiefs, who were explicitly "Government officials" within OSRD. Clark wrote to the vacationing Fred Wiselogle on 2 May 1944, that things were "looking-up." Clark's newly positive outlook stemmed "from a very nice conversation I had the other day with Dr. Bush, Director of OSRD. I learned 'from the horse's mouth,' as they say, that there is in the works a basic organizational plan which seems to meet the requirements. Instead of insisting that I be a Government official, as some of the underlings thought I must be, Bush is perfectly sure that I can fit in somewhere under NRC. Bush agreed that it was perfectly proper for me not to make any commitment until I saw the whole line-up."[53] The conniving "underlings" might have included Richards or at least OSRD general counsel John Connor. Clark assured Wiselogle that whatever the realignment, Clark would remain as a buffer between CMR and the survey. Clark did not resign but continued on in his NRC capacity.

Coup de Grâce

That said, Clark's early fears proved correct and government bureaucracy won out. In 1945, Bush and Richards reorganized the CMR along the lines of the NDRC. As the Board for the Coordination of Malarial Studies was largely a creature of OSRD and CMR, and as the committees subsidiary to the board were dedicated to advice and coordination, administration was largely lacking even as the antimalarial program grew in scale, cost, and complexity.

By late 1944, this distinction between advisory and administrative duties had begun to fray. As Clark wrote, "It became necessary in several instances for these committees or for officers of the Council to exercise administrative functions in minor but vitally important details. By late winter of 1944, this situation had caused considerable concern because final responsibility for the expenditure of federal funds lay in OSRD." Bush and Richards applied the National Defense Research Council model to CMR. At first, only five CMR divisions were created. Malaria held out briefly, as the Malaria Division under George A. Carden Jr. was CMR's last. Carden headed both this CMR division and served as secretary of the board, bringing the two organizations into intimate contact.[54] The reorganization of the CMR along the lines of NDRC was a clear move away from the professional advising and encouraging of research—for which the NRC had been founded—to a supervisory, formalized government bureaucracy. Bush, for his part, completed his reorganization of the malaria program into Division 6 of the CMR and instructed its new chief, George Carden Jr., to review the whole "in confidence" matter with an eye to revising it in the government's favor.[55]

A year after his crisis with Richards, the mollified Clark was still grappling with federal encroachments on the prerogatives of the NRC. A letter addressed to George Carden by Clark, but never sent, gives a nice window onto Clark's rigidity and his obsession with the delicate handling of the "in confidence" material. Clark wanted two items clarified with regard to organizational principles. Clark's first item dealt with a report from Wiselogle "that you requested him to eliminate from the first page of the recently prepared special tables the letterhead of the National Research Council. May I remind you that the Survey was organized by the Division of Chemistry of the National Research Council and that the solicitation of information from suppliers was in the name of two Divisions of NRC and CMR."[56] Clark also worried about his own prerogatives. "I previously pointed out the distinct advantage of soliciting information in the name of a non-government organization, and I would think that it might be advantageous to avoid confusion in the minds of suppliers by continuing the Survey under the Division of Chemistry rather than to make a change." Clark's survey was ever a creature of NRC, a protector of professional chemists. His second item dealt specifically with the containment of "in confidence" materials: "Fred [Wiselogle] received a request from you [George Carden] to deliver to you not less than 75 copies of the special tables containing 'in confidence' information . . . Fred proceeded to put into these tables 'in confidence' information without having in writing, or indeed in any other definite form, the names of the people who are to receive these tables according to the information which Richards doubtless gave to the firms which he contacted . . . as far as the Survey goes, it has skated on very thin ice in its efforts to be accommodating. . . . Again, lest we get our lines of authority tangled, will you please put such requests through me." A new element of restraint can be seen in Clark the spring of 1945: Clark marked this letter as "not sent" but kept it in his files anyway. Perhaps, so late in the war, he had resigned himself to abandoning this battle.

The reorganization of the CMR brought its publicly funded research more under government control. It was one move, among several, to curb the rights and responsibilities of independent scientists and firms. Meeting with an OSRD lawyer, Oscar M. Ruebhausen, to discuss the "protection of public interest," the CMR recommended "that no further testing of compounds submitted by independent organizations be conducted by the Government and that no further information not available to the public be made available to such organizations unless the firms agree to extend to the Government a non-exclusive, royalty-free license under any and all patents pertaining to an antimalarial drug, and to license others on reasonable terms whenever the Director of OSRD may require such licenses as necessary to insure the availability to the public of adequate quantities of high quality antimalarials at reasonable prices." The only caveat was that this policy might be flexible if its exercise might "seriously jeopardize the effectiveness of the antimalarial program."[57] This caveat brought back a suggestion of urgent national emergency, but victory in Europe had already been achieved, and the government was seeking to secure the rights to inventions funded with taxpayer dollars. The target of this change was Clark's gentleman's agreement to share information for the sake of U.S. fighting men. As the guns fell silent, accounting for what belonged to whom became a priority. The CMR saw a huge public investment in the testing and development of therapeutic agents and did not wish to see the public or the government pay twice for these: first in the development costs and then in excessive prices supported by the exclusivity of patent rights.

This change in constitution from a band of dedicated researchers striving together in a time of shared emergency to a set of actors divided by conflicting interests of ownership and property meant that Clark's brokerage of fair dealing would be overturned. The fracture between the public weal and private profits left little room for Clark's good word and NRC as a professional body. Whatever Vannevar Bush's reassurances had been, the government lawyers were, at Bush's request, on the move. By May 1945, Ruebhausen—who had replaced John Connor at the OSRD legal division—had reviewed the antimalarial program and outlined the legal status of all the players. He also developed a plan to bolster the staff of the Division of Malaria so that CMR could "give affirmative direction to the malaria program."[58] After the war, Clark continued to muse over the potential conflict between public funding and private gain: "In any event there is sure to be reencountered the perpetual conflict in men's minds between reliance on faith, hope and charity on the one hand and reliance on the sterner safeguards of the law on the other. Actually, in the whole malaria program, the dominant attitude of all concerned, in Government, Council, private laboratory and commercial company, leaned toward faith, hope and charity."[59] In Clark's view, the record would reveal that the operation of these virtues was "not so bad after all."

Clark was an advocate of common sense over rules (laws) and bureaucracy. The issues with Richards—his being overburdened by administration, for example—suggest that common sense and personal understandings worked well at smaller social scales but that the increasing scale of the project and the desire to consistently compromise between competing interests—military secrecy, proprietary knowledge, scientific openness, and getting on with the work—required impersonal bureaucratic solutions to maintain the peace and the perception of fairness. Clark had not wanted to become a government official, to cross over from NRC to OSRD. He did not want to give up the freedom to act or to abandon the scientific values of NRC. In one dimension, this was a conflict between the power of government and that of the professions. It might strike some as odd that the proponent of science and freedom was the advocate for commercial interests, intellectual property rights, and control of information. Clark pushed for classified (government) data to be shared with commercial firms but felt the firms had the abiding interest in data on their own compounds. Clark defended this ethos with reference to the chemists of America, and he may have been correct that these apparent contradictions were indeed the values of a large segment of practicing scientists of the period. Whatever the case, Clark had given his word to these firms, and he believed that confidentiality actually *improved* cooperation, so long as coordination and communication prevented duplication. This confidentiality contrasted with the open policies pursued in the synthetic rubber and penicillin programs. Clark's inner thoughts remain his own, but he summed up his intentions nicely in an undated draft of a letter that he saved but never sent: "My entire policy has been founded on the faith that we all have our eyes fixed on the fellow in the fox-hole with malaria in his blood."[60]

For the fellow with malaria in his blood, the final year of the war would bring a new hope in the form of chloroquine. Chloroquine and new drugs for the prevention and treatment of malaria would come become widely available in the postwar years.

Chapter 7

Chloroquine, Wonder Drug

The emergence of chloroquine as the first-line drug for malaria prophylaxis and treatment was the great medical accomplishment of the antimalarial program's later years. Chloroquine's path from a failed drug in the Bayer interwar program to a wonder drug of the postwar world merits attention in its own right and also illustrates the networks of relationships that evolved during the U.S. antimalarial program. For U.S. soldiers and marines, chloroquine would emerge from testing programs too late to impact combat operations. With chloroquine and the insecticide DDT, another wartime development, in hand, the old Ross-Koch public health debate about whether mosquitoes or parasites were the proper target for disease intervention entered a new era: these chemicals were deadly weapons against both. DDT and chloroquine would later founder in the face of resistance—pesticide resistance and drug resistance, respectively. But for millions of people living in malarious areas, cheap, effective chloroquine would be a lifesaver.

Chloroquine rose just as the sun was setting on the CMR program itself. Recall sontochin from chapter 3. A chemical cousin of chloroquine developed by Bayer, it appeared more than once early in the U.S. antimalarial program and showed good activity in avian screens.[1] It was one of number of compounds provided to the program by the Winthrop Chemical Company. W. Mansfield Clark's staff gave it Survey Number SN-183, indicating that it was one of the first compounds that they processed. Later in the war, sontochin was thrust into the spotlight when it was captured with an enemy prisoner of war in North Africa. Sontochin, however, had been in the possession of the program even before the formation of the Survey Office. In 1940, Justus B. Rice, vice president for medical research at the Winthrop Chemical Company, had given the compound to Lowell Coggeshall, then still working at the Rockefeller Institute. Though they had the Winthrop compound in 1940, the Rockefeller team did not test it until John Maier picked it up in January 1941. Maier found the compound active against his avian malaria, *P. cathemerium*. In due course, Winthrop released Maier's testing data to the Survey in December 1942, where it rested in the Survey's open files until its North African appearance. Testing by chemists at the Rockefeller Institute in New York revealed that the German sontochin was identical with SN-183. For security reasons, the Survey issued the compound a new survey number, SN-6911. After testing at Hopkins and Chicago, E. K. Marshall reported sontochin to be four to eight times as active as quinine against the duck malaria, *P. lophurae*.[2] The Subcommittee on Coordination of Malarial Studies was especially keen to move forward on sontochin as they already had in their possession a report by a French military doctor in Tunis on field trials of sontochin in the French army, a report they had received courtesy of the U.S. Army Surgeon General's Office.[3] By the spring of 1944, sontochin was moving on in toxicology trials in humans.[4]

Sontochin pointed back to chloroquine. As soon as sontochin had reemerged from the Survey and the North African desert, the CMR solicited all of Winthrop's records on sontochin and related compounds. The program began a reexamination of these 4-aminoquinolines. Readers will recall the sontochin differed from chloroquine by only a methyl group (fig. 3.13). NRC interest in chloroquine originally derived from its inclusion in Bayer antimalarial patents—specifically U.S. Patent 2,233,970—assigned to Winthrop Chemical.[5] Apparently, the company had never produced the compound before Clark and Kenneth Blanchard of the Survey Office requested them to do so in November 1943. With no regard for their prewar ties to Bayer, Winthrop was consistently helpful and compliant with government requests. They assisted with chloroquine voluntarily and under contract, and worked on other wartime chemical problems. In July 1944, the War Production Board received from Winthrop Chemical Company its plasmochin pilot plant.[6]

By July 1944, Marshall and others were convinced that chloroquine, SN-7618, was the drug they had been looking for: Marshall wrote that the board "had as its primary objective the discovery of a drug that is a true causal prophylactic in both falciparum and vivax malaria or a drug which consistently cures both of these infections." He went on to express the recommendation of the board that the military should "welcome" any drug that was better than atabrine in having an improved therapeutic index, lowered relapse rates for vivax malaria, or "such pharmacological and therapeutic properties that 'breakthroughs' on suppressive therapy" were fewer than with atabrine. Chloroquine showed promise in all three areas: "One drug, SN-7618, now appears from available evidence to be significantly superior to quinacrine in having a wider spread between therapeutic and toxic doses." The board required a swift response from the surgeons general as to whether they were interested "in the exploitation of such a drug for the following reasons: 1) if the answer is yes, arrangements must be made at once for development-work and pilot plant studies and 2) if the answer is no, the Board must inform the Committee on Medical Research of this decision as, a reorientation of the malarial research program may be necessary."[7] Chloroquine moved ahead, although subsequent research, as we will see, would show that it could not prevent relapse in vivax malaria.

Testing Chloroquine

Expanding interest in chloroquine meant increased demand for material. Winthrop Chemical and a number of OSRD synthesis contractors worked on the problem. As chloroquine production was scaled up to produce kilograms at a time, bottlenecks appeared, particularly in the availability of the chemical intermediate, dichloroquinoline. Academic contractors at Columbia University, the University of Illinois, and other universities produced this intermediate, which was necessary for the synthesis of chloroquine, sontochin, and related compounds.[8] In September 1944, Robert C. Elderfield, a professor of chemistry at Columbia University and member of the Panel of Review, reported to the panel on the state of chloroquine manufacture.[9] He and Charles C. Price, a University of Illinois organic chemist, had spoken to the chemists at Winthrop: The company would submit a contract for the synthesis of chloroquine to the Panel on Synthesis. Elderfield and Price were well positioned to advise on such a matter as they both had held OSRD synthesis contracts for antimalarial compounds and intermediates for several years.[10] Price himself was an innovator in the synthesis of dichloroquinoline.[11] The industrial and academic chemists worked together to overcome emerging problems.

Technical issues aside, intellectual property rights needed to be addressed. James Shannon was concerned over the "propriety of granting funds and priority privileges to a commercial firm in order to permit that firm to exploit a compound for which they have patent coverage."[12] These concerns were not Shannon's alone. The OSRD lawyers who were involved with William Clark and the Survey weighed in on the patent issues with chloroquine, sontochin, and two related compounds (SN-7373 and SN-8137). The lawyers uncovered little that would give the government claim to these drugs. None of these compounds was found to be patentable by the U.S. government: all four were covered under Winthrop's patents, and sontochin had been captured from the enemy. Some of the processes for their manufacture, such as the synthesis of dichloroquinoline, might be patentable, but overall the government found that it was funding the development of drugs that it did not own.[13] The board, in general, was more communitarian in their approach to intellectual property as indicated by their postwar recommendation to CMR on filing foreign patents: They did not believe that any individual or institution should earn royalties from these patents. In all fairness, "the closely knit, integrated efforts of the various groups under the Board made it impossible to assign with certainty the source of thought, i.e., true inventorship, concerning the development of these compounds."[14] For the most important compounds to emerge from the program such as chloroquine, the government, through its OSRD legal department, entered into nonexclusive, royalty-free license agreements with patent-holding firms. These agreements granted the government rights to the compounds for military, naval, and national defense purposes.[15]

These future commercial and legal arrangements aside, war made the testing and manufacture of chloroquine a vital matter. Whatever the board or the lawyers would come to decide about patents, Carl Marvel, professor of organic chemistry at the University of Illinois and chairman of the Panel on Synthesis, maintained that urgency required unfettered cooperation with the industrial chemists at Winthrop. Because of their familiarity with specific synthetic intermediates, simple expediency demanded that the board enroll their synthetic expertise.[16] As noted after the war, "Under the pressure of wartime conditions it was imperative that production of this drug proceed at the greatest possible speed to supply the OSRD with sufficient material for controlled clinical tests. . . . Operations could not await the design and fabrication of special equipment: production and development had to follow the direction dictated by the available plant equipment, in August 1944, which was pressed into immediate service."[17] The cooperation of academic and industrial chemists produced a hybrid process where scale-up and synthesis were done in diverse locations. Thus in the early days of production, Nathan L. Drake's group at the University of Maryland pooled the dichloroquinoline of the various academic laboratories and added the side chain to yield chloroquine, while the Allied Chemical and Dye Corporation made dichloroquinoline by Charles Price's method and used it to make chloroquine (fig. 7.1). Drake's group, for its part, had hoped to produce up to ten kilograms of chloroquine by 1 October 1944, but a shortage of dichloroquinoline caused delays.[18] Nevertheless, starting in August, enough chloroquine was available to test for toxicity on conscientious objectors at the Massachusetts General Hospital. No adverse toxic symptoms were observed in these preliminary trials. Trials in malaria therapy at the Boston Psychopathic Hospital soon followed.[19] The tests in Boston were just a few of many.[20]

Animal research had expanded into testing in mental patients and prisoners and into testing on soldiers.[21] At Hopkins, E. K. Marshall continued comparative toxicity studies of SN-7618 and other 4-aminoquinolines in monkeys.[22] Testing for efficacy in humans progressed as well. Lowell Coggeshall, now a commander in the U.S. naval reserve, already had chloroquine in patients at the marine barracks at Klamath Falls, Oregon.[23] The army, represented on the board by Lieutenant Colonel Oliver R. McCoy, wanted to move ahead with "a fairly large-scale field study" of the suppressive capability of chloroquine as soon as positive results in prisoner volunteers became available.[24] Alf Alving's University of Chicago group was testing compounds at Illinois's Stateville penitentiary. For chloroquine, the next big milestone would be trials conducted on Australian soldier volunteers, supervised by Neil Hamilton Fairley, about whom more below. The CMR sent the Australian Army 2,500 chloroquine tablets with which to begin this program.[25] Over time this large-scale test grew larger still: CMR's malaria chief, George A. Carden Jr., arranged that five hundred pounds of chloroquine be delivered to the Australians.[26]

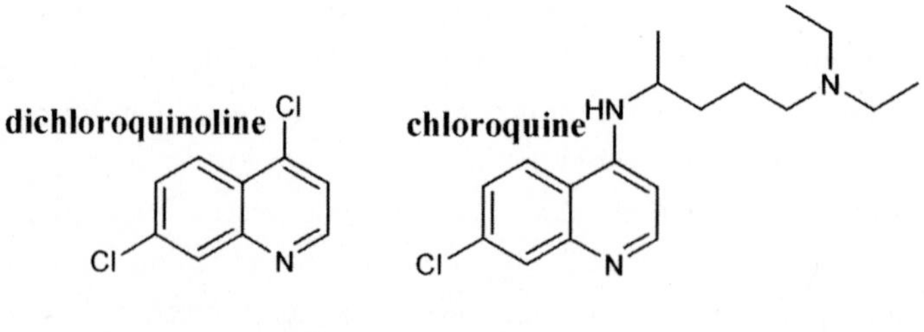

Figure 7.1 Chloroquine

For chloroquine, the Australian clinical work was definitive. Back in September 1944, the board had first decided to initiate studies on chloroquine with Australians based at Cairns.[27] N. Hamilton Fairley oversaw these testing efforts as he had the previous work on atabrine and sontochin.[28] For the Australians, separated from the Japanese advance into Southeast Asia by the island of New Guinea, malaria was a serious problem.[29] According to Fairley, "In 1942 and early 1943 malaria casualities in the South West Pacific had been very grave, amounting in a period of 4 months to some 90% of the forces involved." Fairley's unit was soon called upon to determine effective protocols for quinine, atebrine, and plasmochin. "In New Guinea questions were continually being raised by field commanders and staff officers regarding the efficacy of the antimalarial measures . . . and whether suppressive or prophylactic drugs could control the repeated and heavy malaria infection contracted in jungle warfare." Fairley's malaria group experimentally infected "some 850 healthy volunteers."[30] The Australians ran numerous series of trials with healthy military volunteers in Australia and New Guinea. Tests included heavy exercise and high altitude to determine the effectiveness of drugs under the stress of simulated combat. Eventually, the Australian program assessed not just the prewar trio of drugs, but sulfas, biguanides, sontochin, Paludrine—the novel British antimalarial developed during the war—and, of course, chloroquine.

Key to Australian success was their use of transfused blood—subinoculation—and of tropical strains of *vivax* malaria. *Plasmodium vivax* had a hidden form of the parasite that could cause relapse even after the patient's blood had been cleared of parasites. To study the ability of a drug to prevent this sort of relapse, researchers had to observe subjects after preliminary treatment and discover whether relapse occurred. The Australians determined that, while chloroquine could suppress *vivax* and *falciparum* malarias and provide a radical cure for *falciparum*, it could not prevent relapse in *vivax* since it had no effect on the hidden, non-blood-borne forms of the parasites. This limitation was shared with atabrine, which the Australians had definitively shown, too. Essential to this finding was the subinoculation procedure. To detect latent malaria—to learn if a subject's blood was truly parasite-free—Fairley's Land Headquarters Medical Research Unit transfused the subject's blood into another, previously uninfected, volunteer: "Where a volunteer failed to show a complete break-through after this 5-week period, 200 c.c. of his blood were injected intravenously into a compatible recipient (volunteer)."[31] The failure of the blood recipient to come down with malaria showed that the donor's blood was truly malaria-free. If the donor later relapsed, it was because the drug that had killed all the blood-stage parasites had failed to kill those hidden in his tissues. It is an interesting piece of malaria natural history that tropical strains of vivax relapse much more quickly than their temperate cousins. Therefore the Australians, working with New Guinea strains, could much more rapidly determine activity against relapse than could the U.S. workers who employed local, North American *vivax* strains. Instead of having to wait months for positive relapse results, the Australian trials could expect results in weeks.[32] Again, careful selection of materials brought from the field and into the clinic and lab proved essential to research design and efficiency.

The PHS malaria research group at Columbia, South Carolina—headed by Martin D. Young, the Hopkins trained parasitologist—reported in the prestigious journal *Science* on U.S. acquisition of a tropical New Guinea strain: "An infection of *Plasmodium vivax* was diagnosed in a soldier at Harmon General Hospital in August, 1944. The history of the patient indicated that the infection was contracted in New Guinea during 1944."[33] That same month, Young's group transferred this foreign malaria into local vector mosquitoes, *Anopheles quadrimaculatus*, in the laboratory. With mosquito transmission thus established, they noted "that this *vivax* infection in man reacted differently to certain drugs than did the St. Elizabeth strain of *P. vivax* which has been extensively used for drug testing. This and other characteristics suggest that it might be a strain distinct from some of the American malarias." (The St. Elizabeth, or St. Elizabeths, strain was first isolated at St. Elizabeths Hospital in Washington, DC.) Young knew the value of the new tool he now had and named it after the patient from whom it had been isolated: "the Chesson strain of *Plasmodium vivax*."

G. Robert Coatney—the PHS/NIH researcher who oversaw federal malaria research in human subjects at the Atlanta Federal Penitentiary and in Columbia, South Carolina, for years after the war—echoed Young in his report to the board. He, too, knew it was urgent that U.S. facilities acquire an exotic, New Guinea strain of the disease: "Since the reports of Fairley from Australia had indicated that New Guinea strains possessed different characteristics, and since control of Pacific strains of *vivax* malaria was the major goal of the testing program, comparative studies (with a change of the test strain in mind) were indicated."[34] What proved the critical difference was not so much the strain's response to drugs but its short latency period. It was a good experimental model not just because of its possible similarity to the kinds of vivax malaria with which U.S. soldiers and sailors might return from foreign theaters of war but because its latency period was short and therefore drugs against the hidden, relapsing form of *vivax* malaria could be more quickly tested. Coatney noted this distinction and was using the Chesson strain in his prison studies by the winter of 1944–45.[35] This new strain of vivax malaria was a valuable research tool throughout the remainder of the U.S. program. With it, Alf Alving's group at Chicago showed that chloroquine was better than atabrine and quinine for treating acute *vivax* malaria and that the latency period for relapse was longer for chloroquine than for the other two drugs.[36]

Chloroquine and Public Health

Toward the end of 1944, with the military testing of chloroquine moving along, the board contemplated the field testing of chloroquine in civilian populations. Robert Loeb, chairman of the board, consulted Allan Gregg of Rockefeller's International Health Division, who referred him to IHD officers Lewis Hackett and George Strode. Hackett headed for Peru where he believed "controlled studies under American supervision" could be conducted.[37] Strode concurred. Shannon and Loeb, with the board's support, both pursued the matter with IHD. At this time, Rockefeller operatives had unique knowledge and infrastructure for public-health field testing, especially in civilian populations.[38] On 21 September 1944, the board had "agreed that a number of new anti-malarial drugs had reached the stage in their development which would make it essential that they be given wide-spread trial as therapeutic and suppressive agents." Furthermore, the board believed "that for very obvious reasons it was essential that one of these agents should be tried in a civilian population over a long period of observation in a hyperendemic area and that the drug should be used both as a suppressive and for the termination of acute attacks of malaria."[39] They wanted a study that would give information about the tolerability and ease of use of the new drugs—especially chloroquine—in comparison to atabrine. The Rockefeller IHD group in Peru and their superiors in New York were eager to pursue such studies and felt Peru offered some unique field-research opportunities.

　　The board and IHD worked closely together on the Peruvian tests. The IHD directed the study with the help and cooperation of the Peruvian Department of Health "including the full-time services of the Deputy Director General and Epidemiologist of the Malaria Service, Dr. Alberto Valderrama."[40] Through Shannon and Loeb, the board provided the protocol and advised on the project, while CMR provided the chloroquine and arranged its transport.

Dr. Osler L. Peterson was IHD's man in the field. Peterson, Valderrama, and three technicians conducted the clinical research.

Site selection and logistics in the field were not simple. Peterson reached Lima only in the first week of May 1945. His supply of chloroquine arrived two weeks later. "The opportunity to conduct a suppressive study under ideal conditions—blanket suppression throughout the season of active transmission with appropriate control groups—was therefore lost for this year." The malaria season on the west coast of Peru began in March and peaked in May. Nevertheless, Peterson and Valderrama proceeded with their study, selecting a site north of Lima in the Napeña Valley, the Hacienda San Jacinto. The hacienda's absentee owners, a British family, left their 4,000 acre sugar cane plantation in the care of a "British colonial with a life-long experience in plantation management." The hacienda was, "in fact, a small feudal state employing more than 500 laborers."[41] San Jacinto and two other, smaller villages housed many of these laborers. The hacienda and its workers had a number of characteristics that seemed favorable to the researchers:

In the latter part of May, the malaria rate was still very high at San Jacinto; 300–500 cases reporting for treatment each week. Drs. Peterson and Valderrama were received cordially and assured of all possible assistance and cooperation from the management. The population is conveniently centralized. Most of the laborers and their families live in a small village a few hundred yards from the hospital where the laboratory is situated, and from the headquarters of the malaria unit where the records are kept and the malaria staff housed. The children attend school in this village. In addition to this relatively stable population, a more or less continuous flow of contract labor enters the village from the non-malarious Sierras. These Indians arrive in groups of 20 to 50 and are housed in a large dormitory in the village. They remain a few months and are replaced by others from the Sierras. However, a number return year after year. They are exceedingly primitive, speak only Quechua (an unwritten Indian language) and are almost universally addicted to cocaine (coco leaves).[42]

CMR and IHD had found a compliant and stable civilian population in which to further explore chloroquine's abilities and foibles. As with much contemporary work on human subjects, the sources are silent on matters such as informed consent.

Peru yielded some good data with the promise of more to come. In August 1945, Robert Briggs Watson, MD, principal malariologist of the Tennessee Valley Authority, and George Carden Jr., MD, chief of the Division of Malaria of CMR, spent a week together in a Peru observing the IHD testing of chloroquine.[43] The study had begun in earnest on 11 June 1945, but the data that Carden and Watson saw on their visit were only "hurriedly assembled the night before our arrival." Some toxicity was observed with the drug—toxicity in excess of that seen in atabrine or placebos (aspirin or cascara, a natural laxative). The chloroquine dosage for suppressive therapy was 0.5 grams administered once a week. Overall, the researchers were surprised "that there have been no more severe or frequent evidences of toxicity, since the average weight of the adults receiving the drug is about 45 kilos [99 lbs.]."[44] The toxicity conclusions were favorable. From them, Carden and Watson inferred that chloroquine was safe, even at twice the effective dosage for suppression. They felt confident that "a dose of 0.25 gram once weekly or 0.5 gram every 10 to 15 days would give good suppression without the appearance of toxicity."[45] In comparison to house spraying with DDT, "efficient suppressive therapy certainly offers the most immediate solution to the plantation owner or government health officer, since it will tend to reduce or eliminate the reservoir of infected mosquitoes and in addition permit a population to remain free of clinical attacks during the period of active transmission."[46]

These civilian studies and the references to house spraying suggest that the board was actively interested in extending their military research into the broader public health arena. In September 1945, Osler Peterson wanted to continue the Peruvian studies, but the board was already on its way out. By the end of the month, the deadline for war work on malaria was clearly looming. As George Carden wrote to George Strode, seeking help from Rockefeller with ongoing research, "It has recently been settled that the O.S.R.D. malaria-research program will terminate on 30 June 1946 and Dr. Loeb has elected to dissolve the Board for the Coordination of Malarial Studies at the same time."[47] If malaria research in Peru and elsewhere were to continue, it would not be under OSRD auspices.

Chloroquine performed well and displayed no consistent or widespread side effects. The military's interest continued. According to CMR minutes from June 1945, Lieutenant Colonel O. R. McCoy reported that Army and Navy testing showed chloroquine was superior to atabrine, and that "extensive field tests" were underway overseas. McCoy felt that chloroquine "should be produced in large quantities." But the CMR minutes show that commercial suppliers of intermediates were unwilling to build additional manufacturing capacity without the reassurance of postwar demand. CMR itself was would not move forward unless expressly prompted by the Army surgeon general.[48] By the end of 1945, the board summarized two years of effort with chloroquine (SN-7618) as an "intensive exploration" in both animals and humans. This "included an evaluation of the activity of this compound in avian infections, a study of the pharmacology and toxicology in animals and man and finally of its potentialities as an antimalarial against *vivax* and *falciparum* infections in man." Human testing was categorized into two modes: first, "Extensive studies on its prophylactic activity against domestic and Southwest Pacific strains of *P. vivax* malaria, on its curative activity against sporozoite-induced infections when administered alone and in combination with other compounds, and its suppressive activity," and second, "Extensive investigation in Service installations of the potentialities of this drug for use in the termination of the acute attack and in the suppression of the disease."[49] Finally, the board summarized "fairly extensive" work on chloroquine's pharmacology in "mice, rats, dogs, monkeys, and man," primarily employing atabrine as a control. The board had successfully put chloroquine over many hurdles, but they were looking to get out of the game.

With the war over, OSRD was winding down and CMR had bad news for chloroquine enthusiasts. "OSRD cannot provide funds for the conversion and tableting of the 2000 lbs. of 4,7-dichloroquinoline into SN-7618 for testing by the Public Health Service and others." The committee requested that Dr. Rolla Dyer, director of NIH, seek IHD funds for the chemical conversion and final tableting.[50] And OSRD's lawyers sought to end the close cooperation with foreign programs "because of the opinion of the Legal Division of the OSRD to the effect that a gift of a lot of this drug cannot be made to Australia under existing laws."[51] Loeb, the board chairman, sought a way around this to little avail. The Australians were soon on their own. The board closed out its chloroquine work with a summary medical publication on the use of the new drug in *Journal of the American Medical Association*.[52]

Chloroquine was a drug developed and abandoned in Germany in the 1930s. But the German malaria researchers were not entirely inactive during the war. Two things stand out with regard to U.S. and German antimalarial efforts during World War II. First, the German development of sontochin led to renewed American interest in chloroquine. Without the capture of sontochin in the deserts of North Africa, the 4-aminoquinolines might have languished in the U.S. program. And secondly, conditions for conducting research in Germany grew progressively worse as the war ground on. Beyond conscription and new priorities arising out of war work, shortages of all kinds limited Walter Kikuth and his colleagues at Bayer. Two examples from postwar evaluations of Bayer suggest the degree of difficulty faced there. With regard to the use of *Plasmodium gallinaceum* in chicks—one of the U.S. program's most successful avian malaria models—Kikuth "pointed out that for the past few years it has been impossible to obtain chicks in large numbers in Germany and that even if they had been obtainable, it would have been impossible to obtain an adequate supply of feed."[53] U.S. researchers met similar difficulties, but they had direct access to a nationally mobilized and functioning war economy. When NIH's G. Robert Coatney had trouble getting his hands on chicks and chicken feed or Hopkins' E. K. Marshall needed ducks and duck feed, they had only to ask George Carden to take the matter to the War Food Administration.[54] In contrast, by the closing months of the war, the German scientists had difficulty just feeding themselves: "No work has been carried on in the laboratories at Elberfeld for approximately two months. Kikuth comes to his laboratory irregularly in order to carry on the cultures of various types of parasites with which he has been working. He says that at present it is impossible to carry on active experimental work because of undernourishment of himself and of his staff, because of the time required to maintain a garden to supplement the present rations, and because of the difficulty in obtaining the laboratory assistants, who see little point in working when their income is essentially useless as far as the purchase of food is concerned."[55] Though Bayer made significant contributions to malaria chemotherapy during the war, they did so only indirectly and in the face of great hardship.

Legacies

Along with the development of chloroquine, what were the larger implications of the antimalarial program? A Winthrop Chemical press release suggested at least one rhetorical use for the development of chloroquine: shameless propaganda. Winthrop's story of Aralen, their trade name for chloroquine, did not encompass the coordinating board's communitarian viewpoint: "While the same chemical formula lay dormant in Nazi laboratories, stifled by German regimentation, individual initiative, judgment and the production power of free enterprise in the United States has produced what is known as Aralen, a new potent drug for the war against malaria which afflicts 800,000,000 annually throughout the world, according Dr. Justus B. Rice, vice president in charge of medical research of the Winthrop Chemical Company, Inc." The Winthrop press release quoted Dr. Rice: "The keynote of the story, the fact that is putting the United States ahead of the rest of the world in the development of medicines and pharmaceutical preparations, is individual initiative and judgment." Winthrop and Rice gave credit for chloroquine first and foremost to the lone inventor, who happened also to be a Winthrop employee: "Unrestricted by government control, Dr. Alexander B. Surrey, young chemist on the Winthrop staff, began his own individual experiments on the particular chemical chain that eventuated in the synthesis of Aralen. . . . The same drug was in Nazi hands but its importance was overlooked."[56] According to Winthrop's public relations, individual initiative—in the corporate setting— outfoxed both Nazi regimentation and stifling government control. Others would take away different lessons from the wartime program.

Pearl Harbor and U.S. declarations of war had muted discussions about research freedom and administrative structures—debates begun before the war. Some, such as William H. Taliaferro of the University of Chicago, asserted that progress would be best served if specialists pursued their own lines of research unfettered by bureaucracy. Urging more fundamental research, "Dr. Taliaferro believed that there should be no attempt at regimenting research . . . but that individuals and organizations with special ability and equipment should attack phases of the problem for which they were best suited."[57] Research regimentation versus the individual pursuit of fundamental lines of research was part of broader public debate about the role of war and government in research. Warren Weaver, the director of the Natural Sciences Division of the Rockefeller Foundation, supported the case for unfettered intellectual pursuit. He wrote to the *New York Times* at the end of August 1945 to weigh in on matters of planning and science. Weaver accused the *Times* of supporting "the position that all science should be mapped out and the gaps discovered, and that an all-high, all-embracing central organization, presumably set up by the Federal Government, should plan and direct scientific activities." In Weaver's view, great gains in scientific understanding had been made "by free scientists, following their curiosities, their hunches, their special prejudices, their undefended like and dislikes." This was a contention with which William Taliaferro surely agreed. Weaver also gave a nod to the lone genius: "Free scientists—sometimes working in austere isolation to develop some deep and subtle ideas, sometimes choosing to work in closer contact with other scientists, sometimes electing to work in cooperative teams. But in any case, freely and voluntarily following the procedures that seem to them natural and desirable."[58] The debates continued, particularly with regard to the establishment of the National Science Foundation.[59] Indeed, these discussions lasted for years before the agency came together in the early 1950s.

Though William Mansfield Clark had described the antimalarial program as kaleidoscopic, characterized by much that was ad hoc, the progression of the research was viewed differently in other contexts. For example, a *New York Times* editorial on 13 April 1946, cited the new antimalarial drugs as "proof that war accelerates the progress of science and technology."[60] The key to this accomplishment was "organized research." The editorial concluded, "We have an example of what can be done when scientists work together. . . . Freedom of research is not incompatible with organization. When competent men work together in a common cause more progress can be made in five years than in fifty . . . by the haphazard method. The case of malaria proves it." A letter printed six days later, supporting the editorial and debunking the "Myth of the Lonely Scientist," put the case, if possible, more strongly, emphasizing "how highly organized investigations on a vast scale involving large groups of scientists working as teams, can substantially accelerate scientific progress."[61] Concluding that such scientific organization was a "Twentieth Century" method, the letter asserted that it was "surely preferable to the . . . hit-or-miss, jigsaw puzzle methods, so frequently characterized by waste, repetition, emphasis on the trivial, and the hasty publication of half-baked findings." In contrast, Clark was surely asserting the value of jigsaw puzzle methods when he wrote that "changes in organization were sufficiently kaleidoscopic to give the impression of an unstable pattern. Indeed, a person concerned only with the superficial aspects of organization might be tempted to use the record in support of the contention that a similar emergency in the future had best be handled by a predetermined body in accordance with a pre-formed plan. But this would be to misread the record. It is a record of research in which organizational matters were continually adjusted to meet the demands of scientific advances."[62] While the example of the antimalarial program did not end such debate, it was clearly and repeatedly invoked in the cause of increased scale and coordination in research efforts.[63]

With a surfeit of resources, the program had pursued malaria down many avenues in many disciplines. Faced with a choice between two research problems, it did both. Beyond drug screening and clinical investigation, it examined pharmacology, metabolism, microbiology, and even funded Michael

Heidelberger's unsuccessful malaria vaccine work (more on this in chapter 8).[64] From a drug-discovery standpoint, the program screened compounds at random *and* followed up rationally on lead compounds. These were value-laden choices. Some, such as E. K. Marshall, had valued a move away from random screening to more rational methods of discovery with regard to the testing and synthesis of novel compounds. The program's inclusive procliv-ity was manifested in many areas. It often embraced both the innovative and the routine. For example, some participants, by Clark's account, accorded lower status to routine work such as the development of dosage regimens for atabrine compared with the chemical synthesis of new compounds. In the atabrine area, researchers such as James Shannon, who also chaired the Clinical Panel, addressed questions such as the use and potential toxicity of atabrine, the major preventive/suppressive drug employed in the field. The work on atabrine, whatever its status relative to the search for new and bet-ter drugs, was one of the major practical—military—accomplishments of the wartime program, and, in fact, an area of innovation. Somewhat paradoxi-cally, the highly valued innovations in the synthesis of new compounds did not yield much in the way of clinical advances during the war. The NRC and CMR committees also labeled certain types of work routine. These were endeavors that they deemed less rational, less science-based, less innovative, or more repetitive. This reflected a scientific culture that valued innovation while having a more ambiguous valuation for routine investigations or even clinical research.

The antimalarial program met specific military and emergency goals in such a way as to produce the promise of more to come. For the narrowest military needs, Robert Coatney noted that the

cooperative wartime effort produced four important advances:

1. New and important data on the general biology of the disease;
2. Reliable methods for appraisal of antimalarial activity;
3. A better understanding of Atabrine, i.e., its worth, and its limitations;
4. Discovery of synthetic compounds better than Atabrine.[65]

Under number 4, atabrine's successor was, of course, chloroquine, the older drug's colorless, less-toxic cousin. Another improved compound was one related to plasmochin that showed promise of preventing relapse in vivax malaria: an 8-aminoquinoline, pentaquine (fig. 7.2). The project had screened its thousands of compounds—many synthesized for this purpose—for

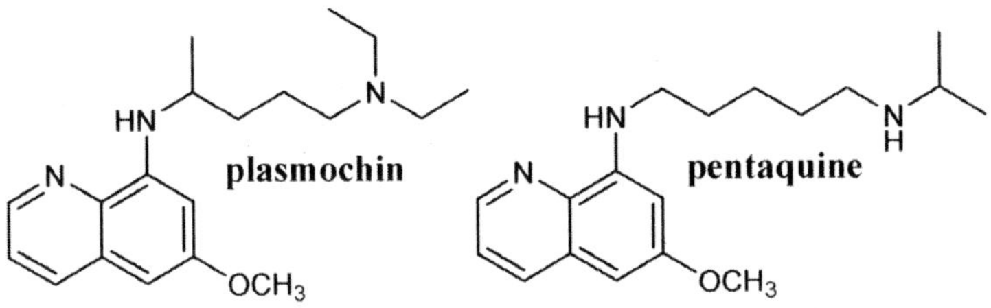

Figure 7.2   Pentaquine

antimalarial activity, and many of these had proceeded to further testing for toxicity and metabolic fate. In the end, however, the U.S. military had relied on atabrine throughout the war, with U.S. production in 1943 reaching an estimated 300 tons, or 2.5 billion tablets.[66]

Even after years of research, the project had not identified a new class of compound for the treatment of malaria, as the smaller British program had done with its development of Paludrine.[67] What NRC and CMR had done was to establish a large-scale, consistent process for testing compounds, keeping records, standardizing biological data, and establishing meaningful structure-activity relationships. Antimalarial research during World War II provided good value. From 1941 to 1947, the CMR spent a total of about $25 million, with malaria receiving $5.6 million.[68] As James Phinney Baxter III wrote in 1946, "During its existence the Committee expended some $24,000,000—a sum which would have supported our [U.S.] share in the war for only four hours—in approximately 600 contracts with 133 universities, foundations, and commercial firms."[69] From a strictly military perspective, medical research and development were also a success. World War II was the first major U.S. "conflict in which fewer of our troops died of disease than of battle injuries and wounds."[70] The manufacture and use of atabrine kept the total number of cases of malaria in the U.S. military below half a million: "Altogether, during the period of 1942–45, there were 494,299 cases of malaria, 410,7272 of these occurring overseas," with an estimated "8 to 9 million man-days" lost during this period.[71] The antimalarial program improved combat effectiveness and saved lives.

Beyond these practical wartime outcomes, Clark and his Survey staff, particularly Fred Wiselogle, left another legacy for postwar malaria workers: They published a massive summary of the program's findings. The board approved this endeavor, as it did not seem realistic to try and fit all their results into the standard literature. The Survey monograph contained all their data and methods, along with "a simple discussion of the general philosophy underlying the program."[72] A circular letter went out to all the contributors to allow the publication of all the data gathered. The responses were positive. A typical commercial response was this one from E. I. du Pont de Nemours and Company (Dupont), thanking Clark and Wiselogle for their efforts maintaining confidentiality: "We have been most gratified by the care exerted by the Survey Office under the guidance of Dr. Wiselogle in handling the large number of chemicals supplied by this Company. Because of the faith we have had in the operation of the Survey Office, we have felt free to supply any research samples that might in any way assist in this important undertaking. All in all we have found the collaboration a most happy one."[73] Having thanked the Survey for its care, the letter proceeded to grant them permission to publish all the data on the du Pont compounds. Within a year, the two-part, three-volume, 2,500-page atlas of factual material appeared under Wiselogle's editorship with the title *A Survey of Antimalarial Drugs, 1941–1945.*[74] It served to relieve the backlog of publishable findings that wartime secrecy had created and remains a fitting monument to the program's efforts.

In June 1946, with OSRD and CMR winding down operations, the Survey had a final party. Wiselogle sent Clark an invitation typed up as a fictitious entry on a data sheet from the Survey with the following data entered:

Amount submitted	70 kg.
Molecular formula	inhomogeneous; 6.25 % N.
Name	Dr. W. Mansfield Clark
Information available	

Your presence is requested at the Johns Hopkins Club, Ladies Wing (east entrance), Saturday, 29 June, 1946 at any time between 8:30 and 11 P.M. for assistance in the completion of the following program:

1. Disposition of remaining official rubber stamps.
2. Classification of all nonessential information.
3. Determination of physiological activity of SN 9,592.

The meeting will be most informal.[75]

On this data sheet, Clark himself was the material submitted, weighing in at 70 kilos and comprised, as we all are, of 6.25 percent nitrogen. SN-9592 was ethyl alcohol—the kind we drink—whose effect on the tired staff of the Survey would be tested that evening. Clark, however, could not make it to the party and sent Wiselogle his regrets: "I should like to smell the burning rubber stamps to see if they make more of a stink than my History did." Clark had had to cleanse his official history of all mention of his conflict with Richards. At his retreat in Lakeville, Connecticut, Clark was feeling a bit better. "As to testing SN 9,592 I need it not now that cool New England air is blowing away the Washingtonian fog. Indeed it might be said that I have run away and I hope that all of you can the same very soon."[76]

With the party and the program behind them, Frederick Wiselogle cited his own reasons for the publication of *A Survey of Antimalarial Drugs, 1941–1945*: "(1) to expedite the search for still better antimalarial drugs and (2) to serve as an established pattern for systematic chemotherapeutic studies of other infections."[77] Wiselogle was not alone. Because of the many medical successes, by war's end, leaders at OSRD and CMR saw a need for still more medical research. The promise of further success was there, and some still wanted to pursue it in the area of malaria research.

With the clock due to run out on CMR funding on 30 June 1946, a core of board members and others interested in continuing the wartime work met under NIH auspices. The Malaria Study Section convened on 3 June 1946. Present, among others, were Arthur Cope of the Panel on Synthesis; Clay G. Huff from Taliaferro's Chicago group; Robert Loeb, chairman of the coordinating board; E. K. Marshall of Johns Hopkins; Paul F. Russell of the Rockefeller Foundation; Captain James J. Sapero of the U.S. Navy and member of the board; Colonel Thomas Wayne of the U.S. Army; and G. Robert Coatney of the NIH. The chairman of the study section was James A. Shannon, who had run clinical and pharmacological endeavors for the program.[78] Shannon introduced Rolla E. Dyer, director of NIH, to the group, and Dyer in turn explained how the NIH study sections and their grants-in-aid worked. NIH was poised to grow exponentially as a funder of biomedical research during the postwar period. At Shannon's request, Sapero also explained how the similar navy research grants worked. The navy would become a critical bridge for research funding in the postwar years, notably through the Office of Naval Research, with Rockefeller's Warren Weaver chairing its Naval Research Advisory Committee.[79] Wayne, the Army's representative, explained that the army's research efforts would be funded through its Epidemiological Board and that "the set-up would probably be very much like that outlined by Doctor Dyer for the Public Health Service and by Capt. Sapero for the Navy." Sapero, in turn, "suggested that there should be a group to act as a clearing house for the interchange of information on malaria inasmuch as the three Services all expect to foster work in the field." Shannon appointed Coatney, Sapero, and Wayne to a committee charged with "giving a concrete proposal as to how a clearing house for malaria might be set up." To all appearances, this meeting seemed to recapture the early days of the wartime program.

With an uncanny air of recapitulation, the "discussion then turned to the freedom of research by the individual investigator. It was the feeling that some group should attempt to judge the products of research and give some direction." [80] These were some of the same concerns aired in the earliest days of the wartime programs. Sapero sought to enroll the study section in a nonbinding advisory capacity for the navy. Following a "general feeling that a decision could not be made at this time," the possibility of establishing a survey office at NIH "was discussed at some length." The meeting gradually moved on to detailed discussion of chemotherapy and new facilities for the testing of antimalarials in prison populations, specifically ongoing research at Alf Alving's Chicago prison project and Coatney's new facility at Seagoville, Texas. Before adjourning, the section discussed and voted on five proposals. Four were approved for NIH funding, and one was rejected. The section would continue through 1948. In this year, infectious disease research at NIH would be reorganized into the new National Microbiological Institute (later the National Institute for Allergy and Infectious Disease), and Shannon would come to NIH full time as head of the new National Heart Institute.

Beyond drawing such leading lights as James Shannon to the NIH, what was the antimalarial program's role in connecting prewar biomedicine to postwar biomedicine? And how did its innovations carry forward? While the deterministic rise of today's biomedical research institutions could not be known from state of the malaria research in 1946, it was a building block of the postwar landscape. The wartime program grew in a specific historical context with particular resources and constraints. Its successes and failures, its innovations and discoveries, and its plans and organizations altered the possibilities, resources, and constraints facing future biomedical programs. Certainly, all malaria workers in the United States in 1939, and many outside these communities, were aware of the work of Roehl and coworkers on plasmochin and atabrine, just as they were aware of and in many cases participated in the malaria control efforts of the Rockefeller Foundation. When war in Asia and Europe brought new urgency to the malaria problem, these modes of research—Bayer's centralized, innovative, industrial-cum-academic-consulting, and Rockefeller's mix of centralized institutes with external academic and industrial partners—were the natural starting points for the scaling up of research efforts. Neither Bayer nor Rockefeller—nor even Clark's beloved National Research Council—needed to be a direct model, merely transcribed by government bureaucrats. All were among the resources—scientific and institutional—that illustrated the possibilities and combinations that kaleidoscopically might form new postwar research models.

For all these programs—before, during, and after the war—interconnectedness mattered. More important than the source of funds were the relationships that existed between different researchers, laboratories, and disciplines. Clark and others had to extend the preexisting networks—as a consciously controlled medium and not as a spontaneous outgrowth of individual interactions—to hundreds of workers in spite of the draft and wartime labor market. The key to their success lay in the building of trust that Clark had pointed to: "There was good will on both sides, and its maintenance was essential."[81] Against this was the model of the independent researcher: William Taliaferro, for example, could receive Rockefeller funding for decades so long as he published good work in the program area, yet he did not want a committee to oversee—to administer—his work. The committee may have been comprised of experts, but he was the expert in the subdiscipline of his specific problem, and he desired to steer his work independently. Clark's reference to the need for committees to occasionally engage in administration was one key to a new mode of research. The growth of research laboratories in the pharmaceutical industry during the postwar period is an example of the growth of research administration. The consultation and exchange networks of the 1930s and early 1940s were not equivalent to the mandated coordination and administration that emerged late in the war.

After 1945, the military and the Public Health Service sought to build on wartime investments. The management and administration of science changed during the war. The scale of projects—in dollars, in hours worked, in disciplinary contributions—grew, and proper communication and the distribution of information supported this change in administration and scale. These innovations—communication between disciplines and across large networks of academic, government, and industrial workers—were the sine qua non of postwar biomedicine, and the antimalarial program was a nexus for the successful deployment of these resources. This successful process would become a model for biomedical research and drug discovery in the postwar period. The final form(s) of the antimalarial program did not emerge in a controlled and planned manner but as an evolution in response to military needs and scientific and technological capabilities. The program was a crossroads for essential elements of scientific research traditions and for organizational and pharmacological innovation. It was also the foundation for all malaria work after the war.

Chapter 8

Lessons Learned

In November 1945, Paul F. Russell, a Rockefeller malariologist who had spent much of the war in the U.S. Army Medical Corps, addressed the annual meeting of the American Society of Tropical Medicine. He began with a lament for the horror and loss of war and a tribute to what had been done to advance science, technology, and medicine, especially with regard to malaria: "Man's net losses from World War II are so enormous that it would be illogical indeed to refer to war-produced scientific advances as dividends or to point to them with thoughtless pride. Rather, such progress constitutes salvage which, to be sure, sometimes has considerable value because conditions of war while they rarely permit classical research do present an urgency which demands, and often obtains, quick answers to difficult problems. New lessons are learned and others re-learned, painfully and at great expense." New lessons learned, and old lessons relearned: a common refrain for those who have worked on malaria. Russell concluded his address to the society with optimistic words: "One may reasonably hope that, with suitable organization, malaria will be eradicated from the United States within the next decade, and that in many tropical areas, even though economically depressed, this disease, now of the greatest importance, may become in the next half century one of the least of public health problems."[1] Read some sixty years later these words prompt two responses. For the United States, malaria was nearly eradicated even as Russell spoke.[2] For the developing world, in harsh contrast, malaria remains one of the greatest public health problems. If the destruction of malaria throughout the world remains before us, what is the deeper legacy of the wartime work?

The U.S. antimalarial program left legacies in three areas: malaria chemotherapy, general biomedical research, and the ongoing need to seek new and creative ways to attack malaria. First and most obviously, the treatment and control of malaria changed with the introduction of chloroquine and several other drugs immediately following the war. And subsequent years saw a number of additional drugs developed, some emerging from leads that wartime researchers had pursued, others emerging from natural products chemistry. Beyond the specific locus of malaria research, the program shaped researchers and altered expectations about what biomedical research could do and how it might be organized and funded.[3] The public and private debates discussed in the previous chapters point up these changed expectations among those who lived through the war and participated in OSRD projects.[4] Malaria has once more emerged into the public consciousness in the developed world during the last decade of the twentieth century. Global advocates for public health and funders of public health investigations and interventions, such as the World Health Organization (WHO) and the Bill and Melinda Gates Foundation, have raised the call for new research into this age-old scourge.

Antimalarials after 1945

Antimalarial research, rooted in the wartime project, continued in the postwar period. The Committee on Medical Research clearly saw two drugs—both developed under CMR contracts—as significant contributions: pentaquine (SN-13276) and chloroquine (SN-7618).[5] Wartime antimalarial drugs and research methods continued and evolved. For example, G. Robert Coatney's group at NIH's National Microbiological Institute continued to screen thousands of compounds against *P. gallinaceum* (chicken malaria).[6] By the 1950s, such avian malarias began a rapid decline as laboratory materials.[7] In the second half of the twentieth century, rodent malarias—especially *Plasmodium berghei,* discovered in 1948—became the dominant research models. Capable of infecting mice and rats, rodent malaria could in principle be extrapolated to simian models and thence to human disease.[8] Of course, other new technologies in biomedicine impacted malariology as well. New microscopic techniques, advances in immunology, and the rise of molecular biology all yielded new tools for infectious disease research.

Chemists continued to innovate even as the importance of malaria research in the United States diminished and attention turned to chronic disease research in areas such as heart disease and cancer. New malaria drugs attacked the previously hidden form of *vivax* malaria. Wartime pentaquine, as we will see, led to primaquine, which killed the newly discovered liver stage of *Plasmodium vivax* and helped to prevent relapse in *vivax* malaria. Even by the early 1950s, with the experience of treating malaria during the Korean War behind them and the novel drug pyrimethamine in hand, Robert Coatney and his NIH collaborators seemed quite sanguine: "It seems likely, however, that satisfactory measures are now at hand for suppression, treatment, and cure of all human malarias. This remarkably favorable position of malaria therapy is in marked contrast to the uncertainty of pre–World War II. It is a tribute to all who took part in the OSRD and postwar malaria researches."[9] Pyrimethamine was a modification of proguanil (also called Paludrine or chlorguanide), the drug developed by the British wartime program. Clever chemical thinking led to its evolution: George Hitchings of Wellcome Research Laboratories in New York State thought that proguanil was active in a cyclic form. This insight led to pyrimethamine, which contained two cyclic structures (fig. 8.1).[10] Indeed, the promise of chloroquine, primaquine, and pyrimethamine—alongside DDT—inspired new, dramatic plans.

In 1955, the World Health Organization convened a conference and decided that the time was at hand to eradicate malaria throughout the world. Chloroquine and DDT were the cornerstones of the global malaria eradication campaign that was outlined by the WHO Expert Committee on Malaria in 1957.[11] Among the suggestions endorsed by the committee was the use of chloroquine in salt—much as one might find iodine in table salt today. Mario Pinotti, director of the Brazilian National Malaria Service, had pioneered chloroquinized salt in Brazil during the early 1950s, but already by the late fifties he was finding lower than the targeted dose (45 milligrams of chloroquine base) being achieved in all cases. In spite of—or perhaps because of—the mass production and distribution of chloroquine, these subtherapeutic

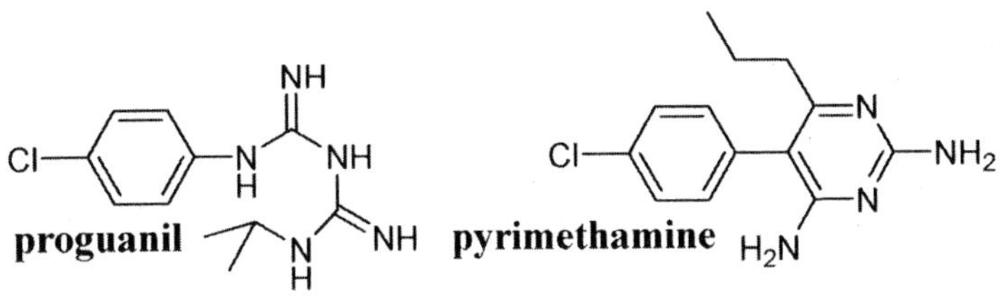

Figure 8.1 Proguanil shown curled around on itself to highlight its structural similarity to cyclic pyrimethamine

doses of the drug were widespread in subject populations. By 1959, WHO was receiving reports of tolerance of, or resistance to, chloroquine and other antimalarials. In northern Nigeria, in the Upper Volta region of Western Africa, in western Venezuela, *P. falciparum* was surviving the drugs. In 1961, two Americans returned from Colombia with a *falciparum* strain that was resistant to chloroquine, amodiaquine, and hydroxychloroquine.

By this time, chloroquinized salt was being used throughout the Amazon region of Brazil, and pilot projects were springing up across the tropics from Guyana to Ghana to New Guinea. The scale of chloroquine use was vast. For example, in 1961, the U.S. International Cooperation Administration (ICA)— the forerunner of the U.S. Agency of International Development (USAID)— provided Brazil with more than 180,000 pounds of chloroquine for use in salt. This was in addition to the 75.5 million chloroquine tablets that the ICA distributed worldwide that year. Chloroquine was being consumed around the world on a massive scale, and the parasites were adapting. Then in 1962, Rachel Carson published her famous attack on chemical insecticides, *Silent Spring*, and DDT became increasingly suspect. By 1966, resistance—in the biological, social, and political sense—was growing, but WHO's Eradication Campaign was pushing harder than ever on the mass distribution and use of chloroquine and other antimalarials: "In some parts of the world with intense and perennial transmission, drugs must be administered on a mass basis, together with the application of residual insecticides, in order to interrupt transmission. Here, chemotherapy must form an essential weapon throughout the attack phase."[12] By the mid-1960s, chloroquine-resistant malaria had emerged in more than one place and was spreading rapidly.

Chloroquine soon seemed less than miraculous, and the foundations of WHO's ill-conceived and ill-fated global malaria eradication campaign were crumbling. Though it remains in use today, chloroquine's efficacy has been severely limited by the rise of drug-resistant strains of malaria. The resilience of malaria parasites in the face of new science and new technology has been remarkable. Wallace Peters of the Liverpool School of Tropical Medicine wrote in 1970, "As biological techniques have developed over the last decades . . . [the] malaria parasite has grown in our minds from the small dot in a red cell on a crudely stained blood film into a complex biological unit with its own highly evolved ultrastructural features, biochemical peculiarities, and remarkable capacity for survival against heavy chemotherapeutic odds. . . . It has been said that the one lesson man learns from history is that he never learns from his mistakes. The history of chemotherapy and drug resistance contains many lessons."[13] Wallace, like Paul Russell before him, saw that the old lessons must be repeatedly relearned. Living creatures, be they protozoans or insects, can and will adapt.

Resistance to drugs in the human bloodstream—to toxins in their natural environment—is one form of adaptation at which malaria parasites have proven adept. And knowledge of the ability of microorganisms to evolve resistance is as old as chemotherapy itself. Paul Ehrlich suggested in 1907, the same year he coined the term chemotherapy, that the use of single agents at subcritical doses would lead to drug-resistant organisms:

> The importance of combined treatment is shown, lastly, in the phenomena of resistance already discussed. The fact that by frequently repeated administration of not completely sterilising doses, there is gradually acquired a resistance to the substance in question, makes it especially desirable that the first onslaught should be as complete as possible. This object, from what I have previously said, may probably best be achieved by a suitable combination of substances. I would like here to call your attention to the fact that two decades ago I discovered a considerable efficacy of methylene blue against certain forms of malaria. This dye had not, however, obtained any extensive employment, since its effect is inferior to that of quinine. On the ground of our recent experience one would, I think, be perfectly justified in attempting to reinforce the attack on the malaria parasites by employing combined doses of quinine and methylene blue.[14]

In many infectious diseases, the use of single-agent therapeutics has rapidly produced resistance. And when another drug is tried after one fails, multidrug-resistant organisms evolve. This is true today for the three biggest killers among infectious disease: HIV/AIDS, tuberculosis, and, of course, malaria. In each case, the use of so-called drug cocktails came only after resistance to one or more drugs had already arisen.[15] With the lessons of combination drug therapy forgotten, chloroquine, miracle drug or not, was seemingly doomed from the beginning.

Drug resistance and war in malarial regions such as Korea and Vietnam kept antimalarial drug discovery moving forward, if at a less frantic pace than during World War II. Behind much of the U.S. military's continued pursuit of malaria in the postwar period was the Armed Forces Epidemiologic Board.[16] Though chloroquine was the dominant drug into the 1960s, other novel antimalarials had their roots in the active series and lead compounds

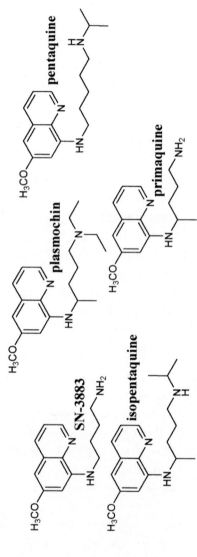

Figure 8.2 Some 8-aminoquinolines, illustrating the structural similarities of later drugs to plasmochin

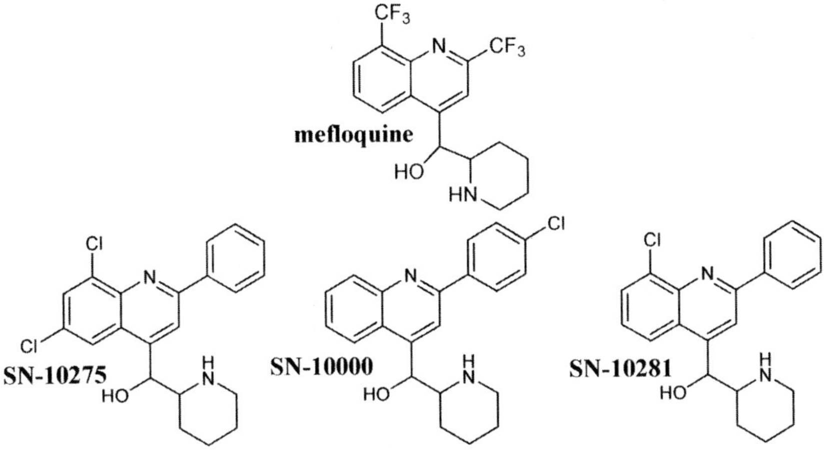

Figure 8.3 Mefloquine, above, and some of its chemical cousins from the wartime program

identified during the war. In the 8-aminoquinoline series, plasmochin itself (SN-971) led to a series of related compounds, from which primaquine (SN-13272) emerged during the Korean War as a drug of choice (fig. 8.2).[17] In the 1970s, mefloquine (Larium, Mephaquine) emerged from a large-scale antimalarial project based at the Walter Reed Army Institute of Research in Washington, DC. Mefloquine, too, had chemical relatives in the Survey data (fig. 8.3).[18] And today's Malarone is a combination of atovaquone (BW-566c) and the older British drug Paludrine (SN-12837, proguanil).[19] Atovaquone is a naphthoquinone, a chemical series well explored during the war, most notably by Louis Fieser at Harvard.[20] Fieser had argued for further clinical testing of the naphthoquinone series, but he made little progress against James Shannon's and Robert Loeb's concerns over toxicity.[21] In the end, the series had to wait for others to take it up again (fig. 8.4). The sulfa drugs, cousins of Promin and other compounds on which Lowell Coggeshall worked in the late 1930s and 1940s (see chapter 4),[22] remain a standard part of antimalarial chemotherapy, sulfadoxine being the most prominent.[23] Against malaria, the sulfas are most often used in combination with other drugs (fig. 8.5).

One major new class of drugs did not emerge from synthetic work but from traditional Chinese medicine. Qinghaosu, or artemisinin, is the active principle found in the plant *Artemisia annua L.*, whose use in China extends back to the second century B.C.E. (fig. 8.6). Starting from this lead, synthetic

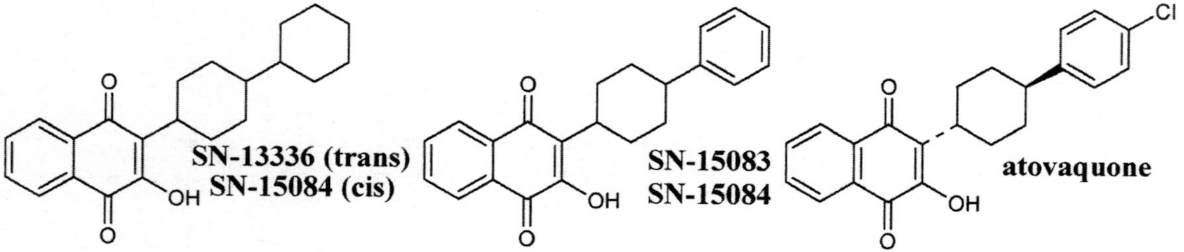

Figure 8.4 Some naphthoquinones from the wartime program and the more recent atovaquone

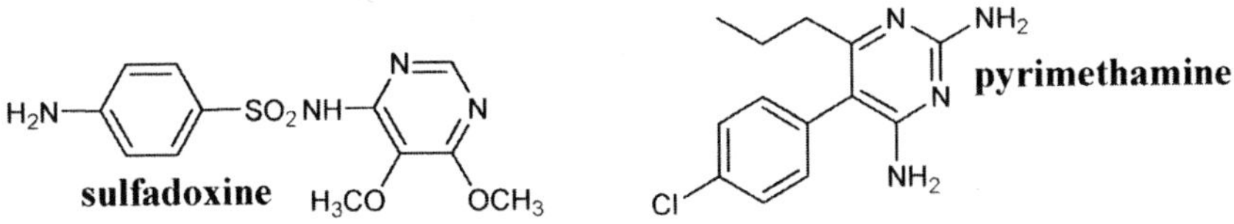

Figure 8.5 Sulfadoxine and pyrimethamine form a combination antimalarial drug known as SP.

chemists have sought to improve the activity and bioavailability of compounds in this series.[24] In many ways, the artemisinin story parallels that of malaria chemotherapy's other famous natural product, quinine. The use of artemisinin is growing, with the encouragement of WHO. In its problems and its promise, one can hear echoes from the nineteenth century: the *Economist* magazine in 2004 might well have been citing August Hofmann's words of 1849, when they wrote, "But the great hope is to find a way of synthesising artemisinin in the laboratory, thereby freeing drugmakers from the vagaries of nature."[25] Hofmann, you might recall from chapter 1, wrote about quinine, "Everybody must admit that the discovery of a simple process for preparing artificially the febrifuge principle of the Cinchona-bark, would confer a real blessing upon humanity."[26] These twenty-first-century reporters remind us of Clements Markham's nineteenth-century declarations when they write, "The WHO is also keen to see *Artemisia* farmed elsewhere in the world. There are pilot projects to do this in Tanzania, Kenya, and Mozambique." Markham, who established economically questionable cinchona plantations in Indian and Ceylon, wrote in 1862, "For these reasons the incalculable importance of introducing the chinchona-plant into other countries adapted for its growth, and thus escaping from entire dependence on the South American forests, has long occupied the attention of scientific men in Europe."[27] Such parallels do little to quell fears of malaria's continued scourge. Paul Russell may have

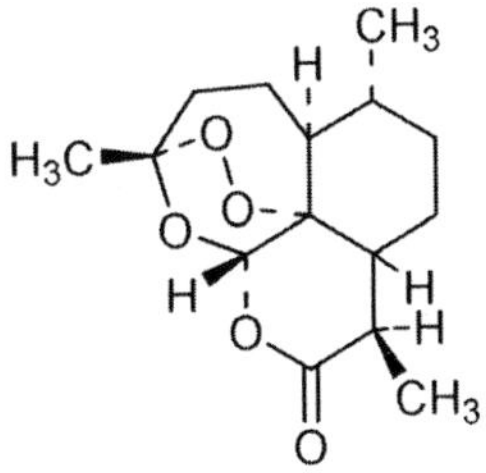

Figure 8.6 Artemisinin

been right that "new lessons are learned and others re-learned, painfully and at great expense." Indeed, today preserving the efficacy of artemisinin antimalarials remains a struggle as many drug makers in China and elsewhere continue to produce single-drug medicines and not the combination pills recommended by the WHO's public health experts.[28]

Scientifically and clinically, the wartime program's legacy extended beyond chemotherapy and pharmacology to parasite biology, animal models of the disease, and the immunology of malaria. As part of the wartime reorganization of science and industry, the program also contributed to organizational shifts in biomedical R&D.

Biomedical Research after 1945

Beyond malaria and after the war, the antimalarial program during World War II contributed to the building of new research structures for the organization and funding of biomedicine. These structures shared at the very least the malaria project's properties of rapid growth and large scale. The postwar growth of the National Institutes of Health under James Shannon was a prime example. Many of the NIH institutes followed the antimalarial program's model of taking a wide-ranging, interdisciplinary approach to a narrowly defined disease area. The combination of university- and government-based researchers paralleled NIH's mixture of extramural and intramural research. One obvious distinction between OSRD and NIH programs was OSRD's use of research *contracts*, while NIH primarily employed research *grants* in its extramural programs and investigator-driven projects within the intramural program.[29] This was a difference, perhaps, of pull versus push in research funding. Some might suggest that there are significant distinctions between these forms of funding, but the circulation of experts between review committees, grant-making agencies, and universities, as well the tight communities of interest created by members of disciplines and subdisciplines, suggests that these differences are largely cosmetic. The antimalarial research program offered ample illustration of this during the war, with members of various committees being the recipients of government contracts while still offering and making decisions on new areas of research and the extension of existing studies. That this regime continued in the postwar period is supported by the comments of scientist and historian Richard Lewontin: "While the NSF [National Science Foundation] and the extramural programs of the NIH were still in their initial stages, the Atomic Energy Commission (AEC), the Office of Naval Research (ONR), and similar agencies were funding research in universities and university research institutes by a system of contracts. The term 'contract,' conveying the notion of the procurement of a determined product specified by the purchaser, hides the reality. The 'contracts' with academic institutions were, in fact, grants to individual investigators or small groups to carry out research projects generated by intellectual forces internal to the disciplines, provided only that some general relevance to the mission of the federal agency could be established."[30] Funding mechanisms aside, the large-scale, interdisciplinary, disease-based programs of NIH were in part expressly modeled on the wartime malaria program.

James A. Shannon was one substantial connection between the wartime regime and subsequent organizations, but he was not alone. It will be remembered that Shannon was the wartime malaria researcher who oversaw the program's clinical investigations and who went on to become director of NIH. Shannon first came to work in Bethesda in 1948, as director of the National Heart Institute. He was associate director of NIH from 1952 to 1955 and director from 1955 to 1968. Shannon, speaking about his NIH recruitment by Rolla E. Dyer (director, 1942–1950) and Norman H. Topping (associate director, 1948–1952), mentioned that Dyer was director of NIH by war's end, "but more importantly, he was a member of the Committee on Medical Research which was A. N. Richards' committee for the management of American Science for the military during World War II."[31] Dyer was well placed to appreciate Shannon's malaria work. His previous post was head of the Division Infectious Diseases at NIH, a division that included the Malaria Office.[32] In Shannon's words, Dyer and Topping "knew that the wartime enterprises had been outstandingly successful, despite the complexity and breadth of the program. They felt that the Goldwater enterprises [where Shannon had conducted his malaria work] which were sprung up and were developed in a very short period of time, was precisely the thing they wanted done at the new NIH—the post-war NIH."[33] During Shannon's time at NIH, its annual appropriations grew from tens of millions to more than a billion dollars.[34]

More narrowly, historians and scientists have often cited the large-scale screening of compounds collected from many sources, which characterized a major segment of the antimalarial program, as a model for the cancer chemotherapy program established at the National Cancer Institute (NCI) in the postwar years.[35] Charles Gordon Zubrod, a major contributor at NCI, had spent the war working with Shannon on the chemotherapy of human malaria at Goldwater Memorial Hospital. Zubrod's successful career in research and administration included a stint with E. K. Marshall at Hopkins (1947–1953) and many years at NCI, where he held a number of positions.[36] Likewise,

Robert W. Berliner was part of Shannon's malaria team and an early postwar NIH hire, joining Shannon there in 1950. Berliner served in a number of positions including NIH deputy director for science. He left NIH in 1973 to become dean of the Yale School of Medicine. As it was for hundreds of other "wartime malariologists," the malaria chemotherapy program was formative in the careers of Shannon, Zubrod, and Berliner.

Outside of NIH, Shannon, Berliner, and others also had an impact. Extramural research grew and medical research and education evolved. Like his NIH colleagues, Lowell T. Coggeshall went on to eminence after his wartime malaria work. Unlike them, he had been a malariologist before the war, but in the postwar years he was widely influential leader in medical education. He held a number of posts at the University of Chicago from which he leveraged his wartime experience. Most publicly visible was his work with the Association of American Medical Colleges and in particular its 1965 report, *Planning for Medical Progress through Education.*[37] Like many who conducted wartime research, Coggeshall was ready to address the opportunities and problems associated with the growing role of the federal government—especially NIH—in the funding and structure of postwar biomedical research. Knowing the value and potential of biomedical research, Coggeshall successfully advocated a growing role for research in medical education and institutions.

The program's impact extended from NIH to medical schools to the postwar boom in drug discovery. Pharmaceutical development in many therapeutic areas helped to define biomedical research after the war. Major screening programs for new leads and drugs, often distributed to multiple locations and institutions, were a part of the biomedical landscape in antibiotics, anti-cancer drugs, antihistamines, tranquilizers, and even further antimalarial research.[38] Beyond academe and the federal government, the antimalarial program resonated with the rapid growth in the U.S. pharmaceutical industry in the postwar years. The U.S. antimalarial program contained organizational and technological dimensions not necessarily associated with centralized R&D in industrial settings.[39] The program, being multicentered rather than contained in a single facility, showed manifold characteristics. Transmitted through wartime work and displaced across the ocean, these developments can be viewed as continuous with programs like Bayer's interwar antimalarial work. The possibilities for biomedical research in the pharmaceutical industry were certainly impacted by the wartime program. In 1965, while testifying before Congress, James Shannon, then NIH director, characterized the industrial approach as one in which one undertook the search for therapeutic agents without first fully understanding "the mechanisms we are trying to interfere with." Nevertheless, this approach had yielded antibiotics, antihistamines, blood-pressure agents, and tranquilizers, all products of industrial, pharmaceutical research in the postwar period.[40] Redolent of William Mansfield Clark's characterization of one wartime approach as "extreme empiricism,"[41] this was the research tradition of Paul Ehrlich, Wilhelm Roehl, and their corporate sponsors. The malaria program had coupled a major, routinized screening process to more scattered investigations of basic parasite biology, immunology, clinical investigations, and more. This was the shape of biomedical research in the pharmaceutical industry.

In 1957, Kenneth M. Endicott, chief of the Cancer Chemotherapy National Service Center of the NCI, wrote, "It has been possible to bring together the pharmaceutical industry, research organizations, private investigators, and the United States Government, each contributing their varied skills and resources to implement an effective cooperative national program."[42] With these words, Endicott concluded a summary of the accomplishments of the cancer chemotherapy program, but he could have been writing about the malaria program that had ended a decade earlier. These categories—the pharmaceutical industry, research organizations, private investigators, and the U.S. government—echo those mobilized by the earlier program. As mentioned above, an important aspect of the antimalarial research was its distributed nature. This arose from three reinforcing causes. Malaria and tropical medicine have traditionally been distributed research areas because of the geographic divide between the prevalence of disease in the tropics and the laboratories and institutions of Europe and America—a divide defined early on by center and periphery, with a few notable exceptions such as Italy, where patients and research were proximal. Compounding latitude and climate were the frequent divides between the clinic and laboratory, between human subjects and animal models, and between patients and pharmaceutical production. These factors created the need for multicenter or multidisciplinary research programs.

During World War II, the Office of Emergency Management and OSRD had to find research expertise and infrastructure wherever they existed and put them to use. Thus, the U.S. antimalarial program was a distributed project—distributed over hundreds of laboratories, firms, and individuals. This sort of networking of expertise was in principle much like that described by the historians Louis Galambos and Jane Eliot Sewell in their work on vaccine development in the twentieth century.[43] In this regard, the antimalarial program was typical of—and contributed to—broader trends in the expanding pharmaceutical industry. The productive flow of personnel, materials, and information from NGOs (for example, NRC, Rockefeller, Gorgas Memorial Hospital), universities (for example, Hopkins, Harvard, Columbia), companies (for example, Lederle Laboratories, Parke Davis, Winthrop Chemical), and governmental organizations (for example, Goldwater Memorial Hospital, NIH, U.S. Army) did not happen easily despite the urgency of the national emergency. Yet it did happen, facilitated by $5.6 million of U.S. government money, and Rockefeller and NRC networks of experts and collaborators. These accomplishments and shortcomings have resonance even into the twenty-first century.

Malaria Today

While malaria in the developed world all but vanished in the second half of the twentieth century, it continued to kill millions in the developing world. Even today, malaria kills millions every year, mostly children in sub-Saharan Africa. Yet the diseases of rich countries, such as heart disease, stroke, and cancer, had pushed malaria off the list of research priorities. New initiatives have put malaria back on track as a major research area, but so far the biomedical research structures of the second half of the twentieth century—whether in the form of NGOs, the state-sponsored NIH, private pharmaceutical companies, or the World Health Organization—have failed to overcome the deadly and debilitating burden of malaria. New tools such as molecular genetics, old and relatively expensive tools such as chemotherapy, and even much improved tools such as vaccines have only just preserved the ability of elites and military personnel to maintain health in a large portion of the world, especially much of sub-Saharan Africa and the tropics; the twentieth century saw little improvement for the majority of people who live in endemic or hyperendemic areas. For those living on a few dollars a day, drugs and bed nets can pose severe economic hardships. With so much still to be done, novel structures have begun to emerge: new philanthropic enterprises, new initiatives, and new ways to mobilize capital for the betterment of the poor.

  With DDT and chloroquine failing in the 1960s, malaria vaccines emerged as the next silver bullet.[44] The possibility of finding a vaccine against the disease was a major contributor to a decline in other areas of research such as chemotherapy and public health monitoring. Malaria vaccine work began in earnest in the 1970s.[45] Here, too, wartime work provided a foundation for future R&D. The CMR funded Michael Heidelberger's attempts to develop a malaria vaccine in humans: Heidelberger, working at Columbia University, had collaborated during the war with Alf Alving's group at Chicago. Heidelberger was an organic chemist and "founding father" of immunochemistry, who had previously worked with dyes and pneumococcus. Alving ran the CMR-funded prisoner volunteer program at Illinois' Stateville penitentiary. Heidelberger was not alone in his attempts to mobilize the body's immune system against malaria. Several other groups conducted significant vaccine work during the 1940s.[46] Among them were Paul Russell's collaborative work in India, funded by Rockefeller's IHD;[47] Jules Freund's group[48] at New York City's health department laboratories, funded by the John and Mary R. Markle Foundation;[49] and William and Lucy Taliaferros' Chicago group, especially their collaborator Wendell D. Gingrich.[50] Ducks, chickens, and monkeys were all successfully immunized against various malarial parasites, but none of these findings could be translated into humans. Heidelberger's results were uniformly negative: Vaccinated prisoners challenged with malaria displayed no resistance.[51] His findings were some of the only published work on human malaria vaccines between World War II and the 1970s, when interest shifted from chemotherapy to vaccines. Vaccine development, by this time a distinct area of research often distant from chemotherapy, seemed an attractive alternative to public health crusaders at international agencies such as WHO and U.S. AID. Perpetually just around the corner throughout the 1970s, 1980s, and 1990s, a safe and effective vaccine for malaria remains elusive.

As a demand for new thinking and resources, malaria is, unfortunately, not alone as cause of death and human misery. In our century, malaria shares the infamous title of most deadly infectious disease with a newcomer, HIV/AIDS, and an older disease returned with new virulence, tuberculosis, often in a multidrug-resistant form. Pneumococcus, hepatitis B, influenza, and measles are among the other pathogens that dominate the list of most deadly infectious diseases. Many disease-causing organisms that we like to fear, such as West Nile virus, the spirochete of Lyme disease, and the Ebola virus, are as yet either so rare or so benign that they do not merit a place in this grim ranking. Thinking globally, the great cost is from the big three: malaria, HIV/AIDS, and tubuculosis.[52] The poverty that often accompanies these makes it difficult to be precise about how many are killed or made sick, but tuberculosis may infect as many as two billion people worldwide—a third of the human race—and it kills millions every year. HIV afflicts tens of millions today and may kill even more than tuberculosis. The social stigma of HIV/AIDS still leads to underreporting, undertesting, and undertreating.

The human immunodeficiency virus that causes AIDS attacks the immune system, opening its victim to all sorts of infections. And these three killers may share other debilitating and lethal synergies. HIV/AIDS, tuberculosis, and malaria have all developed multidrug-resistant strains. Still more tragically, malaria and tuberculosis are both treatable diseases, despite the rise of drug-resistant strains. Resources, not knowledge, are the critical input that is lacking.

In the closing years of the twentieth century, malaria once again became a major subject for biomedical research in the developed world. In the area of direct chemotherapeutic intervention, a first mover was the pharmaceutical giant Glaxo Wellcome, with their Malarone donation program begun in 1996. Glaxo Wellcome launched an initiative to donate its highly effective but relatively expensive combination drug, Malarone, across Africa. Glaxo Wellcome's intent was to provide a low-cost chemotherapeutic intervention for patients suffering from acute falciparum malaria.[53] Such corporate generosity was not without many pitfalls.[54] As GlaxoSmithKline's (Glaxo Wellcome's post-merger successor) 2001 annual report noted, "In July 2001, it was announced that the Malarone Donation Programme, established in 1997, would end in September 2001 upon completion of the pilot phase. The donation programme proved not to be an efficient and effective use of resources to achieve the objective of reducing suffering and death from malaria."[55] The complexities of public health delivery stymied their good corporate intentions, though GSK continues to participate in other programs to alleviate the burden of malaria among the world's poor.

Others—such as the Bill and Melinda Gates Foundation, the Malaria Vaccine Initiative, Medicines for Malaria Venture, and the Malaria Research Institute—entered the fray in the late 1990s. At the center of all these initiatives is WHO's Roll Back Malaria (RBM). In 1998, Dr. Gro Harlem Brundtland, director general of WHO, launched RBM, intending to "reduce the malaria morbidity by 50% and to reduce the mortality by 75% of the levels in 2000 by the year 2010."[56] RBM nestles comfortably within the goals of a broader program, the UN Millennium Project, which has established development goals—marketed as Millennium Development Goals (MDGs)—in the fight against poverty and disease. RBM's narrow, malaria-reduction targets are a part of these broader MDGs.[57] RBM was WHO's first large-scale, global malaria program since conceding defeat in the eradication campaign in the late 1960s. Though it would attract criticism early in the twenty-first century, RBM created new pressure for action against malaria.

This momentum was to be seen in the NGO realm. In 1999, the Gates Foundation donated $50 million to establish the Malaria Vaccine Initiative, attempting to jump-start ailing vaccine programs. In 2003, the Gates Foundation donated another $100 million to the initiative.[58] Launched in 1999, the Medicines for Malaria Venture is a partnership between NGOs, the pharmaceutical industry, and government agencies. The partnership intends to leverage a "business-like framework" to create economic incentives for research and development in the area of malaria chemotherapy. They hope to balance the corporate sector's desire for return on investment and public-sector scientists' desire for publications in a nonprofit hybrid that can produce new medicines for those too poor to underwrite a modern R&D endeavor.[59] With these programs underway, the twentieth century closed with promise.

The early twenty-first century has already seen its own initiatives against malaria and other killers. One of the largest public health programs is the Global Fund to Fight AIDS, Tuberculosis, and Malaria. Launched by UN Secretary General Kofi Annan in the spring of 2001 amid large financial pledges from around the world, the fund "was constituted as an independent Swiss foundation in January 2002. Work in its first year focused on establishing the systems, infrastructure, and policies necessary to efficiently and accountably commit and disburse funds to approved programs. Fully operational by 2003, this architecture is now the basis of increasing outlays of finance in parallel with continued requests and review of new proposals."[60] The fund is intended to raise money and channel it efficiently to programs around the globe. It is not an operating foundation and does not directly implement programs in the field. Like other such initiatives in this period, the fund is explicitly and proudly a partnership, bringing together sovereign entities, nonprofits, and the private sector.[61]

One final, post-twentieth-century malaria program merits mentioning as it is a biomedical research initiative. This is the Malaria Research Institute at the Johns Hopkins Bloomberg School of Public Health.[62] In 2001, an anonymous donor pledged $100 million over ten years to reinforce and renew efforts to develop drugs and vaccines against malaria.[63] A state-of-the-art program has expanded the school's expertise and output in all areas of malaria research. All the initiatives that survive today form a network of experts, funders, and programs that, in detail, is often too interconnected for one to determine where one program begins and another ends.

The spring of 2007 saw another indication that malaria was breaking into the public consciousness of the West. Following her December 2006

White House Summit on Malaria, Laura Bush, wife of the president, hosted a Malaria Awareness Day in 2007. These events, deploying both the first lady and the president, represented a renewed commitment to aid those suffering from malaria in Africa and to educate Americans about the disease's toll in lives and sickness.[64] While new money and new initiative are sorely needed—and the 2005 President's Malaria Initiative promised some $1.2 billion over five years—it is staggering to ponder just how long this new awareness was in coming. The White House should be applauded for putting the facts and funds out there, but the truth of the situation has been evident for decades. The words at the opening for the 2007 Malaria Awareness Day are, unhappily, timeless: "Americans are fortunate to live in a land that eliminated malaria decades ago. . . . On Malaria Awareness Day, we renew our commitment to helping combat malaria in Africa and around the world. . . . Tragically, one child in Africa dies every 30 seconds from malaria, a disease that is highly treatable and preventable."[65]

Efforts against malaria are also tied to other public health initiatives. The very name of the Global Fund to Fight AIDS, Tuberculosis, and Malaria suggests that the big three killers might share some key features. Certainly in terms of intractability, poverty and poor health infrastructure stand in the way of preventing and treating these diseases. Like malaria, tuberculosis is an old and deadly disease that has only just come back into conscience of the developed world. This disease, too, has seen the rise of new public-private partnerships and NGOs, such as the Global Alliance for TB Drug Development and the Stop TB Partnership.[66] The story of HIV/AIDS differs somewhat from that of malaria and tuberculosis. Because HIV/AIDS impacted populations in rich countries as well as the poor, it was able to attract attention and greater resources a decade earlier than TB and malaria. This was accomplished—often through vocal and aggressive political action—in spite of it being a comparatively new disease. Still, like TB and malaria, the problems of efficient delivery and appropriate interventions hobble efforts to provide help to millions of sufferers in the poorest regions of the world.

What does the sixty-year-old antimalarial project tell us about the massive public health initiatives in the new century? It is, mostly, too soon to know. But some indications are emerging. In the spring of 2005, the *Lancet* was a forum for criticism of the RBM program.[67] An opening editorial observed that "in the 7 years since its inception, malaria rates have increased and the organisation has accumulated an expansive list of missed opportunities and dismal failures."[68] Following up on this editorial, the *Economist,* a keen observer of international development, commented, "It is certainly true that in the recent past RBM was indeed a mess. In 2002, an external report found that its loose organisational structure was failing and, as a consequence, decision-making was inhibited."[69] The historically minded might hear echoes of OSRD lawyers and administrators trying to bring order to unruly academics by establishing the Board for the Coordination of Malaria Studies. Then as now, it remains difficult to guide large-scale projects to good results employing only coordination and not administration. As the *Economist* continued, "In response, a supervisory board was introduced. Jon Liden, a spokesman for the Global Fund to fight AIDS, Tuberculosis and Malaria, an international charity that is one of the partners in RBM, agrees that the organisation has been 'unruly and difficult,' but says that such criticisms are several years out of date." With its supervisory board in place, the fund attributed "the lack of progress on malaria" to natural causes rather than social or institutional problems. Progress was hampered by "the absence of a way to combat the spread of resistance to traditional treatments such as chloroquine and sulfadoxine-pyrimethamine, and also, inevitably, a lack of money." Again, as with eradication in the 1960s and even earlier with Paul Ehrlich's warnings, it is resistance that is blamed for failure. The resistance of the parasites to drugs holds back progress. Artemisinin holds out some hope, but the parasite has enormous capacity to adapt and survive. The only thing that seems certain is that malaria will continue to sicken and kill millions of people. Today malaria produces hundreds of millions of cases and millions of deaths each year. Most of the dead are children in sub-Saharan Africa. Good intentions need to be coupled to suitable organization and reliable funding if another generation is to be spared malaria's scourge. Portions of these malaria policies and interventions parallel other critical health issues and emerging diseases, such as AIDS, tuberculosis, and West Nile virus. Malaria remains with us all. Both innovation and luck will be needed if the twenty-first century is to have a better record than the twentieth.[70]

William Mansfield Clark knew that cooperation between private, public, and nonprofits would be needed again. Clark, writing at the end of the war about the potential tension between public funding and private gain, lamented the negative impact that such conflicts could have on the essential sharing of information in a time of emergency. Clark felt that this issue involved "certain principles of cooperation among the people of our Nation that are likely to be reencountered. If so these principles will require recognition or definition and prompt action in an emergency. . . . In any event there is sure to be reencountered the perpetual conflict in men's minds between reliance on faith, hope, and charity on the one hand and reliance on the sterner safeguards of the law on the other. Actually, in the whole malaria program, the dominant attitude of all concerned, in Government, Council, private laboratory, and commercial company, leaned toward faith, hope, and charity. The record will show that the operation of these was [not] so bad after all."[71] In a world of limited resources, we must pray that faith, hope, and charity can be effectively harnessed once again.

Notes

Abbreviations of Archives Consulted

BAL   Bayer Archives Leverkusen
BNI   Bernard Nocht Institute, Hamburg, Germany
Board, *Bulletin* Board for Coordination of Malarial Studies,
                   Bulletin on Malarial Research: Comprising
                   Minutes of Meeting of the Board and Its Panels
                   and of the Various Malaria Committees which
                   Preceded the Board, 2 vols. (Washington, DC,
                   1943–1946)
Clark Collection   Mansfield Clark Collection, American Philo-
                   sophical Society
RFA   Rockefeller Foundation Archives, Rockefeller
                   Archive Center, Sleepy Hollow, New York

Introduction

1. My analysis of historical possibility and choice is informed by the notion of limits defined by resources and constraints. For more on this, see M. Norton Wise and Crosbie Smith, "Measurement, Work, and Industry in Lord Kelvin's Britain," *Historical Studies in the Physical and Biological Sciences* 17 (1986): 147–73; Thomas P. Hughes, "Model Builders and Instrument Makers," *Science in Context* 2 (1988): 59–75; Timothy Lenoir, "Models and Instruments in the Development of Electrophysiology, 1845–1912," *Historical Studies in the Physical and Biological Sciences* 17 (1986): 1–54; and Timothy Lenoir, "Practice, Reason, Context: The Dialogue between Theory and Experiment," *Science in Context* 2 (1988): 3–22.

2. William N. Hubbard Jr., "The Origins of Medicinals," in *Advances in American Medicine: Essays at the Bicentennial*, ed. John Z. Bowers and Elizabeth F. Purcell, 2 vols. (New York: Josiah Macy Jr. Foundation, 1976), 2: 685–721, 708–9.

3. Alexander M. Moore, "Malaria Chemotherapy," in *Encyclopedia of Chemical Technology*, ed. Raymond E. Kirk and Donald F. Othmer (New York: Interscience Encyclopedia, 1952), 8: 660–80, 660. For more on Bataan and malaria, see Office of the Surgeon General, Department of the Army, *The Medical Department, United States Army Preventive Medicine in World War II*, vol. 6, *Communicable Diseases: Malaria* (Washington, DC: U.S. Government Printing Office, 1963), chapter 9, http://history.amedd.army.mil/booksdocs/wwii/Malaria/frameindex.html (viewed 7 March 2007).

4. For a fine global perspective on the history of malaria, see Randall M. Packard, *The Making of a Tropical Disease: A Short History of Malaria* (Baltimore: Johns Hopkins University Press, 2007).

5. The liver stage of the parasite was first identified in simian malaria. See H. E. Shortt and P. C. C. Garnham, "Pre-erythrocytic Stage in Mammalian Malaria," *Nature* 161 (1948): 126. These observations were soon extended to human malaria.

6. Louis H. Miller, P. H. David, and T. J. Hadley, "Perspectives for Malaria Vaccination," *Philosophical Transactions of the Royal Society, London* B 307 (1984): 99–115, 99.

7. W. Mansfield Clark, "History of Co-operative Wartime Program," in *A Survey of Antimalarial Drugs, 1941–1945*, ed. Frederick Y. Wiselogle (Ann Arbor: J. W. Edwards, 1946), 1–57, 2.

Chapter 1 — Quinine and the Environment of Disease

1. G. Robert Coatney, William E. Collins, McWilson Warren, and Peter Contacos, *The Primate Malarias* (Washington, DC: U.S. Government Printing Office, 1971), 11.

2. For more on the history of cinchona and quinine, see Teodoro S. Kaufman and Edmundo A. Rúveda, "The Quest for Quinine: Those Who Won the Battles and Those Who Won the War," *Angewandte Chemie International Edition* 44 (2005): 854–85; Fiammetta Rocco, *The Miraculous Fever-Tree: Malaria and the Quest for a Cure That Changed the World* (New York: HarperCollins, 2003); and M. L. Duran-Reynals, *The Fever Bark Tree: The Pageant of Quinine* (Garden City, NY: Doubleday, 1946).

3. Saul Jarcho, *Quinine's Predecessor: Francesco Torti and the Early History of Cinchona* (Baltimore: Johns Hopkins University Press, 1993).

4. See, for example, Clements R. Markham, *Travels in Peru and India (While Superintending the Collection of Chinchona Plants and Seeds in South America, and Their Introduction into India)* (London: John Murray, 1862), Markham, *Peruvian Bark, a Popular Account of the Introduction of Chinchona Cultivation into British India* (London: John Murray, 1880), and Donovan Williams, "Clements Robert Markham and the Introduction of the Cinchona Tree into British India, 1861," *Geographical Journal* 128 (1962): 431–42.

5. According to some writers, it was not the countess but the corregidor who, in 1630, became the first European cured of intermittent fever by cinchona bark.

6. Leo Suppan said that although Humboldt relegated the story of the countess "to the limbo of fables, there is no sound reason for rejecting its validity" (Suppan, "Three Centuries of Cinchona," in *Proceedings of the Celebration of the Three Hundredth Anniversary of the First Recognized Use of Cinchona* [St. Louis: Missouri Botanical Garden, 1931], 29–138). Others disagreed. A. W. Haggis details the inconsistencies in, and lack of evidence for, the countess's tale (Haggis, "Fundamental Errors in the Early History of Cinchona," *Bulletin of the History of Medicine* 10 [1941]: 417–59 and 568–92). Likewise Jarcho, the most recent and conscientious of cinchona historians, offers a persuasive argument that the legend of the countess is just that (Jarcho, *Quinine's Predecessor*, 1–4).

7. S. Badus, *Anastasis corticis Peruviae* (1663): 239, cited in Jarcho, *Quinine's Predecessor*, 16.

8. Jarcho, *Quinine's Predecessor*, 64. Also see M. J. Dobson, "Bitter-sweet Solutions for Malaria: Exploring Natural Remedies from the Past," *Parassitologia* 40 (1998): 69–81.

9. Originally published in 1682: Henri Regnier, ed., *Oeuvres de J. de la Fontaine* (Paris: Librairie Hachette et Cie, 1890), 6: 307–57.

10. Jarcho, *Quinine's Predecessor*, 196.

11. Pelletier and Caventou, "Recherches chimiques sur les Quinquinas," *Annales de Chimie et de Physique* 15 (1820): 289–318; and "Suite des Recherches chimiques sur les Quinquinas," *Annales de Chimie et de Physique* 1 (1820): 337–65. Also see Sacha Tomic, "L'analyse Chimique des Végétaux: Le Cas du Quinquina," *Annals of Science* 58 (2001): 287–309.

12. O. Theodor Benfey, *From Vital Force to Structural Formulas* (Philadelphia: Chemical Heritage Foundation, 1992 [1964]), 14–37. Also see D. McKie, "Wöhler's 'Synthetic' Urea and the Rejection of Vitalism: A Chemical Legend," *Nature* 153 (1944): 608–10.

13. Adolph Strecker, "Untersuchungen über die Constitution des Chinins," *Liebigs Annalen der Chemie* 91 (1854): 155–70. For more on the history of organic structure determination, see Leo B. Slater, "Woodward, Robinson, and Strychnine: Chemical Structure and Chemists' Challenge," *Ambix* 48 (2001): 161–89.

14. For more on Perkin and mauve, the first synthetic dye, see Simon Garfield, *Mauve: How One Man Invented a Color that Changed the World* (New York: W. W. Norton, 2002).

15. Fine chemicals are dyes, pigments, drugs, and other low-volume, high-value-added materials, as opposed to high-volume commodity chemicals such as fertilizers and alkalis.

16. Philip D. Curtin, *The Image of Africa: British Ideas and Action, 1780–1850* (Madison: University of Wisconsin Press, 1964), 311–12 and 343–59; Lucile Brockway, *Science and Colonial Expansion: The Role of the British Royal Botanic Gardens* (New York: Academic Press, 1979), chapter 6; Philip D. Curtin, *Death by Migration: Europe's Encounter with the Tropical World in the Nineteenth Century* (New York: Cambridge University Press, 1989); Daniel R. Headrick, *The Tools of Empire: Technology and European Imperialism in the Nineteenth Century* (New York: Oxford University Press, 1981), chapter 3, and *The Tentacles of Progress: Technology Transfer in the Age of Imperialism, 1850–1940* (New York: Oxford University Press, 1988), 231–37; and Markham, *Travels*, 19–20.

17. For more on nineteenth-century medical work, see Dale C. Smith, "Quinine and Fever: The Development of the Effective Dosage," *Journal of the History of Medicine* 31 (1976): 343–67.

18. William H. McNeill suggests that not "until 1854, when the Dutch established quinchona plantations in Java, did Europeans command a reliable supply of the right kind of bark" (*Plagues and Peoples* [Garden City, NY: Anchor Press, 1976]). This date is somewhat early for reliable supplies of bark from plantations.

19. Markham, *Travels*, 46. Markham's comments resonate with the contemporary acclimatization movement in England and France. See Warwick Anderson, "Climates of Opinion: Acclimatization in Nineteenth-Century France and England," *Victorian Studies* 35 (1992): 135–57. Markham went on to cite other reasons for transplanting cinchona out of South America: "The distribution of valuable products of the vegetable kingdom amongst the nations of the earth—their introduction from countries where they are indigenous into distant lands with suitable soils and climates—is one of the greatest benefits that civilization has conferred upon mankind. . . . Centuries after the Ganges canal has become a ruin, and the great Vehar reservoir a dry valley, the people of India will probably have cause to

bless the healing effects of the fever-dispelling chinchona-trees, which will still be found on their southern mountains" (60–61).

20. Gabriele Gramiccia, *Life of Charles Ledger (1818–1905): Alpacas and Quinine* (London: MacMillan Press, 1988), 123–30 and 181–87.

21. Norman Taylor, *Cinchona in Java: The Story of Quinine* (New York: Greenberg, 1945).

22. For an overview of cinchona cultivation in Java, see Pieter Honig, K. W. van Gorkom, P. van Leersum, and Norman Taylor, "Chapters in the History of Cinchona," in *Science and Scientists in the Netherlands' Indies,* ed. Pieter Honig and Frans Verdoorn (New York: Board of the Netherlands Indies, Suriname and Curacao, 1945), 181–207.

23. Markham, *Peruvian Bark,* 415–34.

24. *League of Nations, Quarterly Bulletin of the Health Organisation* 2, no. 2 (1933): 183–285, and no. 3, 514–20.

25. For a view of the bureau's later history, see John M. Blair, "The Quinine 'Convention' of 1959–1962: A Case Study of an International Cartel," in *Recht, Macht und Wirtschaft,* ed. Helmut Arndt (Berlin: Duncker and Humblot, 1968), 123–84.

26. On the United States and Italy, see Margaret Humphreys, *Malaria in the United States: Poverty, Race, and Public Health* (Baltimore: Johns Hopkins University Press, 2001); and Frank M. Snowden, *The Conquest of Malaria: Italy, 1900–1962* (New Haven: Yale University Press, 2006). For an interesting view into parasites in a colonial context, see Bruno Latour, *The Pasteurization of France* (Cambridge, MA: Harvard University Press, 1988). For two other recent malaria control histories in national contexts, see Marcos Cueto, *Cold War, Deadly Fevers: Malaria Eradication in Mexico, 1955–1975* (Washington, DC: Woodrow Wilson Center Press; Baltimore: Johns Hopkins University Press, 2007); and Sandra M. Sufian, *Healing the Land and the Nation: Malaria and the Zionist Project in Palestine, 1920–1947* (Chicago: University of Chicago Press, 2007). Also of interest with regard to power, ideology, and malaria is Timothy Mitchell's *Rule of Experts: Egypt, Techno-Politics, Modernity* (Berkeley: University of California Press, 2002).

27. Daniel Headrick describes how changes in the sciences of chemistry and botany have contributed to the economic imbalances between countries of the temperate zone and the poorer ones of the tropics in "Botany, Chemistry, and Tropical Development," *Journal of World History* 7 (1996): 1–20.

28. August W. Hofmann, *Reports of the Royal College of Chemistry, and Researches Conducted in the Laboratories in the Years 1845–6–7* (London: Royal College of Chemistry, 1849), lx–lxi.

29. For an excellent account of the early synthetic dye industry, see Anthony S. Travis, *The Rainbow Makers: The Origins of the Synthetic Dyestuffs Industry in Western Europe* (Bethlehem, PA: Lehigh University Press, 1993). Also see Georg Meyer-Thurow, "The Industrialization of Invention: A Case Study from the German Chemical Industry," *Isis* 73 (1982): 363–81.

30. For more on the sulfa drugs, see John E. Lesch, ed., *The First Miracle Drugs: How the Sulfa Drugs Transformed Medicine* (New York: Oxford University Press, 2006); Lesch, "Chemistry and Biomedicine in an Industrial Setting: The Invention of the Sulfa Drugs," in *Chemical Sciences in the Modern World,* ed. Seymour H. Mauskopf (Philadelphia: University of Pennsylvania Press, 1993), 158–215; John Pfeiffer, "Sulfanilamide: The Story of a Great Medical Discovery," *Harper's* 178 (March 1939): 386–96.

31. For more on penicillin, see Eric Lax, *The Mold in Dr. Florey's Coat: The Story of the Penicillin Miracle* (New York: Henry Holt, 2004); Richard I. Mateles, ed., *Penicillin: A Paradigm for Biotechnology* (Chicago: Candida Corporation, 1998); Peter Neushul, "Fighting Research: Army Participation in the Clinical Testing and Mass Production of Penicillin during the Second World War," in *War, Medicine, and Modernity*, ed. Roger Cooter, Mark Harrison, and Steve Sturdy (Stroud, Gloucestershire: Sutton, 1998), 203–24; John Patrick Swann, "The Search for Synthetic Penicillin during World War II," *British Journal for the History of Science* 16 (1983): 154–90; National Academy of Sciences, *The Chemistry of Penicillin* (Princeton, NJ: Princeton University Press, 1949).

32. German Patent 29123, 8 June 1883, *Berichte der Deutschen Chemischen Gesellschaft*, 17, 1883, 546; Ludwig Knorr, "Einwirkung von Acetessigester auf Phenylhydrazin," *Berichte der Deutschen Chemischen Gesellschaft* 16 (1883): 2597–99, and "Ueber die Constitution der Chinizinderivate," *Berichte der Deutschen Chemischen Gesellschaft* 17 (1884): 2032–49. Also see Leon A. Greenberg, *Antipyrine: A Critical Bibliographic Review* (New Haven: Hillhouse Press, 1950).

33. David Greenwood, "The Quinine Connection," *Journal of Antimicrobial Chemotherapy* 30 (1992): 417–27.

34. For a history of analgesics and antipyretics, see Jan R. McTavish, *Pain and Profits: The History of the Headache and Its Remedies in America* (New Brunswick, NJ: Rutgers University Press, 2004).

35. For more about later attempts to synthesize quinine, including a controversial claim during World War II, see Jeffrey I. Seeman, "The Woodward-Doering/Rabe-Kindler Total Synthesis of Quinine: Setting the Record Straight," *Angewandte Chemie International Edition* 46 (2007): 1378–1413.

36. P. Ehrlich and P. Guttmann, "Über die Wirkung des Methylenblau bei Malaria," *Berliner klinische Wochenschrift* 28 (1891): 953–56.

37. For more on Ehrlich, see Cay-Rüdiger Prüll, "Part of a Scientific Master Plan? Paul Ehrlich and the Origins of his Receptor Concept," *Medical History* 47 (2003): 332–56; Arthur M. Silverstein, *Paul Ehrlich's Receptor Immunology: The Magnificent Obsession* (San Diego: Academic Press, 2002); Jonathan Liebenau, "Paul Ehrlich as a Commercial Scientist and Research Administrator," *Medical History* 34 (1990): 65–78; Timothy Lenoir, "A Magic Bullet: Research for Profit and the Growth of Knowledge in Germany Around 1900," *Minerva* 26 (1988): 66–88; John Parascandola, "The Theoretical Basis of Paul Ehrlich's Chemotherapy," *Journal of the History of Medicine and Allied Sciences* 36 (1981): 19–43; John Parascandola and Ronald Jasensky, "Origins of the Receptor Theory of Drug Action," *Bulletin of the History of Medicine* 48 (1974): 199–220; and C. H. Browning, "Emil Behring and Paul Ehrlich: Their Contributions to Science," *Nature* 175 (1955, parts 1 and 2): 570–75 and 616–19.

38. Lenoir, "A Magic Bullet," 81–82.

39. For more on the history of late nineteenth-century understandings of drug action, see William F. Bynum, "Chemical Structure and Pharacological Action: A Chapter in the History of Nineteenth Century Molecular Pharamcology," *Bulletin of the History of Medicine* 44 (1970): 518–38; Parascandola and Jasensky, "Origins of the Receptor Theory"; and Andreas-Holger Maehle, "'Receptive Substances': John Newport Langley (1852–1925) and his Path to a Receptor Theory of Drug Action," *Medical History* 48 (2004): 153–74. For a perspective on chemotherapy in the first

decades of the twentieth century, see Walter A. Jacobs, "The Chemotherapy of Protozoan and Bacterial Infections," *The Harvey Lectures* (1923–1924): 67–95.

40. The history of this "disinfectant tradition," which makes historical understandings of antiseptics and drugs more complex, is not well explored in the literature. For an excellent approach to this tradition with regard to immunology and serum therapy, see Jonathan Simon, "Emil Behring's Medical Culture: From Disinfection to Serotherapy," *Medical History* 51 (2007): 201–18.

41. Dr. Roehl's "Plasmochin" report, sent by Winthrop Chemical Company with their letter of 16 December 1926, folder 500, box 50, series 100, Record Group 1, Rockefeller Foundation Archives, Rockefeller Archive Center, Sleepy Hollow, New York (hereafter designated RFA), 8. This report is essentially a slightly annotated translation of Roehl's article, W. Roehl, "Die Wirkung des Plasmochins auf die Vogelmalaria," *Archiv für Schiffs- und Tropen-Hygiene, Pathologie und Therapie exotischer Krankheiten, Beihefte* 30 (1926): 311–18.

42. Dr. Roehl's "Plasmochin" report, 7; emphasis in the original.

43. Dr. Roehl's "Plasmochin" report, 7–8.

44. E. M. Lourie, "Studies on Chemotherapy in Bird Malaria: I.—Acquired Immunity in Relation to Quinine Treatment in *Plasmodium Cathemerium* Infections," *Annals of Tropical Medicine and Parasitology* 28 (1934): 151–69; "Studies on Chemotherapy in Bird Malaria: II.—Observations Bearing on the Mode of Action of Quinine," *Annals of Tropical Medicine and Parasitology* 28 (1934): 255–77; "Studies on Chemotherapy in Bird Malaria: III.—Difference in Response to Quinine Treatment between Strains of *Plasmodium Relictum* of Widely-Separated Geographical Origins," *Annals of Tropical Medicine and Parasitology* 28 (1934): 513–23.

45. William H. Taliaferro and Lucy Graves Taliaferro, "Reduction in Immunity in Chicken Malaria Following Treatment with Nitrogen Mustard," *Journal of Infectious Diseases* 82 (1948): 5–30; William H Taliaferro, "The Role of the Spleen and Lymphoid-Macrophage System in the Quinine Treatment of *Gallinaceum* Malaria: I. Acquired Immunity and Phagocytosis," *Journal of Infectious Diseases* 83 (1948): 164–80; William H. Taliaferro and F. E. Kelsey, "The Role of the Spleen and Lymphoid-Macrophage System in the Quinine Treatment of *Gallinaceum* Malaria: II. Quinine Blood Levels," *Journal of Infectious Diseases* 83 (1948): 181–99; William H. Taliaferro and Lucy Graves Taliaferro, "The Role of the Spleen and Lymphoid-Macrophage System in the Quinine Treatment of *Gallinaceum* Malaria: III. The Action of Quinine and of Immunity on the Parasite," *Journal of Infectious Diseases* 84 (1949): 187–220.

46. E. M. Lourie, "Studies on Chemotherapy in Bird Malaria: II.—Observations Bearing on the Mode of Action of Quinine," *Annals of Tropical Medicine and Parasitology* 28 (1934): 255–77.

47. René J. Dubos, "The Significance of the Structure of the Bacterial Cell in the Problems of Antisepsis and Chemotherapy," in *Chemotherapy* (Philadelphia: University of Pennsylvania Press, 1941), 29.

48. For more on Dubos and the ecological perspective, see Jill Elaine Cooper, "Of Microbes and Men: A Scientific Biography of René Jules Dubos" (PhD diss., Rutgers University, 1998). For a more popular account of Dubos' life, see Carol L. Moberg, *René Dubos, Friend of the Good Earth: Microbiologist, Medical Scientist, Environmentalist* (Washington, DC: ASM Press, 2005).

49. Dubos, "The Significance," 40. Dubos cites P. Ehrlich, *Proceedings of the Royal Society, London* 66 (1900): 432.

50. For recent lead reference on the history of receptor theory, see Cay-Rüdiger Prüll, "Caught between the Old and the New—Walther Straub (1874–1944), the Question of Drug Receptors, and the Rise of Modern Pharmacology," *Bulletin of the History of Medicine* 80 (2006): 465–89; and Viviane Quirke, "Putting Theory into Practice: James Black, Receptor Theory, and the Development of the Beta-Blockers at ICI, 1958–1978," *Medical History* 50 (2006): 69–92.

51. Alaric, who had "destroyed all the roads north of Rome, pulled down the bridges and flooded the country," died of fever shortly after his departure from Rome. Angelo Celli, *The History of Malaria in the Roman Campagna from Ancient Times*, ed. and enl. by Anna Celli-Fraentzel (London: Bale and Danielsson, 1933), 48–49.

52. Angelo Celli, *Malaria According to the New Researches*, trans. by John Joseph Eyre (New York: Longmans, Green, 1900), 117.

53. For more on malaria in Italy, see Lewis W. Hackett, *Malaria in Europe: An Ecological Study* (London: Oxford University, 1937), 309–18; Leonard Jan Bruce-Chwatt and Julian de Zulueta, *The Rise and Fall of Malaria in Europe: A Historico-Epidemiological Study* (New York: Clarendon Press, 1980), 89–105; and Frank M. Snowden, *The Conquest of Malaria: Italy, 1900–1962* (New Haven: Yale University Press, 2006).

54. For a detailed account of the work of both Laveran and Ross, see Gordon Harrison, *Mosquitoes, Malaria, and Man: A History of the Hostilities since 1880* (New York: Dutton, 1978).

55. For more on the Ross-Grassi feud, one can begin with Harrison, *Mosquitoes, Malaria, and Man*, 102–8.

56. Harrison, *Mosquitoes, Malaria, and Man*.

57. Paris green, a pigment called "Vert de Schweinfurt" in Paris, is copper acetoarsenite.

58. Celli, *The History of Malaria in the Roman Campagna*, 172.

59. Celli, *The History of Malaria in the Roman Campagna*, 172. The Italian efforts were more complicated and politicized than suggested here. For a fuller understanding, see Snowden, *The Conquest of Malaria*.

60. The effects of DDT on insects were discovered by Paul Müller at Geigy, Basel, in 1939. For more on Müller and DDT, see Sharon Bertsch McGrayne, *Prometheans in the Lab: Chemistry and the Making of the Modern World* (New York: McGraw-Hill, 2001), 148–67; and Lukas Straumann, *Nützliche Schädlinge: Angewandte Entomologie, chemische Industrie und Landwirtschaftspolitik in der Schweiz, 1874–1952* (Zurich: Chronos, 2005). For more on the history of vector control and DDT, see Peter Brown, "Failure-as-Success: Multiple Meanings of Eradication in the Rockefeller Foundation Sardinia Project, 1946–1951," *Parassitologia* 40 (1998): 117–30; Marcos Cueto, "The Cycles of Eradication: The Rockefeller Foundation and Latin American Public Health, 1918–1940," in *International Health Organisations and Movements, 1918–1939*, ed. Paul Weindling (New York: Cambridge University Press, 1995), chapter 11; Thomas R. Dunlap, *DDT: Scientists, Citizens, and Public Policy* (Princeton, NJ: Princeton University Press, 1981); M. A. Farid, "The Malaria Campaign—Why Not Eradication?" *World Health Forum* 19 (1998): 417–27; John Farley, "Mosquitoes or Malaria? Rockefeller Campaigns in the American

South and Sardinia," *Parassitologia* 36 (1994): 165–73; Margaret Humphreys, "Kicking a Dying Dog: DDT and the Demise of Malaria in the American South, 1942–1950," *Isis* 87 (1996): 1–17; John A. Logan, *The Sardinian Project: An Experiment in the Eradication of an Indigenous Malarious Vector* (Baltimore: Johns Hopkins University Press, 1953); R. M. Packard and P. Gadelha, "A Land Filled with Mosquitoes: Fred L. Soper, the Rockefeller Foundation, and the *Anopheles Gambiae* Invasion of Brazil," *Parassitologia* 36 (1994): 197–213; Edmund Russell, *War and Nature: Fighting Humans and Insects with Chemicals from World War I to Silent Spring* (New York: Cambridge University Press, 2001); Andrew Spielman and Michael D'Antonio, *Mosquito: A Natural History of Our Most Persistent and Deadly Foe* (New York: Hyperion, 2001); Darwin H. Stapleton, "A Lost Chapter in the Early History of DDT: The Development of Anti-Typhus Technologies by the Rockefeller Foundation's Louse Laboratory, 1942–1944," *Technology and Culture* 46 (2005): 513–40; Stapleton, "A Success for Science or Technology? The Rockefeller Foundation's Role in Malaria Eradication in Italy, 1924–1935," *Journal of History of Medicine* (*Medicina nei Secoli Arte e Scienza*) 6 (1994): 213–28; Stapleton, "The Dawn of DDT and Its Experimental Use by the Rockefeller Foundation in Mexico, 1943–1952," *Parassitologia* 40 (1998): 149–58; Stapleton, "The Short-Lived Miracle of DDT," *Invention and Technology* (Winter 2000): 34–41; J. de Zulueta, "Forty Years of Malaria Eradication in Sardinia: A New Appraisal of the Great Enterprise," *Parassitologia* 32 (1990): 231–36.

61. On this historical debate, see Humphreys, *Malaria in the United States.*

62. All these quotes are from Marshall A. Barber, *A Malariologist in Many Lands* (Lawrence: University of Kansas Press, 1946), 23.

63. The sharing of needles by drug users was a way in which malaria could spread without the intervention of mosquitoes. While this sort of transmission was observed, it was never a significant contributor to malaria transmission in the way that it was, and is, for viral diseases like hepatitis and HIV.

64. For a slightly later period, Warwick Anderson makes this "preadaptation" explicit for those who worked in tropical medicine. See Warwick Anderson, "Natural Histories of Infectious Disease: Ecological Vision in Twentieth Century Biomedical Science," *Osiris* 19 (2004): 58.

65. For fine introduction to ecology in the U.S. context, see Gregg Mitman, *The State of Nature: Ecology, Community, and American Social Thought, 1900–1950* (Chicago: University of Chicago Press, 1992). Mitman is also well worth reading on the historiography of ecology and disease: see "In Search of Health: Landscape and Disease in American Environmental History," *Environmental History* 10 (2005): 184–210.

66. Barber, preface to *A Malariologist in Many Lands.*

67. Marston Bates, *The Natural History of Mosquitoes* (New York: Macmillan, 1949), 6.

68. Bates, *Natural History of Mosquitoes,* 7.

69. Hackett, *Malaria in Europe.*

70. Wilbur A. Sawyer, "The Importance of Environment in the Study of Tropical Diseases," Presidential Address of the American Academy of Tropical Medicine, delivered 2 December 1937, *American Journal of Tropical Medicine* 18 (1938): 12.

71. On the tensions between field and laboratory research at the IHD—and the positions of Russell, Sawyer, and Hackett—during the period of 1920 and 1946, see John Farley, "The International Health Division of the Rockefeller Foundation: The Russell Years, 1920–1934," in *International Health Organizations and Movements,*

1918–1939, ed. Paul Weindling (Cambridge: Cambridge University Press, 1995), 203–21. Also see Ilana Löwy, "Epidemiology, Immunology, and Yellow Fever: The Rockefeller Foundation in Brazil, 1923–1939," *Journal of the History of Biology* 30 (1997): 397–417.

72. Paul F. Russell, "Preventive Medicine as Exemplified by Malaria," 10 January 1936, 33 pages, folder 503, box 50, series 100, RG 1, RFA, 10–11. Russell's metaphor was specifically gendered: The seed was "a man," the sower was "a female *Anopheles* mosquito," and the soil was "another man."

73. Russell, "Preventive Medicine," 11.

74. Emphasis in the original. Robert Hegner, "Parasite Reactions to Host Modifications," *Journal of Parasitology* 23 (1937): 5. Hegner listed his investigators: "Those who took part in the investigations on which this discussion is based are as follows: Justin Andrews, G. H. Boyd, L. R. Cleveland, M. S. MacDougall,. Lydia Eskridge, Arnoldo Gabaldon, Robert Hegner, E. C. Nelson, H. L. Ratcliffe, Eugene Schumaker, K. S. Shah, L. G. Taliaferro, and W. H. Taliaferro" (1).

75. Myron L. Simpson, "Studies on the Reproduction of the '3T' Strain of *Plasmodium cathemerium* in Ducks" (PhD diss., School of Hygiene and Public Health of the Johns Hopkins University, 1944), 1.

76. NRC, DMS, CMR, OSRD, minutes of the Conference for a Review of the Malaria Research Program, 29 March 1944, in Board for Coordination of Malarial Studies, *Bulletin on Malarial Research: Comprising Minutes of Meeting of the Board and Its Panels and of the Various Malaria Committees which Preceded the Board*, 2 vols. (Washington, DC, 1943–1946), 253. This *Bulletin* comprises the original mimeographed reports of the program. A. N. Richards donated his two volumes to the medical library at the University of Pennsylvania, where I was able to make use of them. All seven volumes of the *Bulletin* are available at National Archives and Records Administration II, College Park, MD: RG 227 Records of the OSRD, CMR, NC-138, entry 167, Boxes 1–4, NND937001. Hereafter referred to as Board, *Bulletin*.

Chapter 2 — Avian Malaria

1. The use of laboratory animals in biomedicine has a rich and growing historiography. One might begin with these works: Richard M. Burian, "How the Choice of Experimental Organism Matters: Biological Practices and Discipline Boundaries," *Synthese* 92 (1992): 151–66; Burian, "How the Choice of Experimental Organism Matters: Epistemological Reflections on an Aspect of Biological Practice," *Journal of the History of Biology* 26 (1993): 351–67; W. F. Bynum, "'C'est un malade': Animal Models and Concepts of Human Diseases," *Journal of the History of Medicine and Allied Sciences* 45 (1990): 397–413; Bonnie Tocher Clause, "The Right Organism for the Job," *Journal of the History of Biology* 26 (1993): 233–367; Otniel E. Dror, "The Affect of Experiment: The Turn to Emotions in Anglo-American Physiology, 1900–1940," *Isis* 90 (1999): 205–37; Gerald L. Geison and Angela N. H. Creager, "Introduction: Research Materials and Model Organisms in the Biological and Biomedical Sciences," *Studies in the History of Biology and Biomedical Sciences* 30 (1999): 315–18; Gerald L. Geison and Manfred D. Laubichler, "The Varied Lives of Organisms: Variation in the Historiography of the Biological Sciences," *Studies in History and Philosophy of Biological and Biomedical Sciences* 32 (2001): 1–29; Frederic L. Holmes, "The Old Martyr of Science: The Frog in Experimental Physiology," *Journal of the History of Biology* 26 (1993): 311–28;

Robert E. Kohler, *Lords of the Fly: Drosophila Genetics and the Experimental Life* (Chicago: University of Chicago Press, 1994); Ilana Löwy, "From Guinea Pigs to Man: The Development of Haffkine's Anticholera Vaccine," *Journal of the History of Medicine and Allied Sciences* 47 (1992): 270–309; Löwy and Jean-Paul Gaudillière, "Disciplining Cancer: Mice and the Practice of Genetic Purity," in *The Invisible Industrialist: Manufacturers and the Production of Scientific Knowledge,* ed. J. Gaudillière and I. Löwy (New York: St. Martin's, 1998), 209–49; Harry M. Marks, *The Progress of Experiment, Science, and Therapeutic Reform in the United States, 1900–1990* (New York: Cambridge University Press, 1997); Karen A. Rader, *Making Mice: Standardizing Animals for American Biomedical Research, 1900–1955* (Princeton: Princeton University Press, 2004); Jean-Paul Gaudillière and Hans-Jörg Rheinberger, "Essay Review: Life Stories," *Studies in History and Philosophy of Biology and Biomedical Science* 35 (2004): 753–64; Daniel P. Todes, "Pavlov's Physiological Factory," *Isis* 88 (1997): 205–46; and Michael Worboys, *Spreading Germs: Diseases, Theories, and Medical Practice in Britain, 1865–1900* (New York: Cambridge University Press, 2000).

2. Neosalvarsan emerged from his lab in 1912.

3. For the text of Ehrlich's lecture, see the Nobel Prize Web site, http://nobelprize. org/medicine/laureates/1908/ehrlich-lecture.pdf (viewed 26 July 2006).

4. Wilhelm Roehl, "Heilversuche mit Arsenophenylglycin bei Trypanosomiasis," *Zeitschrift für Immunitätsforschung und experimentelle Therapie, Jena* 1 (1908–1909): 633–49; Roehl, "Ueber Tryparosan," *Zeitschrift für Immunitatsforschung und Experimentalle Therapie, Jena* 2 (1909): 70–76; Roehl, "Paraminophenylarsenoxyd contra Trypanotoxyl," *Zeitschrift für Immunitätsforschung und experimentelle Therapie, Jena* 2 (1909): 496–500; Roehl, "Ueber den Wirkungsmechanismus des Atoxyls," *Berliner Klinische Wochenschrift* 46 (1909): 494–97.

5. Paul Ehrlich, "Experimental Researches on Specific Therapy III: Chemotherapeutic Studies on Trypamosomes," in *The Collected Papers of Paul Ehrlich,* vol. 3, *Chemotherapy,* ed. F. Himmelweit (New York: Pergamon Press, 1960), 130–34, reprinted from *The Harben Lectures for 1907 of the Royal Institute of Public Health* (London: Lewis, 1908), 130.

6. Percy C. C. Garnham, "Reflections on Laveran, Marchiafava, Golgi, Koch, and Danilewsky after Sixty Years," *Transactions of the Royal Society for Tropical Medicine and Hygiene* 61 (1967): 753–64, 759–60. For a lovely historical discussion of Koch's postulates, see Victoria A. Harden, "Koch's Postulates and the Etiology of AIDS: An Historical Perspective," *History and Philosophy of the Life Sciences* 14 (1992): 249–69.

7. Robert Hegner, Edwin H. Shaw Jr., and Reginald D. Manwell, "Methods and Results of Experiments on the Effects of Drugs on Bird Malaria," *American Journal of Hygiene* 8 (1928): 564. Hegner was born in 1880 and educated at the University of Chicago and the University of Wisconsin where he received his PhD in zoology in 1908.

8. Paul F. Russell to V. G. Heiser, 10 August 1931, p. 3, folder 501, box 50, series 100, RG 1, RFA.

9. Reginald D. Manwell, "Avian Malarial Infections as Classroom Material," *Science* 79 (1934): 545. As Manwell suggested in this *Science* article, geography and complexity made avian disease attractive as a teaching tool. William Taliaferro of the University of Chicago, who had spent time at Hopkins in the 1920s, also appreciated avian and other animal malarias as research materials, as he commented in 1939: "A major

portion of the attention of workers in parasitology at the University of Chicago is devoted to the malarial organisms not only because of their importance to medicine, but also because they are proving to be remarkable material for general biological studies of interest both to medicine and basic science. Among the advantages the following may be mentioned. Their large size, as compared to bacteria and viruses, permits cytological observation of them in both the vertebrate and insect hosts and analysis of the effects of host resistance on the parasite not possible with the smaller invaders." See William H. Taliaferro, "Investigations in Malaria at the University of Chicago, 1925–1939," p. 1, folder 520, box 52, series 100, RG 1, RFA. With regard to teaching and training, malaria was not the only avian disease to be in the right place at the right time. Historian John Farley has pointed out the usefulness of avian schistosomiasis in practicing essential medical techniques, as human schistosomiasis (or bilharzia) was not found in the United States or Canada and migratory birds regularly shed parasites as they traversed the continent. Farley cited William W. Cort, Claude Barlow, J. Allen Scott, and others who were able to gain experience working with schistosome parasites in North America using these avian parasites. See John Farley, *Bilharzia: A History of Imperial Tropical Medicine* (New York: Cambridge University Press, 1991), 105; W. W. Cort, "Schistosome Dermatitis in the United States," *Journal of the American Medical Association* 90 (1928): 1027–29; and Cort "Studies on Schistosome Dermatitis. XI. Status of Knowledge after More than Twenty Years," *American Journal of Hygiene* 52 (1950): 251–307. Today's avian disease of note is often bird flu. On avian influenza and drug development, see Graeme Laver, "From the Great Barrier Reef to a 'Cure' for the Flu: Tall Tales, but True," *Perspectives in Biology and Medicine* 47 (2004): 590–96. The pedagogic use of model systems offers further nuance to discussions of avian malaria models.

10. For more about rodent malarias, see Francis E. G. Cox, "Major Animal Models in Malaria Research: Rodent," in *Malaria: Principles and Practice of Malariology*, ed. W. H. Wernsdorfer and I. McGregor (New York: Churchill Livingstone, 1988), 2: 1503–43; and *Rodent Malaria*, ed. R. Killick-Kendrick and W. Peters (New York: Academic Press, 1978), especially the introduction by L. J. Bruce-Chwatt, xi–xxv.

11. William Trager and James B. Jensen, "Human Malaria Parasites in Continuous Culture," *Science* 193 (1976): 673–75.

12. Alphonse Laveran, "Des hématozoaires des oiseaux voisins de l'hématozoaire du paludisme," *Comptes Rendus de la Société de Biologie (Mémoires)* (1891): 127, my translation.

13. See, for example, Basil Danilewsky, "Zur Parasitologie des Blutes," *Biologisches Centralblatt* 5 (1885–86): 529–37.

14. William Sydney Thayer and John Hewetson, "The Malarial Fevers of Baltimore: An Analysis of 616 Cases of Malarial Fever with Special Reference to the Relations Existing between Different Types of Fever," *John Hopkins Hospital Reports* 5 (1895): 50–53.

15. W. G. MacCallum, "On the Haematozoan Infections of Birds," *Journal of Experimental Medicine* 3 (1898): 125–26.

16. W. G. MacCallum, "On the Flagellated Form of the Malarial Parasite," *Lancet* 2 (1897): 1240–41.

17. Percy Garnham provides background and references for scientific precedence and the establishment of *Plasmodium* species. See P. C. C. Garnham, *Malaria Parasites and Other Haemosporidia* (Oxford: Blackwell Scientific, 1966).

18. For a discussion of the early history of *P. relictum*, see Garnham, *Malaria Parasites*, 522–50.

19. B. Grassi and R. Feletti, "Contribuzione allo Studio dei Parassiti Malarici," *Memoria V, Atti della Accademia Gioenia di Scienze Naturali in Catania* 5, s. 4, Anno 69 (1892): 8–10.

20. Many species of mosquito have been shown in laboratory situations to be competent vectors for *P. relictum*. These include species of the genera *Aedes*, *Culex*, and *Anopheles*.

21. Those interested in the place of canaries in the history of genetics may wish to consult Tim Birkhead, *A Brand-New Bird: How Two Amateur Scientists Created the First Genetically Engineered Animal* (New York: Basic Books, 2003).

22. Phokion Kopanaris, "Die Wirkung von Chinin, Salvarsan und Atoxyl auf die Proteosoma-(Plasmodium praecox-)Infektion des Kanarienvogels," *Archiv für Schiffs- und Tropen-Hygiene, Pathologie und Therapie exotischer Krankheiten* 15 (1911): 586.

23. For Roehl's biographical information, I have relied primarily on two sources: G. Olpp, "Roehl," in *Hervorragende Tropenärzte in Wort und Bild* (München: Verlag der Ärztlichen Rundschau Otto Gmelin, 1932), 344–46; and "Lebenslauf: Wilhelm Roehl," Bayer Archives Leverkusen (hereafter BAL), Pharma Produkte A-Z Plasmochin 1926.

24. See also Horst-Bernd Dünschede, *Tropenmedizinische Forschung bei Bayer, Düsseldorfer Arbeiten zur Geschichte der Medizin, Beiheft II* (Düsseldorf: Michael Triltsch Verlag, 1971), 146–47.

25. Dr. Roehl's "Plasmochin" report, sent by Winthrop Chemical Company with their letter of 16 December 1926, p. 1, folder 500, box 50, series 100, RG 1, RFA. This report is essentially a slightly annotated translation of Roehl's article, W. Roehl, "Die Wirkung des Plasmochins auf die Vogelmalaria," *Archiv für Schiffs- und Tropen-Hygiene, Pathologie und Therapie exotischer Krankheiten, Beihefte* 30 (1926): 311–18.

26. Roehl, "Plasmochin," 1–2.

27. Roehl, "Plasmochin," 3–4.

28. Roehl, "Plasmochin," 4.

29. Roehl, "Plasmochin," 5.

30. Roehl, "Plasmochin," 9.

31. "Bock-Schweickert," 103/09.1: Walter Kikuth, "Bericht: Die Halteridium-Infektion der Reisfinken als Modellversuch," 16 October 1930; and Walter Kikuth, "Jahres-Bericht 1930," 15 January 1931, BAL, Chemotherapeutisches Labor, Elberfeld, Berichte.

32. W. Schulemann to S. P. James, 14 September 1931, copy, folder 675, box 51, series 401, RG 1.1, RFA.

33. James to Strode, 12 November 1931, p. 2, folder 675, box 51, series 401, RG 1.1, RFA.

34. "Bock-Schweickert," 103/09.1: Walter Kikuth, "Jahres-Bericht 1930," 30 January 1932.

35. James to Strode, 12 November 1931. For James's work at Horton hospital, see S. P. James, "Some General Results of a Study of Induced Malaria in England (and 'Discussion')," *Transactions of the Royal Society of Tropical Medicine and Hygiene* 24 (1931): 477–538.

36. Whole ground mosquitoes could produce general inflammation, so often mosquitoes were dissected and only their sporozoite-containing salivary glands injected.

37. Prophylatic study being distinct from the study of the treatment or suppression of infection. These distinctions would appear again as replacements for quinine continued to be sought. Quinine was not curative and only suppressed infection.

38. James, "Some General Results," 509–16.

39. Paul F. Russell to V. G. Heiser, 22 September 1931, folder 501, box 50, series 100, RG 1, RFA.

40. For certain experiments, Kikuth introduced the use of *Halteridium* and rice finches. See, for example, Walter Kikuth, "Zur Weiterentwicklung der Chemotherapie der Malaria. 'Certuna'—Ein Neues Gametenmittel," *Klinische Wochenschrift* 17 (1938): 524–27.

41. Robert Hegner, "Studies on Bird Malaria," *Southern Medical Journal* 19 (1926): 377–81.

42. Ernest Hartman, "Three Species of Bird Malaria, *Plasmodium praecox, P. cathemerium*, n. sp., and *P. inconstans*, n. sp.," *Archiv für Protistenkunde* 60 (1927): 1–7. Earlier and contemporary work often cites *P. praecox* as a distinct species, but it was most likely in fact *P. relictum*. One must approach much of the prewar literature with caution as the species were not clearly delineated by name; in some instances *praecox* may have been *cathemerium*.

43. Lucy Graves Taliaferro, "Infection and Resistance in Bird Malaria, with special reference to Periodicity and Rate of Reproduction of the Parasite," *American Journal of Hygiene* 5 (1925): 742–89; Clay G. Huff, "Studies on the Infectivity of Plasmodia of Birds for Mosquitoes, with Special Reference to the Problem of Immunity in the Mosquito" (PhD diss., School of Hygiene and Public Health of the Johns Hopkins University, 1927); Reginald D. Manwell, "Relapse in Bird Malaria" (PhD diss., School of Hygiene and Public Health of the Johns Hopkins University; 1928); Khwaja Samad Shah, "Studies on the Sexual Forms of a Malarial Parasite, *Plasmodium cathemerium*, of Canary Birds" (PhD diss., School of Hygiene and Public Health of the Johns Hopkins University, 1933); Redginal I. Hewitt, "Parasite Responses to Normal and Modified Young-Cell Percentages in Infections of *Plasmodium cathemerium*" (PhD diss., School of Hygiene and Public Health of the Johns Hopkins University, 1938); Robert Carlisle Rendtorff, "The Early Development of *Plasmodium cathemerium*" (PhD diss., School of Hygiene and Public Health of the Johns Hopkins University, 1944).

44. A. Laveran, "Des hématozoaires des oiseaux voisins de l'hématozoaire du paludisme," *Comptes Rendus de la Société de Biologie (Mémoires)* (1891): 127.

45. Marion M. Brooke, *Effect of Dietary Changes upon Avian Malaria* (PhD diss., School of Hygiene and Public Health of the Johns Hopkins University, 1942), 1.

46. Brooke, *Effect of Dietary Changes*, 3.

47. Myron L. Simpson, "Studies on the Reproduction of the '3T' Strain of *Plasmodium cathemerium* in Ducks" (PhD diss., School of Hygiene and Public Health of the Johns Hopkins University, 1944), 2.

48. Simpson, "Studies on the Reproduction," 1.

49. Garnham, *Malaria Parasites*, 556.

50. Émile Brumpt, "Paludisme Aviaire: *Plasmodium gallinaceum* n. sp. de la Poule Domestique," *Comptes Rendus de l'Academie des Sciences* 200 (1935): 783, my translation.

51. For more on *gallinaceum*, see Émile Brumpt, "Paludisme Aviaire"; Brumpt, "Réceptivité de Divers Oiseaux Domestiques et Sauvages au Parasite (*Plasmodium*

gallinaceum) du Paludisme de la Poule Domestique. Transmission de cet Hématozoaire par le Moustique *Stegomyia fasciata*," *Comptes Rendus de l'Academie des
Sciences* 203 (1936): 750–52; and Garnham, *Malaria Parasites*, 588–619.

52. Garnham, *Malaria Parasites*, 589.

53. Brumpt, "Paludisme Aviaire," 783.

54. Brumpt, "Réceptivité de Divers Oiseaux," 750.

55. Garnham, *Malaria Parasites*, 590–92 and 609. It was later found that *P. gallinaceum's* natural vector was *Mansonia crassipes*: W. J. Niles, M. Agnes Fernando,
and A. S. Dissanaike, "*Mansonia crassipes* as the Natural Vector of Filarioids,
Plasmodium gallinaceum and Other Plasmodia of Fowls in Ceylon," *Nature* 205
(1965): 411–12.

56. Coggeshall was born in 1901 and educated at Indiana University, where he
received his MD in 1928.

57. Lowell T. Coggeshall, "*Plasmodium lophurae*, a New Species of Malaria Parasite Pathogenic for the Domestic Fowl," *American Journal of Hygiene* 27 (1938):
615–16.

58. William Trager, "A Strain of the Mosquito *Aedes aegypti* Selected for Susceptibility to the Avian Malaria Parasite *Plasmodium lophurae*," *Journal of Parasitology*
28 (1942): 457–65.

59. See, for example, Geoffrey M. Jeffery, "Investigation of the Factors Influencing the
Mosquito Transmission of *Plasmodium lophurae*" (PhD diss., School of Hygiene
and Public Health of the Johns Hopkins University, 1944).

60. H. A. Walker and H. B. van Dyke, "Control of Malaria Infection (*P. lophurae*) in
Ducks by Sulfonamides," *Proceedings of the Society for Experimental Biology and
Medicine* 48 (1941): 368.

61. See, for example, Robert Hegner, Evaline West, Mary Ray, and Marian Dobler, "A New
Drug Effective against Bird Malaria," *American Journal of Hygiene* 33 (1941): 101.

62. Walker and van Dyke, "Control of Malaria Infection," 368.

63. Harry Beckman to L. T. Coggeshall, 22 August, 1940, folder 115, box 11, series 4,
RG 5, RFA.

64. John A. Ferrell to Mark F. Boyd, 6 November, 1941, with "Report of International
Health Division of the Rockefeller Foundation Activities against Malaria through
the Chemotherapeutic Approach, by Doctor John Maier, New York City," attached,
folder 115, box 11, series 4, RG 5, RFA.

65. Manwell, "Avian Malarial Infections as Classroom Material," 545.

Chapter 3 — New Drugs

1. League of Nations, Health Committee, Eighth Session, Fifth Meeting, "Work of the
Malaria Commission," 16 October 1926, 28.

2. Alexander M. Moore, "Malaria Chemotherapy," in *Encyclopedia of Chemical
Technology*, ed. Raymond E. Kirk and Donald F. Othmer (New York: Interscience
Encyclopedia, 1952), 8: 660.

3. Research organization and the "industrialization of invention" at Bayer is discussed by John E. Lesch in "Chemistry and Biomedicine in an Industrial Setting:
The Invention of the Sulfa Drugs," in *Chemical Sciences in the Modern World*, ed.
Seymour H. Mauskopf (Philadelphia: University of Pennsylvania Press, 1993). For
an excellent account of pharmaceutical research in an American context, particularly during the interwar period, see John P. Swann, *Academic Scientists and the*

Pharmaceutical Industry: Cooperative Research in Twentieth-Century America (Baltimore: Johns Hopkins University Press, 1988).

4. The legal relationship between the Winthrop Chemical Company and Bayer was complicated. Fundamentally, Winthrop was a 50/50 venture between Bayer and Sterling Products, Inc. Sterling, in turn, was former U.S. subsidiary that had been taken over by the Alien Property Custodian during World War I. For more detail, see Gerhard Kümmel, *Transnationale Wirtschaftskooperation und der National-staat: Deutsch-amerikanische Unternehmensbeziehungen in den dreißiger Jahren* (Stuttgart: Franz Steiner Verlag, 1995), 146–50.

5. For an understanding of chemical structure determination in this period and a discussion of structures as chemical shorthand, see Leo B. Slater, "Woodward, Robinson, and Strychnine: Chemical Structure and Chemists' Challenge," *Ambix* 48 (2001): 161–89.

6. For more on the status of chemical structures, see Leo B. Slater, "Organic Chemistry and Instrumentation: R. B. Woodward and the Reification of Chemical Structures," in *From Classical to Modern Chemistry: The Instrumental Revolution,* ed. P. T. Morris (Cambridge, UK: Royal Society of Chemistry, 2002), 212–28; Joachim Schummer, "The Impact of Instrumentation on Chemical Species Identity," in *From Classical to Modern Chemistry,* 188–211; Slater, "Instruments and Rules: R. B. Woodward and the Tools of Twentieth-Century Organic Chemistry," *Studies in History and Philosophy of Science* 33 (2002): 1–33; and Slater, "Woodward, Robinson, and Strychnine."

7. Dr. Roehl's "Plasmochin" report, sent by Winthrop Chemical Company with their letter of 16 December 1926, p. 4, folder 500, box 50, series 100, RG 1, RFA. This report is essentially a slightly annotated translation of Roehl's article, "Die Wirkung des Plasmochins auf die Vogelmalaria," *Archiv für Schiffs- und Tropen-Hygiene, Pathologie und Therapie exotischer Krankheiten* 30 (1926): 311–18.

8. Among these were Julius Morgenroth, Gustav Giemsa, W. Weise, Fritz Schönhöfer, and C. Tropp.

9. Lead compounds serve as chemical models in biomedicine in parallel to the biological models of, for example, malarial canaries or mice with sleeping sickness. For more on chemical models, see Slater, "Organic Chemistry and Instrumentation"; Eric Francoeur, "The Forgotten Tool: The Design and Use of Molecular Models," *Social Studies of Science* 27 (1997): 7–40; Jacopo Tomasi, "Models and Modeling in Theoretical Chemistry," *Journal of Molecular Structure (Theochem)* 179 (1988): 273–92; Carl Trindle, "The Hierarchy of Models in Chemistry," *Croatica Chemica Acta* 57 (1984): 1231–45; and Colin Suckling, Keith Suckling, and Charles Suckling, *Chemistry through Models* (New York: Cambridge University Press, 1978).

10. August Wingler, "Dyes and Methylene Blue in Medico-Chemical Research," in *Medicine in Its Chemical Aspects* (Leverkusen: I.G. Farbenindustrie A.G., 1934), 2: 225.

11. Werner Schulemann, "Synthetic Anti-Malarial Preparations: A Discussion of the Various Steps which Led to the Synthesis and Discovery of 'Plasmoquine' and a Brief Account of Its Use in Tropical Medicine," *Proceedings of the Royal Society of Medicine* 25 (1932): 897–905, 898.

12. Wingler, "Dyes and Methylene Blue," 224–25.

13. Similar structure activity investigations on a smaller scale were pursued by Harold King and his coworkers in Great Britain. See A. Cohen and Harold King,

"Antiplasmodial Action and Chemical Constitution: Part I. Cinchona Alkaloidal Derivatives and Allied Substances," *Proceedings of the Royal Society of London, Series B* 125 (1938): 49–60; and A. D. Ainley and Harold King, "Antiplasmodial Action and Chemical Constitution: Part II. Some Simple Synthetic Analogues of Quinine and Cinchonine," *Proceedings of the Royal Society of London, Series B* 125 (1938): 60–92.

14. P. Ehrlich and P. Guttmann, "Über die Wirkung des Methylenblau bei Malaria," *Berliner klinische Wochenschrift* 28 (1891): 953–56.

15. For more detail on the Bayer this work, also see Schulemann, "Synthetic Anti-Malarial Preparations"; and Wingler, "Dyes and Methylene Blue," 224–25.

16. Published accounts of Bayer's contributions to synthetic antimalarials can be found in *From Germanin to Acylureidopenicillin: Research that Made History, Documentation of Scientific Revolution*, ed. Rosemarie Alstaedter (Leverkusen: Bayer AG, 1980), 18–24; Horst-Bernd Dünschede, *Tropenmedizinische Forschung bei Bayer, Düsseldorfer Arbeiten zur Geschichte der Medizin, Beiheft II* (Düsseldorf: Michael Triltsch Verlag, 1971), 55–82; Fritz Mietzsch, "Beiträge zur Entwicklung der Chemotherapie aus den Laboratorien der Farbenfabriken Bayer," *Arzneimittel-Forschung* 6 (1956): 503–8; Fritz Mietzsch, "Entwicklungslinien der Chemotherapie (Vom chemischen Standpunkt gesehen)," *Klinische Wochenschrift* 29 (1951): 125–34; and Schulemann, "Synthetic Anti-Malarial Preparations."

17. Fritz, Schönhöfer, "40 Jahre Plasmochin," *Arzneimittel-Forschung* 15 (1965): 1256–58.

18. After Schulemann, "Synthetic Anti-Malarial Preparations," 900.

19. Wingler, "Dyes and Methylene Blue," 226–27.

20. For more on malaria therapy, see Margaret Humphreys, "Whose Body? Which Disease? Studying Malaria while Treating Neurosyphilis," in *Useful Bodies: Humans in the Service of Medical Science in the Twentieth Century*, ed. Jordan Goodman, Anthony McElligott, and Lara Marks (Baltimore: Johns Hopkins University Press, 2003), 53–77; Joel T. Braslow, "The Influence of a Biological Therapy on Doctor's Narratives and Interrogations: The Case of General Paralysis of the Insane and Malaria Fever Therapy, 1910–1950," *Bulletin for the History of Medicine* 70 (1996): 577–608; and William H. Kupper, *The Malaria Therapy of General Paralysis and Other Conditions* (Ann Arbor, MI: Edwards Brothers, 1939).

21. For more on the introduction of malaria therapy, see Erna Lesky, "Julius Wagner von Jauregg," *Dictionary of Scientific Biography* (New York: Scribner, 1976), 14: 114–16.

22. F. Sioli, "Prüfung des Plasmochins bei der Impfmalaria der Paralytiker," *Archiv für Schiffs- und Tropen-Hygiene Pathologie und Therapie exotischer Krankheiten, Beihefte* 30 (1926): 319–24.

23. Peter Mühlens, "Die Behandlung der natürlichen menschlichen Marlariainfektionen mit Plasmochin," *Archiv für Schiffs- und Tropen-Hygiene Pathologie und Therapie exotischer Krankheiten, Beihefte* 30 (1926): 325–35; P. Mühlens and Otto Fischer, "Die Behandlung der natürlichen menschlichen Marlariainfektionen mit Plasmochin," *Archiv für Schiffs- und Tropen-Hygiene Pathologie und Therapie exotischer Krankheiten* 31 (1927): 7–42; P. Mühlens, "Die synthetischen Malariamittel Plasmochin und Atebrin," *Münchener Medizinische Wochenschrift* 79 (1932): 537–40; Otto Fischer, "Über Malariaprophylaxe mit Plasmochin," *Archiv für Schiffs- und Tropen-Hygiene Pathologie und Therapie exotischer Krankheiten* 31 (1927): 43–47.

24. W. Roehl, "Malariatherapie mit Plasmochin in Spanien," *Archiv für Schiffs- und Tropen-Hygiene Pathologie und Therapie exotischer Krankheiten, Beihefte* 31 (1927): 48–58. Roehl's letters from Spain can be found in BAL, Pharma Produkte A-Z, Plasmochin 1933–1937, 166/8, though they are dated from 1925.

25. Werner Schulemann and Guglielmo Memmi, "Plasmochin, ein synthetisches, gegen die Malariainfektion wirksames Chinolinderivat," *Archiv für Schiffs- und Tropen-Hygiene Pathologie und Therapie exotischer Krankheiten* 31 (1927): 59–88. Schulemann's reports from Italy can be found in BAL Pharma Produkte A-Z, Plasmochin 1933–1937, 166/8, though they are dated from 1926.

26. Their first result with plasmochin appeared in their 1926 report: "Experiences with Plasmochin in Malaria (Preliminary Reports)," United Fruit Company, Medical Department, *Fifteenth Annual Report* (Boston: United Fruit Company, 1926), 66–71.

27. Typed translation of letter, 21 October 1926, from United Fruit Company to I. G. Farbenindustrie Atkiengesellschaft, in response to their letter of 1 October: Box 2–1 S-Z, Bernard Nocht Institute, Hamburg, Germany (hereafter BNI) 352–8/9, Prof. Nocht Korrespondenz, folder "U 1900–1930."

28. United Fruit Company, Medical Department, *Thirteenth Annual Report* (Boston: United Fruit Company, 1924), 57.

29. The plasmochin literature is quite large, but another example of interest is perhaps that of the British army in India: see J. A. Manifold, "Report on a Trial of Plasmoquine and Quinine in the Treatment of Benign Tertian Malaria," *Journal of Royal Army Medical Corps* 56, no. 5 (1931): 321–38 and no. 6, 410–23. In the United States during the 1920s and 1930s, standards for the testing and prescription of drugs was evolving. For more on this, see Harry M. Marks, *The Progress of Experiment, Science, and Therapeutic Reform in the United States, 1900–1990* (New York: Cambridge University Press, 1997); and Jan R. McTavish, *Pain and Profits: The History of the Headache and Its Remedies in America* (New Brunswick, NJ: Rutgers University Press, 2004).

30. See, for example, War Department, Army Service Forces, Office of the Surgeon General, Circular Letter No. 153 of 19 August 1943; War Department, Services of Supply, Office of the Surgeon General, Circular Letters No. 135 of 21 October 1942, No. 22 of 16 January 1943, and No. 33 of 2 February 1943. All of these are from Martin Young Files, file "Plasmodium—Human War Malaria" 252–1–13, provided by William E. Collins, CDC, Chamblee, GA. Also see Office of the Surgeon General, Department of the Army, *The Medical Department, United States Army Internal Medicine in World War II*, vol. 2, *Infectious Diseases* (Washington, DC: U.S. Government Printing Office, 1963), chapters 17 and 18, http://history.amedd. army.mil/booksdocs/wwii/infectiousdisvolii/frameindex.html (viewed 12 September 2006).

31. George F. Strode to Frederick F. Russell, 17 November 1931, folder 675, box 51, series 100, RG 1, RFA.

32. James to Strode, 12 November 1931, p. 2, folder 675, box 51, series 401, RG 1.1, RFA.

33. James to Strode, 12 November 1931, 2.

34. James to Strode, 12 November 1931, 1.

35. "Der grundlegende chemische Unterschied zwischen Plasmochin und Atebrin . . . ," 12 April 1934, page 2, BAL Pharma Produkte A-Z, Atebrin 1932–1939, 166/8.

36. Hans Mauss and Fritz Mietzsch, "Atebrin, Ein Neues Heilmittel Gegen Malaria," *Klinische Wochenschrift* 12 (1933): 1276–78; Mauss and Mietzsch, "Notiz zur

Arbeit von O. J. Magidson und A. M. Grigorowski: Acridin-Verbindungen und ihre Antimalaria-Wirkung (I. Mitteil.)," *Berichte der Deutschen-Chemischen Gesellschaft* 69 (1936): 641; and Hans Mauss, "Acridinverbindungen als Malariamittel," in *Medizin und Chemie* (Berlin: Verlag Chemie, 1942), 4: 60–72. Fritz Mietzsch was also involved with the synthesis of the first sulfa drug, Prontosil, which came directly out of a dye program.

37. Atabrine was the U.S. name for the generic drug quinacrine. It was marketed in Germany as Atebrin, in Britain as mepacrine, and in the United States as Atabrine or Chinacrin. A number of spelling variations can be found in different sources. One may also find it referred to as acrichin or acrichine.

38. For Kikuth's account of atabrine in the avian model systems, see Walter Kikuth, "Zur Weiterentwicklung synthetisch dargestellter Malariamittel: I. Über die chemotherapeutische Wirkung des Atebrin," *Deutsche medizinische Wochenschrift* 58 (1932): 530–31.

39. H. Mauss and F. Mietzsch "Atebrin," 31 January 1933, 30 pages, BAL Pharm. wiss. Labor Elberfeld, Berichte, Mietzsch, 103/17.E.2.c.

40. F. Sioli, "Zur Weiterentwicklung synthetisch dargestellter Malariamittel: II. Über die Wirkung des Atebrin bei der Impfmalaria der Paralytiker" *Deutsche medizinische Wochenschrift* 58 (1932): 531–33.

41. F. M. Peter, "Zur Weiterentwicklung synthetisch dargestellter Malariamittel: III. Über die Wirkung des Atebrin gegen natürliche Malaria" *Deutsche medizinische Wochenschrift* 58 (1932): 533–35.

42. Mühlens, "Die synthetischen Malariamittel"; P. Mühlens and O. Fischer, "Über Malaria behandlung mit Atebrin," *Archiv für Schiffs- und Tropen-Hygiene Pathologie und Therapie exotischer Krankheiten* 36 (1932): 196–207.

43. For more about the council and it relationship to drug companies, see Swann, *Academic Scientists and the Pharmaceutical Industry*, especially 146.

44. F. J. Stockman to I. G. Farben, Leverkusen, 9 June 1934, "Plasmochin," BAL Pharma Produkte A-Z, Atebrin, 1931–1939, 166/8; and Winthrop report to Bayer, "3. Atabrine: Council on Pharmacy," 23 November 1932, BAL Pharma Produkte A-Z, Atebrin, 1932–1939, 166/8.

45. See, for example, M. M. van Riemsdijk, M. C. Sturkenboom, L. Pepplinkhuizen, and B. H. Stricker, "Mefloquine Increases the Risk of Serious Psychiatric Events during Travel Abroad: A Nationwide Case-Control Study in the Netherlands," *Journal of Clinical Psychiatry* 66 (2005): 199–204; and Mark Benjamin and Dan Olmsted, "Second Soldier Took Malaria Drug," 9 August 2002, UPI, http://www.upi.com/archive/view.php?archive=1&StoryID=20020809–030540–1747r (viewed 11 October 2006).

46. League of Nations, Health Organization, "Treatment of Malaria: Study of the Therapeutics and Prophylaxis of Malaria by Synthetic Drugs as Compared with Quinine. Fourth General Report of the Malaria Commission," C.H./Malaria./252, 9 December 1937, 7, http://whqlibdoc.who.int/hist/malaria/malaria242(a)-259.pdf (viewed 17 July 2007). The Malaria Commission of the League of Nations Health Organization reports for the years 1924 to 1932 are available at http://www.who.int/library/collections/historical/en/index4.html.

47. League of Nations, Health Organization, Malaria Commission, "Work of the Malaria Commission of the League of Nations since 1930," by Edmond Sergent, president of the Malaria Commission, C.H./Malaria./268, 16 September 1938, 14, http://whqlibdoc.who.int/hist/malaria/malaria260–278.pdf (viewed 17 July 2007).

48. League of Nations, Health Organization, "Agenda for the Meetings of the Reporting Committee and of the Malaria Commission to be held in Amsterdam on Wednesday, September 28th, 1938. Note by the Secretariat," C.H./Malaria./263, 30 August 1938, 3, http://whqlibdoc.who.int/hist/malaria/malaria260–278.pdf (viewed 17 July 2007).

49. Marshall A. Barber, *A Malariologist in Many Lands* (Lawrence: University of Kansas Press, 1946), 138–39.

50. League of Nations, "Work of the Malaria Commission of the League of Nations since 1930," 13.

51. For more on malaria control and the testing of synthetic antimalarials in Georgia, see M. E. Winchester, "The Use of Atabrine in the Control of Malaria," *International Journal of Medicine and Surgery* 48 (1935): 265–67.

52. Report dated 24 November 1933, Section 3. Atabrine, subsection Propaganda, BAL Pharma Produkte A-Z Atebrin 1932–1939 166/8.

53. Report dated 24 November 1933, Section 3. Atabrine, subsection Propaganda.

54. H. Vogel (Winthrop Chemical Co.) to I.G. Farben Pharmaceutical Department, Leverkusen, 23 November 1934, Subject Atabrine Publication, BAL, Pharma Produkte A-Z, Atebrin 1931–1939, 166/8.

55. "Malaria Control: Report by Mr. Hart," 23 December 1933, BAL Pharma Produkte A-Z Atebrin 1932–1939 166/8. This material also appears in BAL Pharma Produkte A-Z, Atebrin 1932–1947, 166/8.

56. Report dated 24 November 1933, BAL. Also see Daniel L. Seckinger, "Atabrine and Plasmochin in the Treatment and Control of Malaria," American Journal of Tropical Medicine 15 (1935): 631–49.

57. "Malaria Control: Report by Mr. Hart," 23 December 1933, BAL. For a summary of some of Komp's Panama work, see Herbert C. Clark and William H. W. Komp, "A Summary of Ten Years of Observations on Malaria in Panama with Reference to Control with Quinine, Atabrine, and Plasmochin, without Anti-Mosquito Measures," in *A Symposium on Human Malaria: With Special Reference to North America and the Caribbean Region*, ed. Forest Ray Moulton, Publication of the American Association for the Advancement of Science No.15 (Lancaster, PA: Science Press Printing Company for the AAAS, 1941), 273–84.

58. "Malaria Control: Report by Mr. Hart," 23 December 1933, BAL.

59. Report of Dr. Lasersohn and Mr. Hart on the Annual Session of the Southern Medical Association and National Malaria Committee (Nov. 14–17, 1933), BAL Pharma Produkte A-Z, Atebrin 1932–1947, 166/8.

60. Report of Dr. Lasersohn and Mr. Hart (Nov. 14–17, 1933), BAL.

61. Report of Dr. Lasersohn and Mr. Hart (Nov. 14–17, 1933), BAL.

62. William N. Bispham, "A Report on the Use of Atebrin in the Prophylaxis of Malaria," *American Journal of Tropical Medicine* 16 (1936): 547–62; and "Final Report on the Use of Atabrine in Prophylaxis and Treatment of Malaria," *American Journal of Tropical Medicine* 18 (1938): 545–64.

63. Memorandum, Winthrop Chemical Company, Inc. (F. J. Stockman), to I.G. Farbenindustrie A.G., "League of Nations' Malaria Congress: Madrid," 2 February 1935, BAL Pharma Produkte A-Z, Atebrin, 1931–1939, 166/8.

64. Bayer to Winthrop Chemical Company, Inc., "Dr. Hackett, Rom," 3 June 1935, BAL Pharma Produkte A-Z, Atebrin, 1931–1939, 166/8.

65. Louis L. William Papers are held by the National Library of Medicine, History of Medicine Division: 1927–1970, MS C 169.

66. Memorandum, Winthrop Chemical Company, Inc. (F. J. Stockman), to I.G. Farbenindustrie A.G., "Malaria Paper by Dr. George Cheever Shattuck," 20 November 1935, BAL Pharma Produkte A-Z, Atebrin, 1931–1939, 166/8.

67. Memorandum, Winthrop Chemical Company, Inc. (F. J. Stockman), to I.G. Farbenindustrie A.G., "Dr. George Cheever Shattuck," 24 January 1936, BAL Pharma Produkte A-Z, Atebrin, 1931–1939, 166/8.

68. Section 13 Atabrine, "Research," [1937, p. 22], BAL Pharma Produkte A-Z Atebrin, 1932–1939, 166/8.

69. "Auszuge aus Akt. Dr. Weiss 1939," p. 25, BAL Pharma Produkte A-Z, Atebrin, 1932–1947, 166/8.

70. "Auszuge aus Akt. Dr. Weiss 1939," 25, BAL.

71. Section 13 Atabrine, "Sales," [1937, p. 21], BAL Pharma Produkte A-Z, Atebrin, 1932–1939, 166/8.

72. Section Personal Injury Claims, "Atabrine," [1937, p. 21], BAL Pharma Produkte A-Z, Atebrin, 1932–1939, 166/8.

73. Section 13 Atabrine, "Psychosis," [1937, p. 21], BAL Pharma Produkte A-Z, Atebrin, 1932–1939, 166/8.

74. Section 13 Atabrine, "Psychosis," [1937, pp. 21–22], BAL.

75. Section 13 Atabrine, "Psychosis," [1937, p. 22], BAL.

76. Minutes, Conferences held with Dr. Mertens on Research Matters, New York, 20–21 October 1937, BAL Pharma Produkte A-Z, Atebrin 1932–1947, 166/8.

77. Section 13 Atabrine, "Quinine Competition," [1937, p. 22], BAL Pharma Produkte A-Z Atebrin 1932–1939 166/8.

78. "Auszuge aus Akt. Dr. Weiss 1939," 25, BAL.

79. Minutes of the Winthrop pharmaceutical conference held on Wednesday, January 20, 1937 at 170 Varick Street, New York City, at 10:00 A.M., page 21 insert, BAL Pharma Produkte A-Z, Atebrin 1932–1947, 166/8.

80. This and subsequent quotes in this paragraph are from "Auszuge aus Akt. Dr. Weiss 1939," 26, BAL.

81. Some of this work was published during the war. See, for example, Fritz Schönhöfer, "Über die Bedeutung der chinoiden Bindung in Chinolinverbindungen für die Malariawirkung," Hoppe-Seyler's Zeitschrift für physiol. Chemie 274 (1942): 1–8.

82. Combined Intelligence Objectives Sub-Committee, "Clinical Testing of Antimalarials by I.G. Farben," CIOS XXIII-13, 20 May 1945, 11.

83. Walter Menk and Werner Mohr, "Sontochin (Nivaquine) in seiner Therapeutischen Wirkung bei Malaria," Zeitschrift für Tropenmedizin und Parasitologie 2 (1950): 351–61. See also Combined Intelligence Objectives Sub-Committee, "Pharmaceuticals and Insecticides at I.G. Farben Plants Elberfeld and Leverkusen," CIOS XXIII 12, [1945], 30.

84. For more on German antimalarial efforts during World War II, see Wolfgang U. Eckart and H. Vondra, "Malaria and World War II: German Malaria Experiments 1939–45," Parassitologia 42 (2000): 53–58; Marion Hulverscheidt, "Menschen, Mücken und Malaria—Das wissenschaftliche Umfeld des KZ-Malariaforschers Claus Schilling," in Medizin im Nationalsozialismus und das System der Konzentrationslager. Beiträge eines interdisziplinären Symposiums, ed. Judith Hahn, Silvija Kavčič, and Christoph Kopke (Frankfurt am Main: Mabuse-Verlag, 2005), 108–26; Richard L. Kenyon, Jos. A. Wiesner, and C. E. Kwartler, "Chloroquine Manufacture," Industrial and Engineering Chemistry 41 (1949): 655; Combined

Intelligence Objectives Sub-Committee, "Pharmaceuticals and Insecticides at I.G. Farben Plants Elberfeld and Leverkusen," CIOS XXIII-12, [1945]; "Clinical Testing of Antimalarials by I.G. Farben," CIOS XXIII-13, 20 May 1945; "Professor Doctor Werner Schulemann Malariologist," CIOS XXIII-17, [1945]; "Pharmaceutical Targets in Southern Germany," CIOS XXIV-16; "Insecticides, Insect Repellents, Rodenticides and Fungicides: I.G. Farbenindustrie A. G., Elberfeld and Leverkusen," CIOS XXVI-73, 19–30 May 1945, and "Tropical Medicines and Other Medical Subjects in Germany," CIOS XXIX-35; and British Intelligence Objectives Sub-Committee, "Pharmaceuticals: Research and Manufacturing at I.G. Farbenindustrie," BIOS Final Report No. 116, 7–23 August 1945.

85. Leonard Jan Bruce-Chwatt and Julian de Zulueta, *The Rise and Fall of Malaria in Europe* (New York: Clarendon Press, 1980), 82–88; Dünschede, *Tropenmedizinische Forschung*, 51–82; Moore, "Malaria Chemotherapy," 8: 660–80; Frederick Y. Wiselogle, ed., *A Survey of Antimalarial Drugs 1941–1945*, 2 vols. (Ann Arbor: J. W. Edwards, 1946); and A. E. Sherndal, "Chemistry and Development of Atabrine and Plasmochin," *Chemical and Engineering News* 21 (25 July 1943): 1154–58.

86. For more on the British project, see David Greenwood, "Conflicts of Interest: The Genesis of Synthetic Antimalarial Agents in Peace and War," *Journal of Antimicrobial Chemotherapy* 36 (1995): 857–72; F. H. K. Green and Sir Gordon Covell, eds., *Medical Research: History of the Second World War United Kingdom Medical Series* (London: H. M. Stationery Office, 1953), 155–60; F. L. Rose, "A Chemotherapeutic Search in Retrospect," *Journal of the Chemical Society* (1951): 2770–88; and various authors in *Annals of Tropical Medicine and Parasitology* 39, nos. 3 and 4 (1945), Liverpool School of Tropical Medicine.

87. See G. Robert Coatney, "Pitfalls in a Discovery: The Chronicle of Chloroquine," *American Journal of Tropical Medicine and Hygiene* 12 (1963): 121–28. Resochin (chloroquine) and sontochin were designated SN-7618 and SN-6911, respectively, by the U.S. wartime antimalarial program.

88. This and subsequent quotes in this paragraph from Atabrine/Winthrop Report circa 1937, "Organization of Malaria Control Services in the United States," Section 7 "Rockefeller Foundation," 5–6, BAL Pharma Produkte A-Z, Atebrin 1931–1939, 166/8.

89. Paul F. Russell, "Preventive Medicine as Exemplified by Malaria," address to the third year class at the Harvard Medical School, 10 January 1936, p. 30, folder 503, box 50, series 100, RG 1, RFA.

90. Lowell T. Coggeshall, Leonard H. Cretcher, Lyndon F. Small, Torald H. Sollmann, and Marston T. Bogert, "The National Research Council Committee on Chemotherapy," *Journal of the American Medical Association* 115 (1940): 307. This NRC-sponsored piece was published simultaneously in *JAMA*, as just cited, and in *Science*. For simplicity, I will make all subsequent references to the *JAMA* article. The reference in *Science* is "Research Work on Chemotherapy," *Science* 92 (1940): 176–78.

Chapter 4 — Preparing for War

1. Lowell T. Coggeshall, Leonard H. Cretcher, Lyndon F. Small, Torald H. Sollmann, and Marston T. Bogert, "The National Research Council Committee on Chemotherapy," *Journal of the American Medical Association* 115 (1940): 307.

2. On the founding of the NRC, see Rexmond C. Cochrane, *The National Academy of Sciences: The First Hundred Years, 1863–1963* (Washington, DC: National Academy of Sciences, 1978), 200–241.

3. For more on wartime mobilization, see Leo B. Slater, "Chemists and National Emergency: NIH's Unit of Chemotherapy during World War II," *Bulletin for the History of Chemistry* 31 (2006): 75–80; Barry D. Karl, *The Uneasy State: The United States from 1915–1945* (Chicago: University of Chicago Press, 1983); R. J. Overy, *The Air War, 1939–1945* (New York: Stein and Day, 1980); and Robert Cuff, "American Mobilization for War, 1917–1945: Political Culture vs. Bureaucratic Administration," in *Mobilization for Total War: The Canadian, American, and British Experience, 1914–1918, 1939–1945*, ed. N. F. Dreisziger (Waterloo, Ontario: Wilfrid Laurier University Press, 1981).

4. World War II was the font of a number of transformational R&D projects. See, for example, on the development of nuclear weapons, Richard Rhodes, *The Making of the Atomic Bomb* (New York: Simon and Schuster, 1986); on radar, Louis Brown, *A Radar History of World War II* (Philadelphia: Institute of Physics, 1999), and Robert Buderi, *The Invention that Changed the World* (New York: Simon and Schuster, 1996); on synthetic rubber, Peter J. T. Morris, *The American Synthetic Rubber Research Program* (Philadelphia: University of Pennsylvania Press, 1989); and on penicillin, Gladys L. Hobby, *Penicillin: Meeting the Challenge* (New Haven: Yale University Press, 1985), and John C. Sheehan, *The Enchanted Ring: The Untold Story of Penicillin* (Cambridge, MA: MIT Press, 1982).

5. W. Mansfield Clark, "History of Co-operative Wartime Program," in *A Survey of Antimalarial Drugs, 1941–1945*, ed. Frederick Y. Wiselogle (Ann Arbor: J. W. Edwards, 1946), 2.

6. Coggeshall et al., "The National Research Council Committee on Chemotherapy," 307.

7. Coggeshall et al., "The National Research Council Committee on Chemotherapy," 307.

8. Coggeshall et al., "The National Research Council Committee on Chemotherapy," 307.

9. *Public Health Reports*, "A Brief Review of Needed Research in Malaria," 55 (1940): 1804.

10. *Public Health Reports*, "A Brief Review," 1808–9.

11. "Autobiography—Medical Director Louis L. Williams Jr., U. S. Public Health Service," 1948, box 1, folder, Biographical Data, Louis L. Williams Papers, 1927–1970, MS C 169, History of Medicine Division, National Library of Medicine, National Institutes of Health, Bethesda, MD. For more on the history of CDC, see Elizabeth W. Etheridge, *Sentinel for Health: A History of the Centers for Disease Control* (Berkeley: University of California Press, 1992), http://www.cdc.gov/od/oc/media/timeline.htm (viewed 24 November 2006) and http://www.cdc.gov/about/ourstory.htm (viewed 24 November 2006).

12. W. H. Taliaferro to Thomas Parran, 27 June 1940, copy, folder 490, box 50, series 100, RG 1, RFA.

13. Coggeshall et al., "The National Research Council Committee on Chemotherapy," 308.

14. Coggeshall et al., "The National Research Council Committee on Chemotherapy," 308.

15. Coggeshall et al., "The National Research Council Committee on Chemotherapy," 308.

16. Coggeshall et al., "The National Research Council Committee on Chemotherapy," 307.

17. Parran himself was a promoter of both wartime malaria research and of postwar growth in publicly financed medical research. See National Library of Medicine, History of Medicine Division, MS C204, Thomas Parran Papers, Box 1, numerous folders, "Ten-Year Postwar Program of U.S. Public Health Service," 1 November 1944. Parran was also central in the founding and maintenance of the National Cancer Institute during its first decade, 1937–1948. See Nancy Carol Erdey, "Armor of Patience: The National Cancer Institute and the Development of Medical Research Policy in the United States, 1937–1971" (PhD diss., Case Western Reserve University, 1995), 66–104.

18. For more about Coggeshall's life and career, see Joel D. Howell, "Lowell T. Coggeshall and American Medical Education: 1901–1987," *Academic Medicine* 67 (1992): 711–18; and *The Reminiscences of Lowell T. Coggeshall*, oral history interviews conducted by Christopher Kimball for the University of Chicago Archives Oral History Program, 31 August and 1 September 1987.

19. For background on the relationship between the IHD and the Institutes, see John Farley, *To Cast out Disease: A History of the International Health Division of the Rockefeller Foundation, 1913–1951* (Oxford: Oxford University Press, 2004), 157–68.

20. See D. F. Milam and L. T. Coggeshall, "Duration of Plasmodium Knowlesi Infections in Man," *American Journal of Tropical Medicine* 18 (1938): 331–38; Monroe D. Eaton and Coggeshall, "Complement Fixation in Human Malaria with an Antigen Prepared from the Monkey Parasite Plasmodium Knowlesi," *Journal of Experimental Medicine* 69 (1939): 379–98; and Eaton and Coggeshall, "Production in Monkeys of Complement-Fixing Antibodies without Active Immunity by Injection of Killed Plasmodium Knowlesi," *Journal of Experimental Medicine* 70 (1939): 141–46. Precipitin tests were also employed to determine the species on which mosquitoes had fed.

21. See, for example, [William Taliaferro], "Investigations in Malaria at the University of Chicago, 1925–1939," p. 5, folder 520, box 52, series 100, RG 1, Rockefeller Foundation Archives, and William Taliaferro to W. A. Sawyer, 23 July 1938, folder 516, box 51, series 100, RG 1, RFA.

22. Coggeshall et al., "The National Research Council Committee on Chemotherapy," 307.

23. E. H. Volwiler (PhD, Vice-President) to L. T. Coggeshall, 2 July 1940, folder 35, box 32, series 4, RG 5, RFA.

24. L. T. Coggeshall to E. H. Volwiler, 30 July 1940, folder 35, box 32, series 4, RG 5, RFA.

25. L. T. Coggeshall to E. H. Volwiler, 30 July 1940.

26. E. H. Volwiler to L. T. Coggeshall, 16 August 1940, folder 35, box 32, series 4, RG 5, RFA.

27. See, for example, H. B. van Dyke (MD, Squibb Institute for Medical Research) to L. T. Coggeshall, 18 October 1940, and L. T. Coggeshall to H. B. van Dyke, 22 October 1940, folder 350, box 32, series 4, RG 5, RFA; and John Maier to van Dyke, 22 November 1940, folder 350, box 32, series 4, RG 5, RFA.

28. L. T. Coggeshall through J. H. Bauer to Wilbur A. Sawyer, "Malaria program," 10 October 1940, folder 490, box 50, series 100, RG 1, RFA.

29. Coggeshall through Bauer to Sawyer, "Malaria program," 10 October 1940.

30. W. A. Sawyer through Bauer to L. T. Coggeshall, 17 October 1940, folder 490, box 50, series 100, RG 1, RFA.

31. Sawyer through Bauer to Coggeshall, 17 October 1940.

32. Notes on John A. Ferrell's conference with Mr. Warren Weaver and Mr. F. B. Hanson, 27 November 1940, folder 490, box 50, series 100, RG 1, RFA.

33. Notes on Ferrell's conference with Weaver and Hanson, 27 November 1940.

34. For more on Marshall, see Marcel H. Bickel, "Eli K. Marshall Jr. (1889–1966): From Biochemistry and Physiology to Pharmacology and Pharmacokinetics," *Drug Metabolism Reviews* 28 (1996): 311–44; and Thomas H. Maren, "Eli Kennerly Marshall Jr., May 2, 1889–January 10, 1966," in *Biographical Memoirs: National Academy of Sciences* (Washington, DC: National Academy Press, 1987), 56: 313–52.

35. Memorandum from Coggeshall to Ferrell, 2 January 1941, folder 491, box 50, series 100, RG 1, RFA.

36. International Health Division, IH 40065, Harvard University, 23 April 1941, copy, folder 112, box 11, series 4, RG 5, RFA.

37. International Health Division, 23 April 1941.

38. International Health Division, 23 April 1941.

39. Coggeshall to J. A. Ferrell, 24 January 1941, and Ferrell to Coggeshall 27 January 1941, folder 491, box 50, series 100, RG 1, RFA.

40. E. K. Marshall to J. A. Ferrell, 2 December 1940, excerpted, folder 490, box 50, series 100, RG 1, RFA.

41. Coggeshall through J. H. Bauer and W. A. Sawyer to John A. Ferrell, "Dr. E. K. Marshall Jr.," 2 December 1940, folder 115, box 11, series 4, RG 5, RFA.

42. E. K. Marshall to J. A. Ferrell, 2 December 1940, excerpted, folder 490, box 50, series 100, RG 1; and Coggeshall through J. H. Bauer and W. A. Sawyer to John A. Ferrell, "Dr. E. K. Marshall Jr.," 2 December 1940, folder 115, box 11, series 4, RG 5, RFA.

43. Coggeshall through Bauer and Sawyer to Ferrell, "Dr. E. K. Marshall Jr.," 2 December 1940.

44. Coggeshall through Bauer and Sawyer to Ferrell, "Dr. E. K. Marshall Jr., 2 December 1940.

45. For more on the development of the sulfa drugs, see John E. Lesch, *The First Miracle Drugs: How the Sulfa Drugs Transformed Medicine* (New York: Oxford University Press, 2006); and Thomas Hager, *The Demon Under the Microscope: From Battlefield Hospitals to Nazi Labs, One Doctor's Heroic Search for the World's First Miracle Drug* (New York: Harmony Books, 2006). For a contemporary account, see John Pfeiffer, "Sulfanilamide: The Story of a Great Medical Discovery," *Harper's* 178 (1939): 386–96.

46. Paul Fildes, "A Rational Approach to Chemotherapy," *Lancet* 238 (1940): 956–57. This rational approach through metabolism was, in part, a complement to vitamin-type research. Both entailed the determination of essential nutrients or metabolites for an organism, but in the case of antibiotic research the essential nutrients were replaced with altered analogs that might block the proper uptake of similar and essential compounds.

47. Later in the war, at least one rational, antimetabolite approach was attempted: D. W. Woolley, "The Revolution in Pharmacology," *Perspectives in Biology and Medicine* 1 (1958): 174–97, 182.

48. *Rockefeller Foundation Annual Report*, 1945, 147.

49. *Rockefeller Foundation Annual Report*, 1945, 148.

50. The rational approach is emblematic of a move to rational drug discovery, based on a more biochemically sophisticated and mechanistic view of drug activity. Rational drug design is a later concept, encompassing activities such as searching molecular databases using criteria derived from structural understandings of receptors and enzymes. For more, see Ralph Hirschmann, "Medicinal Chemistry in the Golden Age of Biology: Lessons from Steroid and Peptide Research," *Angewandte Chemie, International English Edition* 30 (1991): 1291 and 1296–97.

51. Marshall to Coggeshall, 13 May 1940, folder 223, box 20, series 4, RG 5, RFA.

52. Coggeshall to Marshall, 23 May 1940, folder 223, box 20, series 4, RG 5, RFA.

53. J. H. Bauer to Sawyer et al., Inter-Office Correspondence, 29 March 1941, folder 491, box 50, series 100, RG 1, RFA.

54. Coggeshall through J. H. Bauer and W. A. Sawyer to John A. Ferrell, "Chemotherapeutic Program," 29 January 1941, folder 115, box 11, series 4, RG 5, RFA.

55. Coggeshall through J. H. Bauer and W. A. Sawyer to John A. Ferrell, "Chemotherapeutic Program," 29 January 1941, RAC.

56. See, for example, A. W. Schoenleber, "Malaria in Industry," *Medical Bulletin (Standard Oil Co.)* 3, no. 6 (1938): 201–17.

57. Coggeshall through J. H. Bauer and W. A. Sawyer to John A. Ferrell, "Chemotherapeutic Program," 29 January 1941, RAC.

58. Coggeshall through J. H. Bauer to W. A. Sawyer, "Promin," 13 March 1941, folder 491, box 50, series 100, RG 1, RAC.

59. Coggeshall through J. H. Bauer to W. A. Sawyer, "Promin," 13 March 1941, RAC.

60. L. T. Coggeshall, John Maier, and C. A. Best, "The Effectiveness of Two New Types of Chemotherapeutic Agents in Malaria," *Journal of the American Medical Association* 117 (1941): 1077–81. For an interesting note on the mode of action of the sulfas, see Louis F. Fieser, *The Scientific Method: A Personal Account of Unusual Projects in War and in Peace* (New York: Reinhold, 1964), 164–65.

61. P. J. Crawford to Coggeshall, 5 April 1941, and Coggeshall to W. A. Sawyer, 14 April 1941, folder 491, box 50, series 100, RG 1, RAC.

62. For more on Clark, see Hubert Bradford Vickery, "William Mansfield Clark, August 17, 1884–January 19 1964," in *Biographical Memoirs: National Academy of Sciences* (Washington, DC: National Academy Press, 1968), 39: 1–36.

63. Clark, "History," 4.

64. Clark, "History," 6.

65. NRC, DMS, Conference on Chemotherapy of Malaria, minutes of meeting, 8 July 1941, in Board, *Bulletin,* 7–11.

66. "Investigations in Malaria at the University of Chicago, 1925–1939," 26 June 1939, and "Investigations in Malaria at the University of Chicago, 1940–1941," received 2 September 1941, folder 520, box 52, series 100, RG 1, RAC.

67. NRC, DMS, Conference on Chemotherapy of Malaria, minutes of meeting, 8 July 1941, in Board, *Bulletin,* 3.

68. NRC, DMS, Conference on Chemotherapy of Malaria, minutes of meeting, 8 July 1941, in Board, *Bulletin,* 4.

69. Clark, "History," 5.

70. W.A. Sawyer, diary note, 7 November 1942, folder 492, box 50, series 100, RG 1, RFA.

71. NRC, DMS, acting for the CMR of the OSRD, minutes of the Conference on Chemotherapy of Malaria, 30 December 1941, in Board, *Bulletin,* 36.

72. Maier to L. A. Sweet, 8 April 1941, folder 322, box 29, series 4, RG 5, RFA.

73. L. T. Coggeshall to H. B. van Dyke, 22 October 1940, folder 350, box 32, series 4, RG 5, RFA.

74. See E. K. Marshall Jr., "Chemotherapy of Avian Malaria," *Physiological Reviews* 22 (1942): 190–204, 191; NRC, DMS, Conference on Chemotherapy of Malaria, minutes of meeting, 8 July 1941, E. K. Marshall Jr., "Tentative Methods for Preliminary Testing of Antimalarial Drugs," minutes, in Board, *Bulletin*, 7–11; and E. K. Marshall Jr., "Pharmacological Investigations of Potential Antimalarial Drugs," in *A Survey of Antimalarial Drugs*, 60–61.

75. NRC, DMS, Conference on Chemotherapy of Malaria, minutes of meeting, 3 September 1941, in Board, *Bulletin*, 22.

76. NRC, DMS, Conference on Chemotherapy of Malaria, minutes of meeting, 3 September 1941, in Board, *Bulletin*, 22.

77. "Comments Upon Preliminary Evaluations of New Antimalarial Drugs," Malaria Report No. 72, Survey Bulletin No. 11 (20 January 1944): 2, William Mansfield Clark Collection, American Philosophical Society (hereafter referred to as Clark Collection), B:C547, Series V NRC Antimalarial Drug Program.

78. NRC, DMS, Conference on Chemotherapy of Malaria, minutes of meeting, 3 September 1941, in Board, *Bulletin*, 21.

79. Clark, "History," 5.

80. Clark, "History," 6–7.

Chapter 5 — Cooperation and Coordination

1. Norman Taylor, *Cinchona in Java: The Story of Quinine* (New York: Greenberg, 1945); and Richard L. Kenyon, Jos. A. Wiesner, and C. E. Kwartler, "Chloroquine Manufacture," *Industrial and Engineering Chemistry* 41 (April 1949): 654–62.

2. *New York Times*, 2 March 1942. The Tokyo communiqué was dated 1 March.

3. Clark, "History of the Co-operative Wartime Program," in *A Survey of Antimalarial Drugs*, 2. With regard to dates and committees, I cite Clark's "History" for reasons of simplicity and clarity. I have found no contradictions between it and the committee minutes.

4. John Maier through J. H. Bauer to J. A. Ferrell, "Expansion of Chemical Side of Malaria Chemotherapy Program," 14 May 1942, folder 115, box 11, series 4, RG 5, RFA.

5. John Maier through J. H. Bauer to J. A. Ferrell, "Expansion of Chemical Side of Malaria Chemotherapy Program," 14 May 1942, RAC.

6. John Maier through J. H. Bauer to J. A. Ferrell, "Expansion of Chemical Side of Malaria Chemotherapy Program," 14 May 1942, RAC.

7. Clark, "History," 37.

8. Louis F. Fieser et al., "Naphthoquinone Antimalarials. I. General Survey," *Journal of the American Chemical Society* 70 (1948): 3151. For an account of how these compounds came to Fieser and Abbott, see Louis F. Fieser, *The Scientific Method: A Personal Account of Unusual Projects in War and in Peace* (New York: Reinhold, 1964), 166–69.

9. See, for example, Fieser et al., "Naphthoquinone Antimalarials," 3151–55; Fieser and Russell H. Brown, "Naphthoquinone Antimalarials. XXIII. Bz-Substituted Derivatives," *Journal of the American Chemical Society* 71 (1949): 3615–17; and Fieser and Alfred R. Bader, "Rearrangement of Reduction of Hindered

2-Hydroxy-3-alkly-1,4-naphthoquinines," *Journal of the American Chemical Society* 73 (1951): 681–84.

10. Clark, "History," 36–38.
11. Clark, "History," 7–8.
12. NRC, DMS, Conference on Malaria Research, Appendix—Meeting, 3 June 1942, William H. Taliaferro, "Report on Experimental Investigations on Malaria Supported by the Office of Scientific Research and Development," 20 June 1942, in Board, *Bulletin*, 41–42.
13. Clark, "History," 7.
14. NRC, DMS, Conference on Malaria Research, Appendix—Meeting, 3 June 1942, William H. Taliaferro, "Report on Experimental Investigations on Malaria Supported by the Office of Scientific Research and Development," 20 June 1942, Board, *Bulletin*, 43.
15. Clark, "History," 15.
16. NRC, DMS, Conference on Malaria Research, Appendix—Meeting, 3 June 1942, William H. Taliaferro, "Report on Experimental Investigations on Malaria Supported by the Office of Scientific Research and Development," 20 June 1942, Board, *Bulletin*, 44, emphasis in the original.
17. Conference on Malaria Research, Minutes of the Sixth Meeting, 1 July 1942, Board, *Bulletin*, 40.
18. Survey of Antimalarials, Malaria Report #719, p. 1, 18 July 1946, NARA, RG 227, Records of the OSRD, entry 165, box 67, folder CMR JHU OEMcmr-186.
19. Annual Report, 1942–1943, p. 10, [1 July 1943], NARA, RG 227, Records of the OSRD, entry 29, box 67, folder CMR JHU OEMcmr-186.
20. NRC, DMS, minutes of the meeting of the Malaria Conference, 25 August 1942, Board, *Bulletin*.
21. Clark, "History," general letter of solicitation from A. N. Richards, Lewis H. Weed, and W. Mansfield Clark, August 1942, appendix 2, 49–50.
22. Clark, "History," 15.
23. For example, "consultants" to the Subcommittee on Coordination of Malarial Studies in 1943 included the following: L. Earle Arnow, Sharp and Dohm, Inc.; M. L. Crossley, Calco Chemical Division, American Cyanamid, Co.; D. D. Irish, Dow Chemical; M. E. Krahl, Eli Lilly and Co.; Marlin T. Leffler, Abbott Laboratories; John V. Scudi, Merck and Co., Inc.; L. A. Sweet, Parke, Davis and Co.; and H. B. van Dyke, Squibb Institute for Medical Research. List from "Subcommittee on Coordination of Malarial Studies," 27 September 1943, Clark Collection, B:C547, Series II NRC, Antimalarial Drug Program, ca. 1943–1947.
24. Clark, "History," 15.
25. "Clark, W. Mansfield," 11 February 1943, NARA, RG 227, Records of the OSRD, Committee on Medical Research, entry 162, box 14, minutes of the CMR, January 3, 1941—September 28, 1946, Index 1, A—G.
26. "Clark, W. Mansfield," 11 February 1943.
27. Annual Report, 1942–1943, p. 10, [1 July 1943], NARA, RG 227, Records of the OSRD, entry 29, box 67, folder CMR JHU OEMcmr-186.
28. Annual Report, 1942–1943, p. 11, [1 July 1943], NARA, RG 227, Records of the OSRD, entry 29, box 67, folder CMR JHU OEMcmr-186.
29. Survey of Antimalarials, Bulletin #3, pp. 20–24, 4 May 1943, NARA, RG 227, Records of the OSRD, entry 165, box 67, folder CMR JHU OEMcmr-186.

30. Annex 1, Committee on Medical Research of the OSRD, Memorandum, 15 June 1943, Clark Collection, B:C547, Series II NRC Antimalarial Drug Program, ca. 1943–1947.
31. Clark, "History," 16.
32. Clark, "History," 15.
33. Clark to Andrus, 15 June 1943, folder "Clark, Dr. William M., 1943," NARA, RG 227, entry 165, box 22, Records of the OSRD, Committee on Medical Research.
34. Clark, "History," 16.
35. E. K. Marshall Jr., "Pharmacological Investigations of Potential Antimalarial Drugs," in *A Survey of Antimalarial Drugs*, 62–63.
36. See also Kenneth C. Blanchard and Leon H. Schmidt, "Chemical Series of Potential Interest," in *A Survey of Antimalarial Drugs*, 73–75.
37. Clark, "History," 17.
38. James H. Williams, *Chemotherapy of Malaria: A Review of the Biological and Statistical Background of Malaria, and of the Literature on Anti-Malarial Chemotherapeutic Agents* (New York: Lederle Laboratories, 1941); and Harry S. Mosher, *Confidential Report: Antimalarials: Natural and Synthetic* (Ann Arbor, MI: Edwards Brothers, 1942).
39. Clark, "History," 17.
40. Clark, "History," 8.
41. See Wiselogle, ed., *A Survey of Antimalarial Drugs*, 1: 309–12, 2: 304; and Clark, "History," 9.
42. Clark, "History," 9.
43. Survey of Antimalarials, Bulletin #3, p. 1, 4 May 1943, NARA, RG 227, Records of the OSRD, entry 165, box 67, folder CMR JHU OEMcmr-186.
44. James A. Shannon, "Report on a Consideration of the Rationale of the Clinical Testing Program (Antimalarials), Made to the Board for the Coordination of Malarial Studies and Its Civilian Consultants," 29 March 1944, Board, *Bulletin*, 849.
45. Clark, "History," 7–9.
46. Clark, "History," 12.
47. Alfred E. Sherndal, "Chemistry and Development pf Atabrine and Plasmochin" *Chemical and Engineering News* 21 (25 July 1943): 1154–58.
48. Clark, "History," 13.
49. Clark, "History," 14.
50. See, for example, James A. Shannon, David P. Earle Jr., Bernard B. Brodie, John V. Taggart, Robert W. Berliner, and the Resident Staff of the Research Service, "The Pharmacological Basis for the Rational Use of Atabrine in the Treatment of Malaria," *Journal of Pharmacology and Experimental Therapeutics* 81 (1944): 307–30.
51. Clark, "History," 14.
52. Atabrine was such a part of military culture in some areas of operation that a book published after the war that humorously complained about the Army's treatment of the ordinary private was titled *Atabrine Time*: Kilroy, *Atabrine Time* (Philadelphia: Kilroy's, n.d.), illustrations by Albert Ricciardelli.
53. Alfred E. Sherndal, "Atebrin and Plasmoquine: Their Chemistry and Development," *Chemical Age* (25 September 1943): 310.
54. For a look at the place of Brodie, Shannon, and Udenfriend in the history of clinical pharmacology, see Colin T. Dollery, "Clinical Pharmacology: The First

75 Years and a View to the Future," *British Journal of Clinical Pharmacology* 61 (2006): 650–65.

55. NRC, Chemistry Division, "Minutes of a Conference on Methods for Determining Atabrine in Plasma and Urine," Board, *Bulletin*, 315.

56. Millimicrons = nanometers.

57. U.S. Navy, "Malaria Report #383: Construction of a Rugged Quinacrine Dermofluorometer for Possible Field Use," and "Malaria Report #384: Use of a Quinacrine Dermofluorometer to Measure Tissue Quinacrine Levels of Subject on Suppressive Therapy," Board, *Bulletin*, vol. 4, NARA, RG 227, Records of the OSRD, Committee on Medical Research, entry 167, box 2.

58. See Robert Kanigel, *Apprentice to Genius: The Making of a Scientific Dynasty* (Baltimore: Johns Hopkins University Press, 1993), 13–30. Also see Sidney Udenfriend, "Development of the Spectrophotofluorometer and Its Commercialization," *Protein Science* 4 (1995): 542–51; R. L. Bowman, "The History and Development of the Spectrophotofluorometer," *Fluorescence News* 8, no. 1 (February 1974): 1–8; and the office of NIH history Web site, http://history.nih.gov/exhibits/bowman/index.html (viewed on 1 December 2006).

59. John Maier to Sweet, 13 November 1942, folder 332, box 29, series 4, RG 5, RFA.

60. James A. Shannon and David P. Earle, "Malaria Report #724: Chemotherapy of the Human Malarias, Final Report," 31 August 1946, Board, *Bulletin*, vol. 7, NARA, RG 227, Records of the OSRD, Committee on Medical Research, entry 167, box 4.

61. G. Robert Coatney and W. H. Sebrell, "Malaria Report #721: Clinical Testing of Antimalarials at the National Institute of Health, Final Report," 30 June 1946, Board, *Bulletin*, vol. 7, NARA, RG 227, Records of the OSRD, Committee on Medical Research, entry 167, box 4.

62. See, for example, Alf S. Alving, "Malaria Report #586: Procedures Used at Stateville Penitentiary Joliet, Ill. for Testing Potential Antimalarial Agents," 21 December 1945, Board, *Bulletin*, vol. 6, NARA, RG 227, Records of the OSRD, Committee on Medical Research, entry 167, box 3; and Alf S. Alving and Lillian Eichelberger, "Malaria Report #723: Clinical Testing of Antimalarial Drugs, Final Report," 31 August 1946, Board, *Bulletin*, vol. 7, NARA, RG 227, Records of the OSRD, Committee on Medical Research, entry 167, box 4.

63. Leopold's account of his work in the malaria program can be found in his memoir: Nathan F. Leopold, *Life Plus 99 Years* (Garden City, NY: Doubleday, 1958), 305–38.

64. The U.S. Army and Navy contributed dozens of reports. See, for example, "Malaria Report #300: Suppression of Malaria in Combat," 6 October 1944, Board, *Bulletin*, vol. 3, NARA, RG 227, Records of the OSRD, Committee on Medical Research, entry 167, box 2; "Malaria Report #353: Study of the Effectiveness of SN-7618 in the Routine Suppression of Malaria: Studies in Army and Navy Installations," 16 March 1945, Board, *Bulletin*, vol. 4, NARA, RG 227, Records of the OSRD, Committee on Medical Research, entry 167, box 2; L. T. Coggeshall, "Malaria Report #404: Status of Studies on the Effectiveness of Antimalarials against Pacific Vivax Malaria at Marine Barracks, Klamath Falls," 11 May 1945, Board for the Coordination of Malaria Studies, vol. 4, NARA, RG 227, Records of the OSRD, Committee on Medical Research, entry 167, box 2.

65. See N. Hamilton Fairley, "Chemotherapeutic Suppression and Prophylaxis in Malaria: An Experimental Investigation Undertaken by Medical Research Teams in Australia," *Transactions of the Royal Society of Tropical Medicine and Hygiene*

38 (1945): 311–65; and Mary Ellen Condon-Rall, "Allied Cooperation in Malaria Prevention and Control: The World War II Southwest Pacific Experience," *Journal of the History of Medicine and Allied Sciences* 46 (1991): 493–513.

66. Lewis H. Weed to Norman T. Kirk, 21 October 1943, p. 1, Clark Collection, B:C547, Series I NRC Antimalarial Drug Program.

67. NRC, DMS, "Minutes of the Meeting of the Board for the Coordination of Malarial Studies," 10 November 1943, in Board, *Bulletin*, 162.

68. Clark, "History," 10.

69. Clark, "History," 21.

70. Clark, "History," 14.

71. Clark, "History," 20.

72. Clark to Loeb, 22 April 1944, Clark Collection, B:C547, Series I NRC Antimalarial Drug Program.

73. Clark to Loeb, 22 April 1944.

74. Loeb to Clark, 2 May 1944, Clark Collection, B:C547, Series I NRC Antimalarial Drug Program.

75. Board for the Coordination of Malaria Studies, minutes of executive session, 11 July 1944, Clark Collection, B:C547, Series II NRC Antimalarial Drug Program, ca. 1943–1947.

76. Richards to Loeb, 4 May 1944, Clark Collection, B:C547, Series I NRC Antimalarial Drug Program, telegram, copy. The copy is annotated in Clark's hand with the following: "Where upon within 3 hrs Loeb phones *virtual* order to appoint Marvel!!"

77. Clark to Loeb, 6 May 1944, Clark Collection, B:C547, Series I NRC Antimalarial Drug Program.

78. Loeb to Clark, 2 May 1944, Clark Collection, B:C547, Series I NRC Antimalarial Drug Program.

79. Clark to Loeb, 6 May 1944.

80. Clark to Loeb, 22 April 1944.

81. Clark, "History," 11.

Chapter 6 — Trust and Transition

1. Stewart Irvin, *Organizing Scientific Research for War: The Administrative History of the Office of Scientific Research and Development* (Boston: Little, Brown, 1948), 101.

2. On the founding of the NRC, see Rexmond C. Cochrane, *The National Academy of Sciences: The First Hundred Years, 1863–1963* (Washington, DC: National Academy of Sciences, 1978), 200–241.

3. Clark's attitude harkens back to a romantic antibureaucratic notion of American volunteerism typical of an earlier Wilsonian ideal. For more on the tensions between nineteenth-century liberalism and state bureaucratization in the twentieth century, see Robert Cuff, "American Mobilization for War, 1917–1945: Political Culture vs. Bureaucratic Administration," in *Mobilization for Total War: The Canadian, American, and British Experience, 1914–1918, 1939–1945*, ed. N. F. Dreisziger (Waterloo, Ontario: Wilfrid Laurier University Press, 1981).

4. For more on Clark, see Hubert Bradford Vickery, "William Mansfield Clark, August 17, 1884–January 19 1964," *Biographical Memoirs of the National Academy of Sciences* 39 (1968): 1–36; and http://www.amphilsoc.org/library/mole/c/clarkwm. pdf (viewed on 28 December 2006).

5. Clark to Norman H. Cromwell, 4 May 1943,Clark Collection, B:C547, Series I NRC Antimalarial Drug Program.

6. Lewis H. Weed to Norman T. Kirk, 21 October 1943, Clark Collection, B:C547, Series I NRC Antimalarial Drug Program.

7. W. Mansfield Clark, "History of Co-operative Wartime Program," in *A Survey of Antimalarial Drugs, 1941–1945*, ed. Frederick Y. Wiselogle (Ann Arbor: J. W. Edwards, 1946), 9.

8. Irvin, *Organizing Scientific Research for War*, 101.

9. Clark, "History," 2.

10. For an introduction to "gentlemanly" science and communities of trust, see Steven Shapin, *A Social History of Truth: Civility and Science in Seventeenth-Century England* (Chicago: University of Chicago Press, 1994); Bruno Latour and Steve Woolgar, *Laboratory Life: The Construction of Scientific Facts* (Princeton: Princeton University Press, 1979); Jack Morrell and Arnold Thackray, *Gentlemen of Science: Early Years of the British Association for the Advancement of Science* (Oxford: Clarendon Press, 1971); and Robert E. Kohler, "Place and Practice in Field Biology," *History of Science* 40 (2002): 189–210.

11. Clark, "History," 14.

12. Clark, "History," 16.

13. Clark to Shannon, 9 October 1944, Clark Collection, B:C547, Series I NRC Antimalarial Drug Program.

14. Clark to Loeb, 11 November 1944, Clark Collection, B:C547, Series I NRC Antimalarial Drug Program.

15. Clark to members of the Panel on Synthesis of Antimalarial Drugs, 19 January 1944, Clark Collection, B:C547, Series I NRC Antimalarial Drug Program.

16. See, for example, the "December 19th agreement" of 1941: Peter J. T. Morris, *The American Synthetic Rubber Research Program* (Philadelphia: University of Pennsylvania Press, 1989), 9. On rubber and penicillin and the role of the War Production Board, see Peter Neushul, "Science, Technology, and the Arsenal of Democracy: Production Research and Development during World War II" (PhD diss., University of California, Santa Barbara, 1993).

17. Clark to members of the Panel on Synthesis of Antimalarial Drugs, 19 January 1944, Clark Collection, B:C547, Series I NRC Antimalarial Drug Program.

18. Clark to members of the Panel on Synthesis of Antimalarial Drugs, 19 January 1944.

19. Memorandum from Clark to Richards, "Decision on Policy of Disclosure of Information on Antimalarial Drugs," 31 January 1944, Clark Collection, B:C547, Series I NRC Antimalarial Drug Program.

20. The NDRC bureaucracy was threatening to others at the NAS. For example, see Larry Owens, "The Counterproductive Management of Science in the Second World War: Vannevar Bush and the Office of Scientific Research and Development," *Business History Review* 68 (1994): 561.

21. Memorandum from Clark to Richards, "Decision on Policy of Disclosure of Information on Antimalarial Drugs," 31 January 1944, Clark Collection, B:C547, Series I NRC Antimalarial Drug Program.

22. Bush to Jewett, 18 March 1944, Clark Collection, B:C547, Series I NRC Antimalarial Drug Program.

23. An excellent lead reference on wartime transition and Bush is Owens, "The Counterproductive Management of Science in the Second World War," 515–76.

24. Clark to Loeb, 22 April 1944, Clark Collection, B:C547, Series I NRC Antimalarial Drug Program.

25. "Recommendation Regarding Exchange of Information between OSRD Contractors and Commercial Firms," memorandum from Lt. L. W. Dibble to Dr. A. N. Richards, NRC, DMS, CMR, OSRD, Board for the Coordination of Malarial Studies, minutes of meeting, 4 March 1944, in Board, *Bulletin*, 248. Lt. Dibble, whose name is not clear from these documents, was presumably one of the many attorneys working for Capt. Lavender, on whose behalf Dibble seems to have written this memo.

26. "Recommendation Regarding Exchange of Information," memorandum from Dibble to Richards, Board, *Bulletin*.

27. Clark to Richards, 6 March 1944, Clark Collection, B:C547, Series I NRC Antimalarial Drug Program.

28. Clark to Richards, 6 March 1944.

29. Bush to Jewett, 18 March 1944, Clark Collection, B:C547, Series I NRC Antimalarial Drug Program.

30. Clark to Dochez, 27 March 1944, Clark Collection, B:C547, Series I NRC Antimalarial Drug Program.

31. Clark to Jewett, 27 March 1944, Clark Collection, B:C547, Series I NRC Antimalarial Drug Program.

32. For more on penicillin, see Eric Lax, *The Mold in Dr. Florey's Coat: The Story of the Penicillin Miracle* (New York: Henry Holt, 2004); Richard I. Mateles, ed., *Penicillin: A Paradigm for Biotechnology* (Chicago: Candida Corporation, 1998); Peter Neushul, "Fighting Research: Army Participation in the Clinical Testing and Mass Production of Penicillin during the Second World War," in *War, Medicine, and Modernity*, ed. Roger Cooter, Mark Harrison, and Steve Sturdy (Stroud, Gloucestershire: Sutton, 1998), 203–24; John Patrick Swann, "The Search for Synthetic Penicillin during World War II," *British Journal for the History of Science* 16 (1983): 154–90; Chester S. Keefer, "Part Nine: Penicillin," in *Science in World War II*, vol. 2 of Office of Scientific Research and Development, *Advances in Military Medicine* (Boston: Little, Brown, 1948). Nicolas Rasmussen has suggested that information sharing was more controlled in the penicillin project than other historians have, but it is clear that Clark and other chemists saw it as differing on this point from the malaria work: see Nicolas Rasmussen, "Of 'Small Men,' Big Science, and Bigger Business: The Second World War and Biomedical Research in America," *Minerva* 40 (2002): 121–25.

33. Clark to Adams, 7 April 1944, Clark Collection, B:C547, Series I NRC Antimalarial Drug Program.

34. Adams to Clark, 17 April 1944, Clark Collection, B:C547, Series I NRC Antimalarial Drug Program.

35. Bush to Jewett, 7 April 1944, Clark Collection, B:C547, Series I NRC Antimalarial Drug Program.

36. Loeb to Clark, 19 and 21 April 1944, with handwritten note on Hay-Adams House stationery, dated 21 April and typed enclosure, dated 19 April, Clark Collection, B:C547, Series I NRC Antimalarial Drug Program. Following his meeting with Clark, Loeb had written a letter to his wife, and, finding it expressed his true feelings about Clark, he had it typed and sent it on to Clark.

37. Bush to Clark, 18 April 1944, Clark Collection, B:C547, Series I NRC Antimalarial Drug Program.

38. Clark to Bush, 19 April 1944, Clark Collection, B:C547, Series I NRC Antimalarial Drug Program.

39. Irvin, *Organizing Scientific Research for War*, 186.

40. Clark to Jewett, 19 April 1944, Clark Collection, B:C547, Series I NRC Antimalarial Drug Program. .

41. Clark to Bush, 19 April 1944, Clark Collection, B:C547, Series I NRC Antimalarial Drug Program.

42. Clark to Jewett, 19 April 1944.

43. Bush to Clark, 21 April 1944, Clark Collection, B:C547, Series I NRC Antimalarial Drug Program.

44. Clark to Loeb, 22 April 1944.

45. Clark to Loeb, 22 April 1944.

46. See, for example, Leo B. Slater, "Industry and Academy: The Synthesis of Steroids," *Historical Studies in the Physical and Biological Sciences* 30 (2000): 457–58. For a revisionist view of this matter, see Nicolas Rasmussen, "Steroids in Arms: Hormones of the Adrenal Cortex and U.S. Military Research, 1940–1945," *Medical History* 46 (2002): 299–324; Rasmussen, "Of 'Small Men,' Big Science, and Bigger Business"; and Rasmussen, "The Moral Economy of the Drug Company-Medical Scientist Collaboration in Interwar America," *Social Studies of Science* 34 (2004): 161–85.

47. Clark to Loeb, 22 April 1944.

48. Clark to Dochez, 27 March 1944.

49. Clark to Loeb, 22 April 1944.

50. Clark to Loeb, 22 April 1944.

51. Clark to Loeb, 22 April 1944.

52. Bush to Richards, 26 April 1944, and enclosed Memorandum for Reorganizing the Administration of OSRD Medical Research Program of the same date, Clark Collection, B:C547, Series I NRC Antimalarial Drug Program.

53. Clark to Wiselogle, 2 May 1944, Clark Collection, B:C547, Series I NRC Antimalarial Drug Program.

54. Clark, "History," 11–12.

55. Bush to Carden, Inter-Office Memorandum, "OSRD Antimalarial Program," 21 May 1945, NARA, RG 227, Records of the OSRD, entry 165, box 53, folder "Malaria 1945–1946."

56. Clark to Carden, not sent, 27 March 1945, Clark Collection, B:C547, Series I NRC Antimalarial Drug Program.

57. "Malaria" file card, 17 May 1945, NARA, RG 227, Records of the OSRD, Committee on Medical Research, entry 162, box 15, minutes of the CMR, Jan. 3, 1941—Sept. 28, 1946, Index 2, H—P.

58. Memorandum, Ruebhausen to Bush, re: OSRD Antimalarial Program, 14 May 1945, NARA, RG 227, Records of the OSRD, entry 165, box 53, folder "Malaria 1945–1946 [b]."

59. "A Survey of Antimalarial Drugs, 1941–45: History of the Organizations," early manuscript of "History," not dated, 40–41, Clark Collection, B:C547, Series IV.

60. Clark Collection, B:C547, Series I NRC Antimalarial Drug Program, folder 4, not dated. A number of undated and partial drafts of letters exist in this folder. Many show quite a bit more emotion than Clark's other extant correspondence. A scan of these pages reveals a high degree of homology with the letter Clark wrote to Frank B. Jewett on 27 March 1944.

Chapter 7 — Chloroquine, Wonder Drug

1. Panel on Pharmacology, 20 January 1943, in Board, *Bulletin*, 60a.
2. Minutes of the meeting of the Subcommittee on the Coordination of Malarial Studies, 4 November 1943, Board, *Bulletin*, 155. Also see Richard L. Kenyon, Jos. A. Wiesner, and C. E. Kwartler, "Chloroquine Manufacture," *Industrial and Engineering Chemistry* 41 (1949): 654–62.
3. Minutes of the meeting of the Panel on Pharmacology of Antimalarials, 16 September 1943, Board, *Bulletin*, 127; and minutes of the meeting of the Subcommittee on the Coordination of Malarial Studies, 4 November 1943, Board, *Bulletin*, 155.
4. Minutes of the meeting of the Board for the Coordination of Malarial Studies, 4 March 1944, Board, *Bulletin*, 246.
5. Kenneth C. Blanchard to George Carden, 24 July 1944, Board, *Bulletin*, 416.
6. Fred J. Stock, chief, Drugs and Cosmetics Branch, Chemicals Bureau, WPB Dept. 7610 to Chester Keefer, NRC, 22 July 1944, reproduced in Board, *Bulletin*, 413.
7. Minutes of the meeting of the Panel of Review, 31 July 1944, "Meeting of the Board to Determine the Position of the Army and Navy Concerning the Exploitation of SN-7618," Board, *Bulletin*, 406; memorandum drafted by E. K. Marshall and edited by the Panel of Review was "Exhibit F," p. 415.
8. See Kenyon, Wiesner, and Kwartler, "Chloroquine Manufacture," 657.
9. Minutes of the Panel of Review, 16 September 1944, Board, *Bulletin*, 496–97.
10. W. Mansfield Clark, "History of Co-operative Wartime Program," in *A Survey of Antimalarial Drugs, 1941–1945*, ed. Frederick Y. Wiselogle (Ann Arbor: J. W. Edwards, 1946), 36–37.
11. See Charles C. Price and Royston M. Roberts, "The Synthesis of 4-Hydroxyquinolines. I. Through Ethoxymethylenemalonic Ester," *Journal of the American Chemical Society* 68 (1946): 1204–8.
12. Minutes of the Panel of Review, 16 September 1944, Board, *Bulletin*, 496.
13. Benton A. Bull to Robert A. Lavender, memorandum, 8 December 1944, NARA, RG 227, Records of the OSRD, Committee on Medical Research, NC 138, entry 165, box 52. Interestingly, Bull and Dibble were careful to note that this memorandum was confidential not just with regard to the Espionage Act but also with regard to the Board's "in confidence" agreements with commercial firms.
14. Board for the Coordination of Malarial Studies, minutes of meeting, 28 February 1946, in Board, *Bulletin*, 1408.
15. See folder "Malaria—OSRD Relationship with Commercial Firms Division 6," NARA, RG 227, Records of the OSRD, Committee on Medical Research, entry 165, box 56.
16. Minutes of the Panel of Review, 16 September 1944, Board, *Bulletin*, 496.
17. Kenyon, Wiesner, and Kwartler, "Chloroquine Manufacture," 657.
18. Minutes of the Panel of Review, 16 September 1944, *Bulletin*, 497. For more on Drake's chloroquine work, see Nathan L. Drake et al., "Synthetic Antimalarials: The Preparation of Certain 4-Aminoquinolines," *Journal of the American Chemical Society* 68 (1946): 1208–13; and Drake et al., "Synthetic Antimalarials: The Preparation and Properties of 7-Chloro-4-(4-diethyl-amino-1-methylbutylamino)-quinoline (SN-7618)," *Journal of the American Chemical Society* 68 (1946): 1214–16.
19. Minutes of the meeting of the Panel on Clinical Testing, 18 September 1944, Board, *Bulletin*, 421.

20. Toxicity in normal subjects was also studied in Boston. See, for example, Allan M. Butler, MD, Massachusetts General Hospital, OEMcmr 419, 28 October 1944, Exhibit I, "Clinical Manifestations Encountered in the Long-Term Administration of SN-7618," minutes of the meeting of the Board, closed session, 6 November 1944, Board, *Bulletin*, 529–32. For prison studies of toxicity, see, for example, Alf S. Alving, Lillian Eichelberger, Branch Craige Jr., Ralph Jones Jr., C. Merrill Whorton, and Theodore N. Pullman, "Studies on the Chronic Toxicity of Chloroquine (SN-7618)," *Journal of Clinical Investigation* 27 (1948): 60–65; "Malaria Report #436: Long-Term Toxicity Study of SN-7618 at Illinois State Penitentiary, Joliet, Illinois," 13 June 1945, Staff of Malaria Research Unit, Department of Medicine, University of Chicago, Board, *Bulletin*, vol. 5, NARA, RG 227, Records of the OSRD, Committee on Medical Research, entry 167, box 3; and appendix I of "Malaria Report #565: A Lichen-Planus-Like Eruption Occurring in the Course of SN 7618 Administration," 20 December 1945, Board, *Bulletin*, vol. 6, NARA, RG 227, Records of the OSRD, Committee on Medical Research, entry 167, box 3.

21. Before the Nuremberg Code, much of human subject research was run in ways that we today might find highly questionable. For more on the subject, see Susan Lederer, *Subjected to Science: Human Experimentation in America before the Second World War* (Baltimore: Johns Hopkins University Press, 1995); U.S. Advisory Committee on Human Radiation Experiments, *The Human Radiation Experiments: Final Report of the President's Advisory Committee* (Oxford: Oxford University Press, 1996); Jordan Goodman, Anthony McElligott, and Lara Marks, eds., *Useful Bodies: Humans in the Service of Medical Science in the Twentieth Century* (Baltimore: Johns Hopkins University Press, 2003).

22. Executive session, 22 November 1944, minutes, Board, *Bulletin*, 562.

23. Comdr. L. T. Coggeshall (MC) USNR, "Interim Report on SN-7618," 12 November 1944, executive session, 22 November 1944, Board, *Bulletin*, 574.

24. Executive session, 21 February 1945, minutes, Board, *Bulletin*, 815.

25. "Malaria" file card, 29 November 1945, NARA, RG 227, Records of the OSRD, Committee on Medical Research, entry 162, box 15, minutes of the CMR, Jan. 3, 1941–Sept. 28, 1946, Index 2, H–P.

26. "Malaria" file card, 17 January 1946, NARA, RG 227, Records of the OSRD, Committee on Medical Research, entry 162, box 15, minutes of the CMR, Jan. 3, 1941–Sept. 28, 1946, Index 2, H–P.

27. Minutes of the meeting of the Board for the Coordination of Malarial Studies, executive session, 21 September 1944, Board, *Bulletin*, 489.

28. For more on Fairley's life, see E. Ford, "Neil Hamilton Fairley (1891–1966)," *Medical Journal of Australia* 2 (1969): 991–96. Fairley published a number of papers on the wartime malaria work: N. Hamilton Fairley, "Chemotherapeutic Suppression and Prophylaxis in Malaria: An Experimental Investigation Undertaken by Medical Research Teams in Australia," *Transactions of the Royal Society of Tropical Medicine and Hygiene* 38 (1945): 311–65; "The Chemotherapeutic Control of Malaria," *Schweizerische Medizinische Wochenschrift* 76, no. 37/38 (1946): 925–32; "Sidelights on Malaria in Man Obtained by Subinoculation Experiments," *Transactions of the Royal Society of Tropical Medicine and Hygiene* 40 (1947): 621–76; "Malaria with Special Reference to Certain Experimental, Clinical, and Chemotherapeutic Investigations," *British Medical Journal* 2 (1949): 891–97; "Chemoprophylaxis and Chemotherapy of Malaria in Man with Special Reference to

the Life Cycle," *Australasian Annals of Medicine* 1 (1952): 7–17; "Malaria Prophylaxis," *British Medical Journal* 1 (1954): 274; and "Experiments with Antimalarial Drugs in Man. VI. The Value of Chloroquine Diphosphate as a Suppressive Drug in Volunteers Exposed to Experimental Mosquito-Transmitted Malaria (New Guinea Strains)," *Transactions of the Royal Society of Tropical Medicine and Hygiene* 51 (1957): 493–501.

29. For a detailed account of the Australian work and its impact, see Tony Sweeney, *Malaria Frontline: Australian Army Research During World War II* (Carleton, Vic.: Melbourne University Press, 2003). Also see Judith A. Bennett, "Malaria, Medicine, and Melanesians: Contested Hybrid Spaces in World War II," *Health and History* 8 (2006): 27–55, http://www.historycooperative.org/journals/hah/8.1/bennett.html (viewed 7 March 2007); P. F. L. Boreham, "Dreamtime, Devastation, and Deviation: Australia's Contribution to the Chemotherapy of Human Parasitic Infections," *International Journal for Parasitology* 25 (1995): 1009–22; F. Fenner and A. W. Sweeney, "Malaria in New Guinea during the Second World War: The Land Headquarters Medical Research Unit," *Parassitologia* 40 (1998): 65–68; Stanley J. M. Goulston, "The Malaria Frontline: Pioneering Malaria Research by the Australian Army in World War II," (letter) *Medical Journal of Australia* 166 (1997): 672; Sweeney, "The Malaria Frontline: Pioneering Malaria Research by the Australian Army in World War II," (letter) *Medical Journal of Australia* 166 (1997): 316–19; and John H. Pearn, "One Weapon for Victory: Disease and Its Prevention as One Determinant of the Outcome of War," *Medical Journal of Australia* 157 (1992): 637–40.

30. Fairley, "The Chemotherapeutic Control of Malaria," 926.

31. Fairley, "Chemotherapeutic Suppression and Prophylaxis in Malaria," 318.

32. See Sweeney, "The Malaria Frontline: Pioneering Research by the Australian Army in World War II," 318.

33. Frederick C. Ehrman, John M. Ellis, and Martin D. Young, "*Plasmodium vivax* Chesson Strain," *Science* 101 (1945): 377.

34. "Malaria Report #721: Clinical Testing of Antimalarials at the National Institutes of Health, Final Report, OSRD Contract M-3993," G. Robert Coatney and W. H. Sebrell, 30 June 1946, 6, Board, *Bulletin*, vol. 7, NARA, RG 227, Records of the OSRD, Committee on Medical Research, entry 167, box 4. Also see Ehrman, Ellis, and Young, "*Plasmodium vivax* Chesson Strain," 377.

35. "Malaria Report #721: Clinical Testing of Antimalarials," 6.

36. Theodore N. Pullman, Branch Craige Jr., Alf S. Alving, C. Merrill Whorton, Ralph Jones Jr., and Lillian Eichelberger, "Comparison of Chloroquine, Quinacrine (Atabrine), and Quinine in the Treatment of Acute Attacks of Sporozoite-Induced *Vivax* Malaria (Chesson Strain)," *Journal of Clinical Investigation* 27 (1948): 46–50.

37. Executive session, 22 November 1944, minutes, Board, *Bulletin*, 563.

38. For example, see Darwin H. Stapleton, "A Lost Chapter in the Early History of DDT: The Development of Anti-Typhus Technologies by the Rockefeller Foundation's Louse Laboratory, 1942–1944," *Technology and Culture* 46 (2005): 513–40.

39. Robert Loeb to Andrew Warren (IHD), 6 February 1945, Board, *Bulletin*, 818.

40. Watson and Carden, "Malaria Report #500, Current Status of a Field Study with SN 7618 in Peru," 20 August 1945, 3, Board, *Bulletin*, vol. 5, NARA, RG 227, Records of the OSRD, Committee on Medical Research, entry 167, box 3.

41. "Malaria Report #500," 4.

42. "Malaria Report #500," 5.

43. "Malaria Report #500." The IHD also provided the Board with a second, more detailed report: Peterson and Valderrama, "Malaria Report #553: A Field Study of the Suppressive Action, Toxicity, and Therapeutic Value of SN 7618," 28 November 1945, Board, *Bulletin*, vol. 5, NARA, RG 227, Records of the OSRD, Committee on Medical Research, entry 167, box 3.

44. "Malaria Report #500," 8.

45. "Malaria Report #500," 9.

46. "Malaria Report #500," 8.

47. Carden to Strode, 28 September 1945, exhibit 3, meeting of the Panel of Review, 5 October 1945, Board, *Bulletin*, 1312. Also see two other letters included in the minutes: exhibit 1, Peterson to Carden, 6 September 1945, 1308–9; and exhibit 2, Watson to Carden, 28 September 1945, 1310–11.

48. "Mc Coy, Lt. Col. Oliver R." file card, 21 June 1945, NARA, RG 227, Records of the OSRD, Committee on Medical Research, entry 162, box 15, minutes of the CMR, Jan. 3, 1941–Sept. 28, 1946, Index 2, H–P.

49. "Malaria Report #565: Summary of Available Data on SN 7618," 20 December 1945, 1, Board, *Bulletin*, vol. 6, NARA, RG 227, Records of the OSRD, Committee on Medical Research, entry 167, box 3.

50. "Malaria" file card, 21 June 21 1946, NARA, RG 227, Records of the OSRD, Committee on Medical Research, entry 162, box 15, minutes of the CMR, Jan. 3, 1941–Sept. 28, 1946, Index 2, H—P.

51. Minutes of the meeting of the Board for Coordination of Malarial Studies, General Session, 28 December 1945, Board, *Bulletin*, 1377. See also minutes of the meeting of the Board, General Session, 28 February 1946, 1408.

52. Board for Coordination of Malarial Studies, "Activity of a New Antimalarial Agent, Chloroquine (SN 7618)," *Journal of the American Medical Association* 130 (1946): 1069–70.

53. Kenneth C. Blanchard, "Work on Antimalarials, I. G. Farbenindustrie, Elberfeld," CIOS, G-2, SHAEF (Rear) APO 413, visited 30 May–1 June 1945 (Washington, DC: Office of the Publication Board Department of Commerce, [1945?]), courtesy of the Alan Chesney Medical Archives, Johns Hopkins University, 4–5.

54. NRC, DMS, CMR, OSRD, Subcommittee on the Coordination of Malarial Studies, minutes of meeting, 7 October 1943, in Board, *Bulletin*, 140.

55. Blanchard, "Work on Antimalarials, I. G. Farbenindustrie, Elberfeld," 20.

56. Press release, Baldwin and Marmay for Winthrop Chemical Company, Inc., 11 July 1946, NARA, RG 227, entry 165, box 53, folder "Malaria 1945–1946."

57. Minutes of meeting, Conference on Chemotherapy of Malaria, 8 July 1941, Board, *Bulletin*, 4.

58. "Free Science Sought," Warren Weaver, letter to the editor dated 28 August 1945, *New York Times*, 2 September 1945, 58. Also see "The Lesson of the Bomb"—to which, in part, Weaver is responding—*New York Times*, 19 August 1945, section 4, 8.

59. J. Merton England, *A Patron for Pure Science: The National Science Foundation's Formative Years, 1945–57* (Washington, DC: National Science Foundation, 1982).

60. "Control of Malaria," *New York Times*, 13 April 1946, 16.

61. "Myth of the Lonely Scientist," letter to the editor by Joseph Bernstein, *New York Times*, 19 April 1946, 28.

62. Clark, "History," 2.

63. For related historical discussions, see Lily E. Kay, *Molecular Visions of Life: Caltech, the Rockefeller Foundation, and the Rise of the New Biology* (New York: Oxford University Press, 1993), 223–25; and Hans-Jörg Rheinberger, *Toward a History of Epistemic Things: Synthesizing Proteins in the Test Tube* (Stanford, CA: Stanford University Press, 1997), 41–42, specifically, "This was the language of partnership and cooperative individualism that characterized America's early postwar science policy discourse" (41).

64. Heidelberger's results were uniformly negative but were some of the only work published on human malaria vaccines between World War II and the 1970s, when interest shifted from chemotherapy to vaccines.

65. G. Robert Coatney, "Pitfalls in a Discovery: The Chronicle of Chloroquine," *American Journal of Tropical Medicine and Hygiene* 12 (1963): 122.

66. Moore, "Malaria Chemotherapy"; Richard L. Kenyon, Jos. A. Wiesner, and C. E. Kwartler, "Chloroquine Manufacture," *Industrial and Engineering Chemistry* 41 (April 1949): 654–62; and R. C. Elderfield "The Antimalarial Program of the Office of Scientific Research and Development," *Chemical and Engineering News* 24 (10 October 1946): 2598–2602. Also see David P. Earle Jr. and Robert W. Berliner, "Chloroquine," *Proceedings of the Fourth International Congresses on Tropical Medicine and Malaria, Washington, DC, May 10–18, 1948,* 2 vols., publication 3246 (Washington, DC: Department of State, 1948), 725–33.

67. For more on the British project, see David Greenwood, "Conflicts of Interest: The Genesis of Synthetic Antimalarial Agents in Peace and War," *Journal of Antimicrobial Chemotherapy* 36 (1995): 857–72; F. H. K. Green and Sir Gordon Covell, eds., *Medical Research*, History of the Second World War, United Kingdom Medical Series (London: H. M. Stationery Office, 1953), 155–60; F. L. Rose, "A Chemotherapeutic Search in Retrospect," *Journal of the Chemical Society* (1951): 2770–88; and various authors in Liverpool School of Tropical Medicine's *Annals of Tropical Medicine and Parasitology* 39, nos. 3 and 4 (1945).

68. Stephen P. Strickland, *Politics, Science, and Dread Disease: A Short History of United States Medical Research Policy* (Cambridge, MA: Harvard University Press, 1972), 16.

69. James Phinney Baxter III, *Scientists against Time* (Boston: Little, Brown, 1946), 300.

70. W. Paul Havens Jr., preface to *Infectious Diseases*, vol. 2 of *Internal Medicine in World War II*, ed. John Boyd Coates Jr. (Washington, DC: U.S. Govt. Printing Office, 1963), xvi.

71. Fred H. Mowrey, "Statistics of Malaria," in *Infectious Diseases*, 453.

72. Clark, "History," appendix 4, pp. 55–57 (original report approved by the Board, 6 September 1945).

73. J. E. Kirby to Clark and Wiselogle, 20 September 1945, Clark Collection, B:C547, Series I NRC Antimalarial Drug Program.

74. Wiselogle, ed., *A Survey of Antimalarial Drugs*.

75. Wiselogle to Clark, encl. 22 June 1946, Clark Collection, B:C547, Series I NRC Antimalarial Drug Program.

76. Clark to Wiselogle, 22 June 1946, Clark Collection, B:C547, Series I NRC Antimalarial Drug Program.

77. Frederick Y. Wiselogle, preface to *A Survey of Antimalarial Drugs*, v.

78. "Minutes of Meeting of the Malaria Study Section," 3 June 1946, *Malaria Study Section Reports, 1946–1948*, 2 vols., National Institutes of Health Library, Bethesda, MD, RC156.N1.

79. For more on the ONR, see Harvey M. Sapolsky, *Science and the Navy: The History of the Office of Naval Research* (Princeton, NJ: Princeton University Press, 1990); and "Academic Science and the Military: The Years since the Second World War," in *The Sciences in the American Context: New Perspectives*, ed. Nathan Reingold (Washington, DC: Smithsonian Institution Press, 1979), 379–99. Also see David K. Allison, "U.S. Navy Research and Development since World War II," in *Military Enterprise and Technological Change: Perspectives on the American Experience*, ed. Merritt Roe Smith (Cambridge: MIT Press, 1985), 289–328; and S. S. Schweber, "The Mutual Embrace of Science and the Military: ONR and the Growth of Physics in the United States after World War II," in *Science, Technology, and the Military*, vol. 12, ed. E. Mendelsohn, M. R. Smith, and P. Weingart (Dortrecht: Kluwer Academic Publishers, 1988), 3–45.

80. "Minutes of Meeting of the Malaria Study Section," 3 June 1946.

81. Clark, "History," 17.

Chapter 8 — Lessons Learned

1. Paul F. Russell, "Lessons in Malariology from World War II," *American Journal of Tropical Medicine* 26 (1946): 5, 13.

2. See, for example, Margaret Humphreys, "Kicking a Dying Dog: DDT and the Demise of Malaria in the American South, 1942–1950," *Isis* 87 (1996): 1–17.

3. The organization of postwar science and technology is the subject of a rich and growing historiography. See, for example, A. Hunter Dupree, "National Security and the Post-war Science Establishment in the United States," *Nature* 323 (1986): 213–16; Dupree, "The Great Instauration of 1940: The Organization of Scientific Research for War," in *The Twentieth-Century Sciences: Studies in the Biography of Ideas*, ed. Gerald Holton (New York: W. W. Norton, 1972), 223–467; Dupree, "The Structure of the Government-University Partnership after World War II," *Bulletin of the History of Medicine* 39 (1965): 245–51; Henry Etzkowitz, *MIT and the Rise of Entrepreneurial Science* (New York: Routledge, 2002); Peter Galison and Bruce Hevly, eds., *Big Science: The Growth of Large-Scale Research* (Stanford: Stanford University Press, 1992); David Kaiser, "Cold War Requisitions, Scientific Manpower, and the Production of American Physicists after World War II," *Historical Studies in the Physical Sciences* 33 (2002): 131–59; Daniel J. Kevles, "The National Science Foundation and the Debate over Postwar Research Policy, 1942–1945: A Political Interpretation of Science—The Endless Frontier," *Isis* 68 (1977): 4–26; Stuart W. Leslie, *The Cold War and American Science: The Military-Industrial-Academic Complex at MIT and Stanford* (New York: Columbia University Press, 1993); Rebecca S. Lowen, *Creating the Cold War University: The Transformation of Stanford* (Berkeley: University of California Press, 1997). Some areas of postwar science are better studied than others, for example, see the three-volume *A History of the United States Atomic Energy Commission*; vol. 1, Richard G. Hewlett and Oscar E. Anderson Jr., *The New World, 1939–1946* (University Park: Pennsylvania University Press, 1962); vol. 2, Hewlett and Anderson *Atomic Shield, 1947–1952* (University Park: Pennsylvania University Press, 1962); vol. 3, Hewlett

and Jack M. Holl, *Atoms for Peace and War, 1953–1961: Eisenhower and the Atomic Energy Commission* (Berkeley: University of California Press, 1989).

4. For more on how OSRD secured its place during wartime and how it educated a cadre of postwar science and technology leaders, see Carroll Pursell, "Science Agencies in World War II: The OSRD and Its Challengers," in *The Sciences in the American Context: New Perspectives*, ed. Nathan Reingold (Washington, DC: Smithsonian Institution Press, 1979), 359–78.

5. "Malaria, Patents, foreign" file card, 21 March 1946, Major B.A. Bull present, NARA, RG 227, Records of the OSRD, Committee on Medical Research, entry 162, box 15, minutes of the CMR, Jan. 3, 1941–Sept. 28, 1946, index 2, H—P.

6. G. Robert Coatney, W. Clark Cooper , Nathan B. Eddy, and Joseph Greenberg, *Survey of Antimalarial Agents: Chemotherapy of* Plasmodium gallinaceum *Infections, Toxicity, Correlation of Structure and Action*, Public Health Monograph No. 9 (Washington, DC: U.S. Government Printing Office, 1953).

7. Leo B. Slater, "Malarial Birds: Modeling Infectious Human Disease in Animals," *Bulletin of the History of Medicine* 79 (2005): 290–94.

8. For more on simian malarias, see W. E. Collins, "Major Animal Models in Malaria Research: Simian," in *Malaria: Principles and Practice of Malariology*, ed. W. H. Wernsdorfer and I. McGregor (New York: Churchill Livingstone, 1988), 2: 1473–1501.

9. L. H. Schmidt and G. R. Coatney, "Review of Investigations in Malaria Chemotherapy (USA) 1946–1954," *American Journal of Tropical Medicine and Hygiene* 4 (1955): 216.

10. George H. Hitchings, Gertrude B. Elion, Henry VanderWerff, and Elvira A. Falco, "Pyrimidine Derivatives as Antagonists of Pteroylglutamic Acid," *Journal of Biological Chemistry* 174 (1948): 765–66; E. A. Falco, G. H. Hitchings, P. B. Russell, and H. VanderWerff, "Antimalarials as Antagonists of Purines and Pteroylglutamic Acid," *Nature* 164 (1949): 107–8; and E. A. Falco, L. G. Goodwin, G. H. Hitchings, I. M. Rollo, and P. B. Russell, "2:4-diaminopyrimidines: A New Series of Antimalarials," *British Journal of Pharmacology* 6 (1951): 185–200. Hitchings and Elion later shared the Nobel Prize in Physiology or Medicine with James Black for their work on the principles of drug treatment.

11. See Wallace Peters, *Chemotherapy and Drug Resistance in Malaria* (New York: Academic Press, 1970). My account of chloroquine resistance owes much to Peters, particularly the introduction, from which I take many of the following statistics.

12. World Health Organization (WHO), "Expert Committee on Malaria Twelfth Report," *Technical Report Series World Health Organization* 324, 1966, quoted in Socrates Litsios, *The Tomorrow of Malaria* (Wellington, NZ: Pacific Press, 1996), 86.

13. Peters, *Chemotherapy and Drug Resistance*, 1.

14. Paul Ehrlich, "Experimental Researches on Specific Therapy III: Chemotherapeutic Studies on Trypamosomes," in *The Collected Papers of Paul Ehrlich*, ed. F. Himmelweit (New York: Pergamon Press, 1960), 130–34, reprinted from *The Harben Lectures for 1907 of the Royal Institute of Public Health* (London: Lewis, 1908), 134.

15. For a more contemporary view of drug resistance and multidrug combinations, see, for example, N. J. White and W. Pongtavornpinyo, "The De Novo Selection of Drug-Resistant Malaria Parasites," *Proceedings of the Royal Society of London,*

B 270 (2003): 545–54. Nicolas White has been a vocal proponent of combination drugs for malaria chemotherapy.

16. For more on the Armed Forces Epidemiological Board, see Theodore E. Woodward, *The Armed Forces Epidemiological Board: Its First Fifty Years* (Falls Church, VA: Office of the Surgeon General, Department of the Army, 1990), on the Web at http://history.amedd.army.mil/booksdocs/itsfirst50yrs/default.htm (viewed 21 January 2008).

17. See L. H. Schmidt and G. Robert Coatney, "Review of Investigations in Malaria Chemotherapy (U.S.A.) 1946 to 1954," *American Journal of Tropical Medicine and Hygiene* 4 (1955): 213–15.

18. Gordon M. Trenholme et al., "Mefloquine (WR 142,490) in the Treatment of Human Malaria," *Science* 190 (1975): 792–94. Also see David F. Clyde, "Malaria Studies at the University of Maryland, 1964–1975," in *Research on Infectious Diseases at the University of Maryland School of Medicine and Hospital: A Global Experience, 1807–2000,* ed. Theodore E. Woodward (Baltimore: University of Maryland, 1999), 158–65. For a more recent overview of the Walter Reed Army Institute of Research, see Kenneth J. Arrow, Claire B. Panosian, and Hellen Gelband, eds., *Saving Lives, Buying Time: Economics of Malaria Drugs in an Age of Resistance* (Washington, DC: National Academies Press, 2004), 305–11.

19. Malarone is produced and distributed by GlaxoSmithKline, the successor company, in turn, to Hitchings Wellcome; Burroughs-Wellcome, which lent its name to atovaquone's number, BW-566c; and finally to Glaxo Wellcome, which launched the Malarone donation program.

20. For Fieser's account of this work, see Louis F. Fieser, *The Scientific Method: A Personal Account of Unusual Projects in War and in Peace* (New York: Reinhold, 1964), 163–91. Fieser and others published dozens of papers on the naphthoquinones after the war. See, for example, *Journal of the American Chemical Society* 70, no. 10 (1948).

21. Minutes of the meeting of the Panel of Review, 9 June 1944, Item 16, Board, *Bulletin*, 365; appendix B to these same minutes, letter from Fieser to E. K. Marshall, 6 June 1944, Board, *Bulletin*, 368–69; and Fieser, *The Scientific Method*, 184–85.

22. See, for example, L. T. Coggeshall, John Maier, and C. A. Best, "The Effectiveness of Two New Types of Chemotherapeutic Agents in Malaria," *Journal of the American Medical Association* 117 (1941): 1077–81.

23. For more on the development of the sulfas as antimalarials in the postwar period, see H. J. Scholer, R. Leimer, and R. Richle, "Sulphonamides and Sulphones," *Handbook of Experimental Pharmacology (Continuation of Handbuch der experimentellen Pharmakologie),* vol. 68, 2nd ed., ed. W. Peters and W. H. G. Richards (New York: Springer-Verlag, 1984), 123–206.

24. See, for example, Kristina Borstnik, Ik-hyeon Paik, Theresa A. Shapiro, and Gary Posner, "Antimalarial Chemotherapeutic Peroxides: Artemisinin, Yingzhaosu, and Related Compounds," *International Journal for Parasitology* 32 (2002): 1661–67.

25. *The Economist*, 20 November 2004, print edition; online dated 18 November 2004, http://www.economist.com (viewed on 18 July 2007).

26. August W. Hofmann, *Reports of the Royal College of Chemistry, and Researches Conducted in the Laboratories in the Years 1845-6-7* (London: Royal College of Chemistry, 1849), lx–lxi.

27. Clements R. Markham, *Travels in Peru and India, While Superintending the Collection of Chinchona Plants and Seeds in South America, and Their Introduction into India* (London: John Murray, 1862); and *Peruvian Bark, a Popular Account of the Introduction of Chinchona Cultivation into British India* (London: John Murray, 1880), 46.

28. See, for example, Nicolas Zamiska and Betsy McKay, "Global Health, China's Pride on Line in Malaria Clash," *Wall Street Journal*, 6 March 2007, A1+.

29. For more on the history of the NIH, see Buhm Soon Park, "A 'Crucial Seed' for the Development of the Intramural Research Program at the National Institutes of Health after World War II," *Perspectives in Biology and Medicine* 46 (2003): 383–402; Stephen P. Strickland, *The Story of the NIH Grants Program* (Lanham, MD: University Press of America, 1989); Daniel M. Fox, "The Politics of the NIH Extramural Program, 1937–1950," *Journal of the History of Medicine and Allied Sciences* 42 (1987): 447–66; Victoria A. Harden, *Inventing the NIH: Federal Biomedical Research Policy, 1887–1937* (Baltimore: Johns Hopkins University Press, 1986); DeWitt Stetten Jr. and William T. Carrigan, eds., *NIH: An Account of Research in Its Laboratories and Clinics* (Orlando: Academic Press, 1984); Donald S. Fredrickson, "The National Institutes of Health Yesterday, Today, and Tomorrow," *Public Health Reports* 93 (1978): 642–47; G. Burroughs Mider, "The Federal Impact on Biomedical Research," in *Advances in American Medicine: Essays at the Bicentennial*, ed. J. Z. Bowers and E. F. Purcell (New York: Josiah Macy Jr. Foundation, 1976), 2: 806–71; Stephen P. Strickland, *Politics, Science, and Dread Disease: A Short History of United States Medical Research Policy* (Cambridge, MA: Harvard University Press, 1972); and Donald C. Swain, "The Rise of a Research Empire: NIH, 1930–1950," *Science* 138 (1962): 1233–37.

30. Richard C. Lewontin, "The Cold War and the Transformation of the Academy," in *The Cold War and the University: Toward an Intellectual History of the Postwar Years* (New York: New Press, 1997), 1–34, 16. In contrast—on the significance of contracts—see Larry Owens, "The Counterproductive Management of Science in the Second World War: Vannevar Bush and the Office of Scientific Research and Development," *Business History Review* 68 (1994): 515–76. On grants at NIH, see Daniel M. Fox, "The Politics of the NIH Extramural Program, 1937–1950," *Journal of the History of Medicine and Allied Sciences* 42 (1987): 447–66. For more on NIH research in the federal government context, see John P. Swann, "Biomedical Research and Government Support: The Case of Drug Development," *Pharmacy in History* 31 (1989): 103–16.

31. National Library of Medicine, History of Medicine Division, James A. Shannon Collection, OH 86, Interview by Thomas J. Kennedy, 11 January 1984, 51.

32. See L. R. Thompson to Coggeshall, 10 February 1941, folder 324, box 29, series 4, RG 5, RFA.

33. NLM, History of Medicine Division, James A. Shannon Collection, OH 86, interview by Thomas J. Kennedy, 11 January 1984, 51.

34. This was for the period from 1948 to 1968. Congressional appropriations could fluctuate, but the upward trend is clear. For more data, see the National Institutes of Health Web site, http://www.nih.gov/about/almanac/appropriations/index.htm (viewed 22 February 2007).

35. C. Gordon Zubrod, "Origins and Development of Chemotherapy Research at the National Cancer Institute," *Cancer Treatment Reports* 68 (1984): 9–19, 11; Robert F.

Bud, "Strategy in American Cancer Research after World War II: A Case Study," *Social Studies of Science* 8 (1978): 425–59, note 17; C. G. Zubrod, S. Schepartz, J. Leiter, K. M. Endicott, L. M. Carrese, and C. G. Baker, "The Chemotherapy Program of the National Cancer Institute: History, Analysis, and Plans," *Cancer Chemotherapy Reports* 50 (1966): 354. For an excellent account of the NCI, see Nancy Carol Erdey, "Armor of Patience: The National Cancer Institute and the Development of Medical Research Policy in the United States, 1937–1971" (PhD diss., Case Western Reserve University, 1995).

36. See the Association of American Physicians Web site, http://www.aap-online.org/ In_memoriam/InMemZubrod.htm (viewed 26 July 2005).

37. For more on the report and Coggeshall's legacy, see Joel D. Howell, "Lowell T. Coggeshall and American Medical Education: 1901–1987," *Academic Medicine* 67 (1992): 711–18.

38. The program at Walter Reed Army Institute of Research in Washington, DC, mentioned above screened hundreds of thousands of compounds for antimalarial activity in the postwar years.

39. For a wider discussion of the place of the program in the historiography of industrial research, see Leo B. Slater, "Malaria Chemotherapy and the 'Kaleidoscopic' Organization of Biomedical Research during World War II," *Ambix* 51 (2004): 107–34.

40. Shannon quoted in C. Gordon Zubrod, "The Drug Development Program of the National Cancer Institute: Its History, Results, and impact on Marketing," in *Orphan Drugs*, ed. Fred E. Karch, vol. 13 of *Drugs and the Pharmaceutical Sciences* (New York: M. Dekker, 1982), 150.

41. Clark, "History of the Co-operative Wartime Program," in *A Survey of Antimalarial Drugs*, 21.

42. Kenneth M. Endicott, "The Chemotherapy Program," *Journal of the National Cancer Institute* 19 (1957): 293.

43. Louis Galambos and Jane Eliot Sewell, *Networks of Innovation: Vaccine Development at Merck, Sharp and Dohme, and Mulford, 1895–1995* (Cambridge: Cambridge University Press, 1995).

44. For more on the history of vaccines and immunology, see Stanley A. Plotkin and Bernadino Fantini, eds., *Vaccinia, Vaccination, Vaccinology: Jenner, Pasteur, and Their Successors* (Paris: Elsevier, 1996); Galambos and Sewell, *Networks of Innovation*; Susan L. Plotkin and Stanley A. Plotkin, "A Short History of Vaccination," chapter 1 in *Vaccines*, 2nd ed., ed. Stanley A. Plotkin and Edward A. Mortimer Jr. (Philadelphia: W. B. Saunders, 1994), 1–11; Jane S. Smith, *Patenting the Sun: Polio and the Salk Vaccine* (New York: W. Morrow, 1990); and Henry James Parish, *A History of Immunization* (Edinburgh: E. and S. Livingstone, 1965).

45. For some of the sad tale of twentieth-century malaria vaccine research (through the 1980s), see Robert S. Desowitz, *The Malarial Capers: More Tales of Parasites and People, Research and Reality* (New York: W. W. Norton, 1991), 221–76. For a more recent tale of malaria vaccine work, see Mark Honigsbaum, *The Fever Trail: In Search of the Cure for Malaria* (New York: Farrar, Strauss and Giroux, 2001), 234–61.

46. Malaria vaccine research goes back to earlier German work, particularly that of S. W. Konstansoff; see "Malariaimmunität, Malariavakzine, und Vakzination," *Zentralblatt für Bakteriologie, Orig.* 116 (1930): 241–56. Also see Claus Schilling,

"Schutzimpfung gegen Malaria," *Deutsche medizinische Wochenschrift* 65 (1939): 1264–67. For his later work with death-camp inmates, Schilling was found guilty and executed: see Marion Hulverscheidt, "Menschen, Mücken und Malaria: Das wissenschaftliche Umfeld des KZ-Malariaforschers Claus Schilling," in *Medizin im Nationalsozialismus und das System der Konzentrationslager. Beiträge eines interdisziplinären Symposiums*, ed. Judith Hahn, Silvija Kavčič, Christoph Kopke (Frankfurt am Main: Mabuse-Verlag, 2005), 108–26; and Wolfgang U. Eckart and H. Vondra, "Malaria and World War II: German Malaria Experiments 1939–45" *Parassitologia* 42 (2000): 53–58.

47. H. W. Mulligan, Paul F. Russell, and Badri Nath Mohan, "Specific Agglutination of Sporozoites," *Journal of the Malaria Institute of India* 3 (1940): 513–24; Russell, Mulligan, and Mohan, "Specific Agglutinogenic Properties of Inactivated Sporozoites of *P. Gallinaceum*," *Journal of the Malaria Institute of India* 4 (1941): 15–24; Mulligan, Russell, and Mohan, "Active Immunization of Fowls against *Plasmodium Gallinaceum* by Injections of Killed Homologous Sporozoites," *Journal of the Malaria Institute of India* 4 (1941): 25–34; Russell, Mulligan, and Mohan, "Active Immunization of Fowls against Sporozoites of *Plasmodium Gallinaceum* by Injections of Homologous Sporozoites," *Journal of the Malaria Institute of India* 4 (1942): 311–19; Russell and Mohan, "The Immunization of Fowls against Mosquito-Borne Plasmodium Gallinaceum by Injections of Serum and of Inactivated Homologous Sporozoites," *Journal of Experimental Medicine* 76 (1942): 477–95.

48. Jules Freund, Harriet E. Sommer, and Annabel W. Walter, "Immunization against Malaria: Vaccination of Ducks with Killed Parasites Incorporated with Adjuvants," *Science* 102 (1945): 200–202; Jules Freund, K. Jefferson Thomson, Harriet Sommer, Annabel Walter, and Edna Schenkein, "Immunization of Rhesus Monkeys against Malarial Infection (P. Knowlesi) with Killed Parasites and Adjuvants," *Science* 102 (1945): 202–4; Thomson, Freund, Sommer, and Walter, "Immunization of Ducks against Malaria by means of Killed Parasites with or without Adjuvants," *American Journal of Tropical Medicine* 27 (1947): 79–105; Freund, Thomson, Sommer, Walter, and Teresa M. Pisani, "Immunization of Monkeys against Malaria by means of Killed Parasites with Adjuvants," *American Journal of Tropical Medicine* 28 (1948): 1–22.

49. For more about the Markle Foundation, see http://archive.rockefeller.edu/collections/nonrockorgs/marklebio.php and http://www.markle.org/about_markle/foundation_history/index.php (viewed 16 February 2006).

50. Wendell D. Gingrich, "Immunization of Birds to Plasmodium Cathemerium," *Journal of Infectious Diseases* 68 (1941): 46–52; and Gingrich, "The Role of Phagocytosis in Natural and Acquired Immunity in Avian Malaria," *Journal of Infectious Diseases* 68 (1941): 37–45.

51. Michael Heidelberger, Manfred M. Mayer, and Constance R. Demarest, "Studies in Human Malaria: I. The Preparation of Vaccines and Suspensions Containing Plasmodia," *Journal of Immunology* 52 (1946): 325–30; Heidelberger, W. A. Coates, and Mayer, "Studies in Human Malaria: II. Attempts to Influence Relapsing Vivax Malaria by Treatment of Patients with Vaccine (Pl. Vivax)," *Journal of Immunology* 53 (1946): 101–7; Heidelberger, Curtis Prout, Joseph A. Hindle, and Augustus S. Rose, "Studies in Human Malaria: III. An Attempt at Vaccination of Paretics against Blood-Borne Infection with Pl. Vivax," *Journal of Immunology* 53 (1946): 109–12; Heidelberger and Mayer, "Studies in Human Malaria: IV. An Attempt at Vaccination of Volunteers against Mosquito-Borne Infection with Pl. Vivax,"

Journal of Immunology 53 (1946): 113–18; Mayer and Heidelberger, "Studies in Human Malaria: V. Complement-Fixation Reactions," *Journal of Immunology* 54 (1946): 89–102.

52. N.b. I do not want to downplay the deadly toll of diarrheal diseases on young children in the developing world.

53. See the Task Force for Child Survival and Development Web site, http://www.task-force.org/malhome.html (viewed 26 July 2005). Also see Peter B. Bloland, Peter N. Kazembe, William M. Watkins, Ogobara K. Duombo, Okey C. Nwanyanwu, and Trenton K. Ruebush II, "Malarone-Donation Programme in Africa," *Lancet* 350 (1997): 1624–25.

54. For lead reference on the controversy, see R. Shretta, R. Brugha, A. Robb, and R. W. Snow, "Sustainability, Affordability, and Equity of Corporate Drug Donations: The Case of Malarone," *Lancet* 355 (2000): 1718–20.

55. GlaxoSmithKline Web site, http://www.gsk.com/financial/reports/ar2001/annual-report-01/gskrep18.html (viewed 26 July 2005).

56. World Health Organization Web site, http://w3.whosea.org/en/Section10/Section21/Section335.htm (viewed 26 July 2005).

57. For these goals, see UN Millennium Project Web site, http://www.unmillennium-project.org/goals/index.htm (viewed 26 July 2005).

58. See the Gates Foundation Web site, http://www.gatesfoundation.org/Global-Health/GranteeProfiles/SGGHMalariaMVI-011019.htm, and the Malaria Vaccine Initiative Web site, http://www.malariavaccine.org (both viewed 26 July 2005). The foundation was formally founded in January of 2000 with the combination of the Gates Learning Foundation and William H. Gates Foundation.

59. Medicines for Malaria Venture Web site, http://www.mmv.org (viewed 16 February 2006).

60. Global Fund to Fight AIDS, Tuberculosis and Malaria Web site, http://www.theglo-balfund.org/en/files/annualreport_executivesummary.pdf (viewed 26 July 2005).

61. For more about the fund, see http://www.theglobalfund.org/en/ (viewed 28 February 2007).

62. In the interest of disclosure, I should mention that I was funded for two years by the MRI. Their support helped make this book possible.

63. See the 7 May 2001 press release, http://www.jhu.edu/news_info/news/univ01/may01/malaria.html (viewed 26 July 2005).

64. For more on the President's Malaria Initiative, see http://www.whitehouse.gov/infocus/malaria/ (viewed 17 July 2007).

65. http://www.whitehouse.gov/news/releases/2007/04/20070424-11.html (viewed 17 July 2007).

66. See the TB Alliance Web site, http://new.tballiance.org/home/home-live.php, and http://www.stoptb.org (viewed 28 February 2007).

67. Brian M. Greenwood, Kalifa Bojang, Christopher J. M. Whitty, and Geoffrey A. T. Targett, "Malaria," *Lancet* 365 (2005): 1487–98.

68. Editorial, "Reversing the Failures of Roll Back Malaria," *Lancet* 365 (2005): 1439.

69. This and subsequent quotes from the *Economist*, 30 April 2005, 77.

70. For recent glimmers of hope emerging from public-private-NGO partnerships, see Mary Moran, "A Breakthrough in R&D for Neglected Diseases: New Ways to Get the Drugs We Need," *Public Library of Science Medicine* 2, no. 9 (2005): e302.

71. "A Survey of Antimalarial Drugs, 1941–45: History of the Organizations," early draft of "History," not dated, pp. 40–41, Clark Collection, B:C547, series IV.

Index

4-aminoquinolines, 81, 157, 160, 166. *See also* chloroquine; sontachin

8-aminoquinolines, 63–64, 65, 183. *See also* compound VI; isopentaquine; pentaquine; plasmochin; primaquine; SN-3883

acridine, molecular structure of, 69

Aedes aegypti mosquito. *See* mosquitoes

animal models of malaria. *See* avian models

Anopheles mosquito. *See* mosquitoes

antimalarial drugs: 8-aminoquinoline series, 63–64, 65, 183; after 1945, 178–186; acridine, 69; affordability of, 82; artemisinin, 183, 184–185, 185; atabrine, 53, 69–72, 121–126; atovaquone, 183; Chinese medicine and, 183, 185; chloroquine, 80–81, 156–176; clinical development of, 125–126; clinical tests in humans, 64–69; combinations, 181, 186; compound VI, 64; confidentiality and, 116; data, standardization of, 119; development, 18, 59–83; drug screening theory, 96–97; first-generation, 59–64; isopentaquine, 182; latency periods for relapse, 162–163; Lowell T. Cogeshall and, 89–95; malaria strains resistant to, 180; Malarone, 183, 192; marketing of, 72–80; mefloquine, 183; methylene blue and its compounds, 62–63; molecular structures of, as models for biological activity, 60; naphthoquinones, 183; Paludrine, 183; pentaquine, 170–171, 182; plasmochin, 28, 64, 182, 183; primaquine, 182, 183; proguanil, 183; Promin, 102; quinine (*see* quinine); quinoline compounds, 61–64; screening, 105; second-generation, 69–72; secrecy about, per the Malaria Confer-

ence (June 1942), 115; side effects of early, 86; SN-10000, 183; SN-10275, 183; SN-10281, 183; SN-13336 (trans), 183; SN-15083, 183; SN-15084 (cis), 183; SN-3883, 182; sontachin, 156–157; SP, 185; succession of, during wartime, 110; sulfa drugs, 183; sulfanilamides, 56; survey of (1942), 114–120; synthesis, lack of coordination between synthesizers and testers, 127–128; synthetic substitutes for quinine, 58–83; tension between collaboration and protection of proprietary interests, 114, 136–145; third-generation, 80–81; toxicity of, Marshall's position on, 107; trials, 161. *See also* antimalarial research; chemotherapy; U.S. antimalarial program

antimalarial program. *See* U.S. antimalarial program

antimalarial research: 1941 Rockefeller research outline, compared to 1931 Bayer outline, 101; collaborations, 84–108; compared with penicillin and synthetic rubber programs, 154–155; effect of U.S. entry into war on, 110–114; empiricism in, 127–128; issues in drug screening, 105; models, 48, 57, 178 (*see also* avian models); modes, 174–175; novel avian parasites, 50–58; postwar, 174–175; public–private research partnerships, 136–145, 153–155, 190–196; redundancy of efforts, 112–113. *See also* antimalarial drugs; malaria conferences; U.S. antimalarial program

antipyretics, 26–27

antipyrine, molecular structure of, 27

Aralen. *See* chloroquine

artemisinin: development as an antimalarial compound, parallel with quinine, 184–185; molecular structure of, 185

A former pharmaceutical research chemist, Leo B. Slater earned a PhD in history from Princeton University in 1997. His research interest is the history of twentieth-century biomedicine, science, and technology. He has held fellowships at the Chemical Heritage Foundation, the Johns Hopkins Bloomberg School of Public Health, the Max Planck Institute for the History of Science, and the National Institutes of Health. He is a fellow at the Johns Hopkins University's Institute for Applied Economics and the Study of Business Enterprise.